Women's Health and the World's Cities

The City in the Twenty-First Century

Eugenie L. Birch and Susan M. Wachter, Series Editors

A complete list of books in the series is available from the publisher.

Women's Health and the World's Cities

Edited by
Afaf Ibrahim Meleis,
Eugenie L. Birch, and Susan M. Wachter

PENN

UNIVERSITY OF PENNSYLVANIA PRESS

PHILADELPHIA

Published by
University of Pennsylvania Press
Philadelphia, Pennsylvania 19104-4112
www.upenn.edu/pennpress

Printed in the United States of America on acid-free paper
10 9 8 7 6 5 4 3 2 1

Library of Congress Cataloging-in-Publication Data

Women's health and the world's cities / edited by Afaf Ibrahim Meleis,
Eugenie L. Birch, and Susan M. Wachter. — 1st ed.
    p. cm. — (The city in the twenty-first century)
  Includes bibliographical references and index.
  ISBN 978-0-8122-4353-6 (hardcover : alk. paper)
  1. Urban women—Health and hygiene. 2. Urban women—
Social conditions. 3. Urban health. 4. Women's health
services. 5. Urbanization—Environmental aspects. 6. Urbanization—
Social aspects. I. Meleis, Afaf Ibrahim. II. Birch, Eugenie
Ladner. III. Wachter, Susan M. IV. Series: City in the twenty-first
century book series.
  RA564.85.W666524 2011
  362.1082—dc22

                                                2011012391

To Dean Kehler

for inspiring and supporting this initiative
from its inception, and for his unwavering commitment
to healthier communities

Contents

Foreword

Amy Gutmann

> The good we secure for ourselves is precarious and uncertain until it is secured for all of us and incorporated into our common life.
> —*Jane Addams*

Long before the University of Pennsylvania hosted the 18th Congress of the International Council on Women's Health Issues, American suffragist Jane Addams was skillfully integrating her argument for extending voting rights to women with trenchant observations about health, the environment, and nutrition. Writing in 1915, she advocated for women's active involvement in the public sphere, emphasizing that individual action alone could not provide access to transportation, housing, and unpolluted air and water, or ensure the availability of safe and nutritious food.

Nearly a century later, we continue to draw connections between women's opportunities and the places in which they live. Addams would certainly marvel at our progress, but she also would remind us that if we do not continue to broaden the scope of our efforts "we shall fail to go forward, thinking complacently that we have 'arrived' when in reality we have not yet started." Securing voting rights was, indeed, a historic policy breakthrough, but women's journey to control their own destiny is far from being over.

Despite inspiring progress around the world, far too many women and girls continue to suffer abuse and to meet unimaginable fates. They are systematically tortured and raped as a war tactic. They are exploited for profit, forced into marriages as children, and killed for bringing dishonor on their families.

The access of women and girls to education, health care, and employment is grossly unequal to that of their male counterparts, and true gender equality remains a goal for all nations. Since 2006, the three highest ranking countries in the World Economic Forum's *Global Gender Gap Report*—Iceland, Finland, and Norway—have closed a little more than 80 percent of their gender gaps, whereas the lowest ranking country—Yemen—has closed less than half of its gender gap. Societies the world over continue to squander the potential of half of the human race to contribute to economic, political, and social advancement.

We honor the advancement of women's rights most fittingly when we dedicate ourselves to the important work that remains. The future is filled with daunting challenges, but also with thrilling opportunities for world-changing success. To boldly advance human rights and women's health in the twenty-first century, we must continue to increase awareness, to promote action, and to advance assessment of our policies and our practices. Only then will we truly celebrate the end of the journey and share a "common life" distinguished by equality and opportunity for all.

Increasing Awareness

The emergence of new technology and the surging popularity of social media enable us to personalize global issues and to increase awareness of human rights. In 2009, when a 26-year-old Iranian civilian, Neda Agha-Soltan, was shot during a demonstration in Tehran, a bystander recorded her final moments on his cell phone. The footage and news of her death spread rapidly over Facebook, YouTube, and Twitter, drawing international attention to the political protests.

Stories like Neda's increase awareness around the world by connecting statistics and reports with faces and names. The digital age has given us unprecedented access to vast amounts of information, and opportunities abound to learn about and to communicate directly with people who would have been strangers to us a generation ago. By harnessing new technology, we move from abstractions to concrete examples of both tragedy and triumph, and the urgency of the global women's movement crystallizes.

Promoting Action

Over the past decade, grass roots initiatives and partnerships to empower women have sprung up around the world. These collaborations embrace the complexity inherent in globally oriented interventions and promote understanding of cultural differences as a means to achieve progress. Promoting and supporting action in local communities gives rise to successful models that can be modified and replicated.

One of my favorite examples has roots at the University of Pennsylvania. After learning of Muhammad Yunus's work with Grameen Bank and meeting him in person, Wharton alumna Roshaneh Zafar returned to her native Pakistan and started the Kashf Foundation, the country's first specialized microfinance organization. Through Kashf, women from low-income communities have access to loans and insurance. Since 1997, the foundation has worked with more than a million families, providing small sums of money to enable economic growth. In turn, this growth has enabled families to send their children to school, generating a virtuous cycle of education and achievement.

Advancing Assessment

Identifying efforts that produce the most significant change and the most sustainable outcomes will drive the global women's movement forward. To improve the opportunities and choices of urban women, we need an effective coalition of researchers, clinicians, educators, and community advocates to identify the most effective policies and then to push for significant policy changes in the world's cities.

Improving health is among the most effective ways of transforming the lives of women and girls. Better health improves educational outcomes and decreases poverty. Interventions that promote health education, prevent disease and injury, and increase access to health care have a tremendous demonstrable impact in communities around the world. Just as Addams did a century ago, we must continue to demonstrate the connection between women's rights, health, and successful urbanization.

The Journey Ahead

Currently, more than half of the people on the planet—an estimated 3.5 billion women, men, and children—live in urban areas. Over the next two decades, the world's cities will grow, eventually supporting a staggering 5 billion people.

The challenges posed by swelling populations are great. Will our cities buckle under the strain? Or will we work together and develop systems that meet the most basic human needs: unpolluted air, clean water, sanitation, food, and decent health care? Because women face far fewer employment opportunities and assume greater responsibilities as caregivers, they are at special risk of bearing the most costly burdens of urbanization.

What role can today's premier teaching and research universities play in meeting this global challenge?

Ours is an increasingly connected and complex world, and the critical issues of our time demand approaches that crosscut academic disciplines. At the University of Pennsylvania, we encourage the integration of knowledge by supporting centers and institutes—like the innovative Penn Institute for Urban Research—that connect faculty and foster collaboration. Through our Penn Integrates Knowledge initiative, we attract world-renowned scholars who have devoted their careers to interdisciplinary inquiry. All the while, faculty in our twelve schools work with one another to address challenges that do not fit neatly within academic boundaries.

At the same time, we broadly educate our students, encouraging them to pursue their passions and develop their leadership skills inside and outside of the classroom. Young women and men who today are engaged in the movement to empower women and to improve the world for women and men alike will fuel tomorrow's efforts.

Each year at Penn, more than 4,000 of our 9,600 undergraduates engage in sustained service activities in addition to their academic studies. In recognition of our local engagement efforts with the City of Philadelphia, Penn and the University of Southern California tied for number one "best neighbor" among American colleges and universities in 2009.

Many schoolchildren in Philadelphia and other major cities in the United States and around the world have limited access to nutritious food and open spaces. Penn's Agatston Urban Nutrition Initiative provides education programs in twenty public schools and empowers elementary and high school students to take control of their health. Students who go through the program often become nutrition advocates in their communities.

Our commitment to improving the world begins locally but extends globally. Through the Guatemala Health Initiative, Penn students help develop interventions to improve maternal and child health outcomes. Under the direction of a medical anthropologist on our faculty, a junior in our University Scholars Program constructed her own research protocol, tracked the weights of pregnant women, and investigated the major factors that shape Guatemalan women's attitudes about nutrition and the connections among those attitudes, resulting behaviors, and fetal health.

These are just two of the myriad ways in which Penn students are working to empower women and improve the world before they graduate. Imagine what could be accomplished if we unlocked the potential of all university students who are interested in empowering women to improve the world.

Moving Forward

Jane Addams reminds us to reinvent our approaches. We must recognize that the pressing challenges posed by urbanization on the lives of women and girls are lifelong challenges, not only to individuals but also to institutions. Universities must broadly educate the next generation of leaders. We must be models of engagement with local and global communities, and we must identify, support, and share the programs that demonstrate the best results.

Writing in 1786, Penn's founder, Benjamin Franklin, "observe[d] with concern how long a useful truth may be known, and exist, before it is generally received and practiced on." The useful truth is that when we improve health care, education, and employment opportunities for women, they drive their families, their communities, their cities, their nations, and the world forward. The chapters in this volume exemplify the breadth of viewpoints and depth of experience on which we must capitalize to improve our world, not only on the margins but also at the core—with health care, education, and employment for all.

Introduction

Developing Urban Areas as if Gender Matters

Afaf Ibrahim Meleis

The world is becoming more urbanized, and urban populations are growing at an unprecedented pace. More than half of the world's population, approximately 3.5 billion people, live in cities; by 2030 this number is expected to increase to almost 5 billion. People are moving to urban areas seeking new opportunities, new options, freedom in choices, and better resources. Women in particular believe that they can improve their status, position, and their children's opportunities by seeking work and educational opportunities for themselves or their children in the cities. Many even venture beyond their own countries in search of a better quality of life.

Increasing urbanization is not only a U.S. phenomenon; rather, it is a global phenomenon. Although most of this growth in numbers of urban dwellers and in migration to urban areas is occurring in higher income nations, similar migration patterns are occurring in developing nations as well, such as Africa, Asia, and Latin America (ISTED 2010; WHO 2010e). The United Nations has estimated that in the early twentieth century approximately sixteen cities in the world had populations of at least 1 million. By the beginning of the twenty-first century, approximately 400 cities were this size. Megacities, defined by the United Nations as metropolitan areas with a total population of more than 10 million people, are also increasing in number, and many of these will be located in the developing world.

As urbanization increases, the number of urban poor will also continue to rise (United Nations 2008c). Many of these will be women moving from rural to urban areas and across countries with dreams of finding better lives, more educational and health resources, and fewer restrictions on new freedoms. Among these women are the Syrian, Filipina, and Thai maids, nannies, cooks, and housekeepers who work in Saudi Arabia, Egypt, Hong Kong, and Taiwan. They are the mail-order brides from Korea, Lithuania, Estonia, Vietnam, Taiwan, Germany, and the United States. They are the female nurses from all over the world who live and work in Brunei, Kuwait, the United Kingdom, the United States, and other countries far from their homes.

Most, if not all, of these women settle in urban areas that are not designed with their safety in mind; nor is access provided to resources that meet their unique and universal needs. While urbanization comes with new opportunities and many options, it is often hazardous to women and to their health. The process of urbanization contributes to a scarcity of resources, lack of infrastructure, and deprivations in social structure. In urban areas, women face new health risks caused by poor sanitation, lack of electricity, as well as more pollution, stress, crime, and traffic accidents (United Nations 2008c, 2010a). In congested cities, women also face an increased risk of communicable diseases and infections. Women are more compromised than men under these urban conditions due to gender inequities and to a lack of awareness among urban developers and policymakers of their specific needs and concerns.

Urbanization creates new issues for health and health care for women, and although there has been attention to the relationship between urbanization and health, less is known about the intersection of these three subjects: urbanization, gender, and health. A focus on the role of gender in urban health is absent from dialogues about urbanization (Frye, Putman, and O'Campo 2008). Further, limited dialogue exists on the intersection between public spaces and women's health-care needs. Urban environments, with their specific social and structural characteristics, have an undeniable impact on the health and well-being of urban populations, especially on women, who are more at risk because of the prevailing gender divide and limited access to resources and health services.

This book is designed to provide a platform for a robust dialogue about the social and physical environments and space configurations in which women live, and the impact of the urban environment and its planning on the health of women. The goals of the chapters that follow are to stimulate urban planners and women's health professionals to initiate dialogue about, and research into, the intersection between urbanization and women's health.

Broadly, the aim of this book—*Women's Health and the World's Cities*—is to examine urban planning to identify areas with the potential to better support women's health. Far too often, professionals from all fields, from health-care professionals to policymakers to urban planners, assume that structuring a healthy environment for a woman is the same as structuring a healthy environment for a man. In fact, women's needs are unique. Remarkable opportunities to have a profound impact on urban women's lives can result from opening a multidisciplinary dialogue among professionals from all facets of health care, health policy, and urban design, among other areas.

This leading-edge, solution-driven volume is meant to inspire dialogue about contemporary issues that affect urban women's health and life experiences. National and international authors of individual chapters are actively involved in urban development or in researching, planning, and advocating for women's health programs. They are experts in the fields of urban design, health sciences, health policy, law, social policy, education, and sociology, among others. Some of the chapters are more oriented toward research, whereas others integrate scholarship with activism. Resolving issues related to vulnerable and marginalized populations requires integrating empirical, theoretical, and advocacy approaches. This book provides academicians and professionals the opportunity to evaluate frameworks and research evidence about the effect of urbanization on women's health and, conversely, the effect of women's health on urban communities. Women play critical roles in our societies—as mothers, providers, leaders, caregivers, and volunteers—that give them an exponentially powerful role in guiding not only their own health but the health of their children, their families, and their community. With these points in mind, the book's contributors

present models of interdisciplinary and cross-sectoral collaboration among urban women's health researchers, urban planners, policymakers, clinicians, philosophers, and community workers from the Global South and Global North, and encourage further networking and collaboration;

propose an agenda for urban women's health that identifies general crosscutting items as well as strategies for specific localities; and

present strategies and best practices for economically efficient delivery of health promotion, health education, and disease and injury prevention guidelines for urban women in the Global North and Global South.

Authors address common themes, including the properties of urbanization that intersect with women and their health, and the most significant determinants of vulnerability and risk for women. Among these are aging, violence, poverty, and access to health care. All authors offer strategies for improving urban women's health by improving the spaces in which they live.

Urbanization

Life in cities entails negative as well as positive aspects. Urbanization may offer more opportunities overall, such as better educational opportunities, diverse employment options, networks that open doors, more access to resources, better health care, and more advanced transportation. Urbanization may also pose risks for women, such as harassment, violence, costly health care, transportation issues, and changes in lifestyle that put women at risk for disease.

Often, inequality in cities becomes more pronounced as cities develop and expand, particularly when expansion is due to an inflow of already disadvantaged groups such as migrants, immigrants, rural people, women, and minorities. Very often, favelas, Ashish, shanty cities, and slums form to accommodate the newcomers. These accommodations are characterized by poor sanitation, unsafe drinking water, high population density, lack of transportation, violence, and unsafe sex practices. In such environments, women become even more vulnerable than men due to gender inequities. In some urban slums, a third of homes are headed by women (UN-HABITAT 2006). Compared to their male counterparts, these women are even more at risk because they tend to have lower paying jobs and higher illiteracy rates due to lack of education, which cause major financial and social stressors that can profoundly affect their health.

Urban areas are characterized by the nature of their social capital and physical capital. Social capital is the glue that binds members of a community together. It is "the patterns and intensity of connections within and between social networks that combine to create shared value and benefits" (WHO 2008b: 9). A community's social capital is measured by its inhabitants' perceptions of livability and their estimation of the extent to which they feel they can get help from one another. It is also measured by their sense of belonging and the trust they place in their neighbors (Hutchinson et al. 2009). Vulnerable populations such as women, immigrants, migrants, and minorities are in greater need of a social safety net composed of a critical mass of individuals with whom they can develop trust, bond, and form strong ties. Social capital has been associated with preventive behaviors (Hsieh et al. 2008). Communities with strong ties provide information, support, babysitting, elderly care, emergency care, access to car pools, and shared responsibilities when needed (Coogan et al. 2009). Women organize and manage such resources as they need and utilize these resources for themselves and for their families. Communities without strong ties, where individuals are isolated, lack the support and resources women rely on to care for themselves and their families.

The physical capital of urban areas can be characterized in terms of walkability, transportability, aesthetics, and safety. These measures reflect the extent to which the environment promotes exercise and activity, provides access to healthy food, and makes access to health care available. Urban areas designed without attention to safety produce less walkability and tend to increase weight-related chronic conditions as well as self-reported poor health risks (Doyle et al. 2006). The nature and problems of a community's physical capital influence the nature of its social capital. The way an urban area is organized—the safety of its streets, the availability of space for meeting others, the location of resources including how shopping for essential needs is organized, the density in living and the type of housing—affects how and where people meet and the connections they develop with one another.

Women's Health

Women's lives connect to geography and space in many different ways. Among these are women's relationships with their homes, with their kitchens, and with their places of work and the immediate spaces surrounding them. Although women have been influential in the design of private spaces, their influence on public spaces has been relatively absent. Gender and urban development has received minimal attention. Feminist geographers have uncovered and discussed some of the gender spatial segregations that have existed in the private lives of women; similar dialogues on public spaces are still needed.

Urbanization creates physical demands on women due to new waged work, urban stressors, limited convenient transportation, demands on their time, and new complexities in their lives. Employment opportunities have both positive and negative effects on women's health. Although access to waged work can improve women's health by allowing poor urban women to become more independent and by improving their social and economic situations, it can also have negative consequences. These women often find themselves having to work in substandard employment conditions that can be harmful to their health. They often work in underpaid, unsafe jobs in industries where they are exposed to toxic substances and environmentally hazardous conditions that can have profound effects on their physical and mental health (Doyal 2004). Although some women are able to ease their work burdens by obtaining domestic assistance, those who are hired are mostly women whose health is jeopardized by the nature of the work or by the lack of access to health care. Most of these women are migrants or immigrants to urban areas.

Lower paying jobs and fewer employment opportunities create difficulty for women in renting or owning houses, as that requires capital or credit, both of which are more challenging to obtain for vulnerable populations such as women than for advantaged populations, since they face greater poverty. Also, when housing is insecure, so too is the ability to find healthy food due to a lack of access to full-service supermarkets and farmer's markets, which are all made readily accessible in more stable communities; when healthy food is inaccessible, illness may follow (UN-HABITAT 2004b).

In addition, women face a myriad of other health issues that are best served by gender-specific responses; these include cancer, obesity, hypertension, osteoarthritis, diabetes, and depression (WHO 2010e). These issues are often exacerbated by such challenges as air, water, and land pollution; environments that promote sedentary lifestyles due to lack of space and a dearth of opportunities for physical activity; gender-specific marketing campaigns that lead to increases in the consumption of tobacco and alcohol by the targeted audience; traffic accidents; exposure to stress and violence; and limited access to healthy and fresh foods. Lack of access to healthy food with limited support from a network (due to migration or immigration) place women at new risk (Doyal 2004). These all serve as examples of how women often bear the heavier burden of urban development problems due to gender inequities in society, limited education, and a lack of awareness of their needs among urban developers and policymakers.

Health disparities related to gender and poorly conceived approaches to women's health pose a dire threat considering that, in many societies, women are the backbone of families and communities and the keepers of social values and capital. Though recognition of the centrality of women for family, community, and society's health has increased over the years—as manifested by a focus on microfinancing and lending to women—a focus on women and their health and welfare continues to lag in many parts of the world. Lowering women's morbidity and mortality rates, improving their education, and raising their incomes are still at the top of the unachieved Millennium Development Goals (MDGs) (United Nations 2010a). Other challenges include translating research into practice and policy and implementing best practices in community interventions.

Health Risks for Women in Urban Areas

So what are some of the major health risks women face in urban areas? Kettel (1996) argued that women's relationships with their geographical spaces are laden with environmental hazards that put them at risk that is clearly gender-differentiated. Lack of careful gendered planning leads to "disease environments" for women. Lack of access to health care in general and preventive services in particular is one of the major determinants of poor health. Gender differences in health and illness patterns are the product of both biology and the sociocultural context in which people live.

Lack of access to health care translates into increased infant and maternal morbidities and mortalities. Whether or not women's needs are met for reproductive health care is predicated on cost, time, availability, transportation ease, and ability to take time from work—all of which are imbedded in urban planning. The geographical location of women's health clinics becomes more challenging in urban areas due to congestion, population density, and distance. Problems in accessing reproductive health care have been well manifested and addressed in rural areas; similar dialogues and planning need to be addressed in urban areas. Even when data indicate that urban dwellers enjoy better health outcomes than rural dwellers, when income, environment, and other variables are considered, women in urban settings are more vulnerable to mental illness and to infections and are more at risk for cancer, reproductive health problems, and other environmentally related problems than are women in rural areas (Harpham 2009; National Cancer Institute 2010).

Another particularly vulnerable group in urban areas is elderly women. Life expectancy is increasing worldwide as is the proportion of people who are considered old (age 65 and over). Women tend to live longer than men; therefore women are either the caregivers of their spouses or other family members who need care, or they are living alone with limited resources for their own care. Urban areas tend to isolate the elderly, making it difficult to create social networks, particularly in socially disadvantaged areas (Boneham and Sixsmith 2006). Aging in general makes people more vulnerable to chronic illness and other phenomena, and aged women particularly are vulnerable in urban areas due to limited or fixed incomes, isolation, dehydration, limited access to health care, and climate changes, particularly heat and cold waves. Furthermore, they are more vulnerable to harassment, violence, and injuries, particularly when urban areas are not developed with good lighting and easy and accessible transportation. As more elders wish to age at home, urban planning must pay greater attention to their needs.

One of the major health hazards that women and girls face in urban areas is exposure to many forms of violence. They encounter harassment, sexual advances and coercion, rape, intimate partner violence, injury, and murder. Urban environments exacerbate the emotional scars that women suffer from due to their gender. Dating violence is prevalent among urban youth and is associated with suicide attempts among adolescent girls. Accessible screening must be provided as well as mental health services (Olshen et al. 2007).

There is a connection between physical space and greater vulnerability to violent acts. Environments designed with more lighting, better transportation, and more emphasis on density and organization of urban areas may decrease the risk of violence to women. Communities that are safer and more walkable tend to have lower crime rates; individuals who live in these communities tend to have lower body mass, to exercise more, to have healthier eating habits, and to be generally healthier (Doyle et al. 2006).

Another major risk factor for women and their health is poverty. Poverty and economic inequities (which exacerbate health risks for women) exist within cities, and these risks affect women differently in developing and developed countries. Economic poverty is associated with environmental poverty. The urban poor are highly vulnerable to many health hazards. They live at the periphery of cities in shanty communities and in Ashish and favelas. Those who live in these slum areas suffer from lack of hygiene and sanitation, limited clean water, inadequate sewage systems, and insufficient transportation infrastructure, making access to health care and resources even more meager.

As managers of the lives of their families, women also become the managers of systems needed to care for their families, which include water, transportation, social support, and food. As a result of negotiating these systems, women face increased stresses and burdens, making them more vulnerable to the hazards of negotiating these systems as well as to the infections, chronic diseases, and malnutrition that are ubiquitous in impoverished urban areas. Thus transportation planning, for example, needs to be seen as a women's issue.

Recommendations for the Future of Healthy Cities and Healthy Women

Gender matters in urbanization and globalization. In any dialogues about the development of nations, there is a global recognition of the centrality of women. This recognition is manifested in the Millennium Development Goals, which were developed in 2000 by the United Nations and the Organisation for Economic Co-operation and Development to improve the lives of hundreds of millions of people around the world and ensure their basic human rights (the top five of the eight goals address women's issues such as poverty, education, maternal and infant mortality rates, and infections). The designation of the United Nations entity for gender equality and the empowerment of women (UN Women), developed after ten years of dialogues and recommendations to the secretary-general of the United Nations, and the appointment of Melanne Verveer as the U.S. ambassador for global women's issues by President Barack Obama, are indications of recognition of the vital role that healthy and educated women play in developing communities and nations and for how world diplomacy can be enhanced by educating and empowering women through paying attention to designing healthy environments for them.

Urban planners must consider five forces in planning and developing urban areas in order to improve women's lives. The first condition is that there is momentum for improving the situation and status of women through empowering them by providing access to education, health care, healthy lifestyles, and resources in urban areas. This momentum must be the force for continuity in designing urban areas that are responsive to women's needs. That leads to the second important condition—developing cities with women's needs in mind. Women want to live in safe environments with better lighting, lower population density, and spaces that permit connections and allow them to provide the care that their roles demand to meet the needs of their children, friends, partners, elders, and other family members. This means providing access to resources for their children's needs as well as elders' needs. Improving conditions in or replacing slums, where many women newcomers to the city live, must be part of urban planning and development. Urban planning for women must acknowledge the inadequacy of shanty cities, favelas, Ashish, and other low-income areas for black, Latino, and immigrant communities (Day 2006). Gender-sensitive and age-sensitive approaches to urban development should be included. A third condition in planning urban dwellings and infrastructure is to pay attention to the sociocultural context and religious mores that drive, and often dictate, women's movements, educational and working options, and housing needs. Developing urban areas in religiously conservative Muslim or Jewish communities or in socially strict societies requires different criteria and guidelines that determine the physical and social capitals and hence the space configurations. The fourth vital condition is to seek and include women's voices in planning decisions. Women should be key players in the policies and plans used for the development of communities (Boneham and Sixsmith 2006). Involving women in policies related to urban planning and development ensures that their perspectives, needs, and voices are included in designing spaces with women's needs in mind. The fifth and most important condition is to develop a conceptual framework that provides a structure for systematically investigating gender and its impact, or lack of it, on urban environments as well as on health and well-being. This conceptual framework would drive the design and translation of research programs into gender-sensitive urbanization development plans. Questions that should be addressed relate to the differences in urban living between men and women and to differences in health outcomes among those who live in urban areas with differential incomes, and theories should be developed that are sensitive to defining and investigating the nature of gender disparities that are characteristic of those who live in urban areas (Frye, Putman, and O'Campo 2008). Preventing urbanization's spatial, social, and health risks for women through careful advance planning will be far more effective and productive than intervening after the fact.

Conclusion

The MDGs galvanized world leaders to forge global partnerships to achieve these universal objectives by 2015 (Yusuf, Nabeshima, and Ha 2007). These eight goals are:

- Eradicate extreme poverty and hunger.
- Achieve universal primary education.
- Promote gender equality and empower women.
- Reduce child mortality.
- Improve maternal health.
- Combat HIV/AIDS, malaria, and other diseases.
- Ensure environmental sustainability.
- Develop a Global Partnership for Development.

While the top five goals are clearly related to women and their health care, all the goals address the challenges and opportunities of providing quality and accessible health care for women. The disparity between rich and poor countries makes it difficult for poor countries to achieve the MDGs. By all indications, most of these goals have not been achieved in most of the world. In September 2010, world leaders reconvened at the United Nations in New York to review the progress being made in achieving the eight goals. Although some progress has been made in the efforts to reduce poverty, disease, and environmental degradation, much work still needs to be done to successfully attain many of the MDGs by 2015. In 2005, it was estimated that 1.4 billion people were still living below the poverty line. According to the United Nations, today one in four children under the age of 5 are malnourished due to lack of food, lack of clean water, and poor sanitation and health services. The gap between the rich and poor is a major deterrent in achieving the MDGs, particularly those related to women and girls, and it must be eliminated. Girls living in 20 percent of the most impoverished households in developing nations are 3.5 times more likely not to be enrolled in schools than girls in affluent households and four times more likely to be out of school than boys from the richest households. This large gap between the rich and poor also affects the improvement of maternal health due to differences in access to professional health services. For example, in many parts of the developing world, fewer than half of women have access to skilled health personnel when giving birth (United Nations 2010a). The absence of a common framework between rich and poor countries also makes it difficult for the exchange of knowledge and lessons learned, thus hindering progress and widening the gap between them.

Gender equality and the empowerment of women are central to the MDGs and therefore necessary to achieve these goals (United Nations 2010a). Global health problems require global solutions, and global solutions require partnership and better communication. Addressing urbanization and urban development while considering women's needs for safety, education, access to quality health care and support, healthy food, and a healthy environment may be a catalyst for achieving these vital goals for the well-being of nations.

The chapters that follow discuss the issues that women face living in urban areas in the United States, Africa, Asia, and elsewhere, and examples are given of how urbanization can either promote or hinder better health care for women. In addition, authors discuss creative solutions to living in slums and in unsafe environments. Partnerships between private and public organizations as well as governmental, national, and international organizations are vital for developing and implementing gender-sensitive solutions to urbanization; the chapters provide insights into what global agencies, such as the World Health Organization, as well as U.S. agencies, such as the National Institutes of Health's Office of Research on Women's Health and the Department of Health and Human Services, are proposing as strategic goals for the future.

This book examines the risks faced by women in urban areas s well as ways to enhance the health and safety of women by better planning of urban areas. This volume reflects the dialogues among scholars, clinicians, and activists about best practices to advance women's issues. The combination of empirical and tacit knowledge gives the needed support for women's voices to be heard. The integration of the diversity of methods, frameworks, evidence, advocacy, and the required support to reinforce actions in developing models of care and instituting changes is what will make a difference in designing healthy environments for women.

And when women are healthy and safe, so are their families and communities.

PART I

Women's Health in Urban Areas

Chapter 1

Women's Health and the City: A Comprehensive Approach for the Developing World

Julio Frenk and Octavio Gómez-Dantés

Women living in cities in the developing world face an increasingly complex set of health challenges that can be met only through innovative and comprehensive strategies. This chapter discusses the nature of these challenges and some strategies to address them. We begin by examining the impact of urbanization on the health of women in developing nations. Next, we address potential responses to the health needs of women in the developing urban world, building on the lessons from the primary health care (PHC) movement. Following this, we discuss potential obstacles to the implementation of these responses and present examples illustrating how such obstacles can be successfully overcome.

Urbanization and Women's Health

In response to major health threats in European cities in the nineteenth century (cholera, typhoid fever, tuberculosis), modern public health was born and networks of public health offices were established (Hamlin 2009). This progress nourished the sanitary reforms that yielded unprecedented improvements in living and working conditions in urban European centers, which led to the ensuing decline in mortality rates and a steady increase in life expectancy. The image of modern cities as places where order, tranquility, and cleanliness reigned, and where previously deadly diseases were under control, won general acceptance.

This image was challenged by the explosive growth of cities in low- and middle-income countries in the second half of the twentieth century, which was the product of high birth rates, declining infant mortality figures, and massive immigration waves. This uncontrolled growth has resulted in a high exposure to health risks by city dwellers, especially those living in slums, who frequently suffer from higher exposures to these risks than people living in rural areas (Montgomery 2009).

This epidemiological vulnerability is due not so much to a lack of resources as it is to "maldevelopment": a lack of consistency between the needs of a specific population and the responses generated to meet them (Touraine 1992). Many cities in developing nations lack planning procedures and regulatory mechanisms, have adopted inadequate urban models, and suffer from badly implemented policies.

The essential characteristic of maldevelopment is the juxtaposition of problems. In developed societies, new problems tend to replace old ones. In contrast, in maldeveloped societies, old and new problems coexist, fighting for public resources and for a place in the public agenda.

Health reflects better than other fields this pattern of development. Whereas rich countries experience a substitution of old for new patterns of disease, the developing world simultaneously faces a triple burden of ill health: first, the unfinished agenda of common infections, malnutrition, and reproductive health problems; second, the emerging challenges represented by noncommunicable diseases, mental disorders, and the growing scourge of injury and violence; and third, the health risks associated with globalization, including the threat of pandemics like AIDS and influenza, the trade in harmful products like tobacco and other drugs, the health consequences of climate change, and the dissemination of harmful lifestyles leading to the epidemic of obesity.

This protracted health transition is compressed in urban environments, especially in slums. Limited access to safe drinking water, inadequate sewer facilities, and insufficient waste disposal—all common in slums—help disseminate common infections, which are responsible for the more than 3 million deaths in girls under 5 that occur annually worldwide (WHO 2009b; Brocklehurst and Bartram 2010). Health services tend to be understaffed and lack basic resources, a fact that explains many of the 350,000 annual maternal deaths that occur worldwide in pregnancy and childbirth. "Maternal deaths," according to the Web page of the Averting Maternal Death and Disability Initiative at Columbia University, are "symptoms of health systems in crisis" (AMDD 2010).

At the same time, urban lifestyles expose women to risk factors linked to noncommunicable ailments, including heart disease, diabetes, cancer, and mental disorders. Cardiovascular diseases are the main causes of death and disability in women aged 60 years and over in low- and middle-income countries. Annually, 4.5 million women in developing regions die from stroke and ischemic heart disease, the same number as those who die from HIV/AIDS, tuberculosis, and malaria combined (4.6 million women in 2008) (WHO 2009b; Kaiser Family Foundation 2010).

Diabetes is also a major challenge. This disease is responsible for the deaths of almost 400,000 women annually in the developing world. The World Health Organization (WHO) projects that over the next ten years the number of deaths due to this ailment will increase by over 80 percent in upper middle-income countries (WHO 2010d).

Cancer in women in the developing world is increasing as well. Developing countries account for 46 percent of the 1 million new cases of breast cancer diagnosed each year worldwide and for 55 percent of deaths from breast cancer (Garcia et al. 2007). In Latin America, Uruguay and Argentina have reached breast cancer incidence rates similar to those of Canada, which are among the highest in the world (Lozano et al. 2009). Cervical cancer, which has become a rare disease in rich nations, causes more than 200,000 deaths annually in developing regions.

Injuries are also conspicuous in the cities of the developing world, and they increasingly affect women. Six of the ten most common causes of death in females aged 10 to 19 in middle-income countries are road traffic accidents, drowning, self-inflicted injuries, violence, poisoning, and burns (WHO 2009b). Most of these causes of death are more prevalent in urban settings.

Domestic violence is a critical topic. Evidence from health surveys in several developing countries shows a high prevalence of intimate partner abuse: 44 percent in Colombia, 34 percent in Egypt, 42 percent in Peru, and 48 percent in Zambia (Kishnor and Johnson 2004).

The rifts in the social fabric, particularly frequent in excluded urban populations, also create fertile soil for the development of mental problems. In fact, depression is a leading cause of disability among urban women in developing regions (Montgomery 2009).

Finally, we must consider the health risks associated with globalization, such as pandemics, harmful lifestyles, and climate change. Globally, 17 million women aged 15 to 49 are living with HIV/AIDS, 98 percent of whom live in the developing world. Urban prevalence rates of this disease are much higher than rural rates (UNAIDS, UNFPA, UNIFEM 2010). Women 15 to 24 years old are particularly vulnerable to this infection. In this age group, women now constitute more than 60 percent of the total cases of HIV/AIDS.

Today, more than 1 billion adults in the world are overweight. In the developing world this epidemic first affected affluent middle-aged adults, but it has now spread to younger and poorer populations. In Mexico, 70 percent of adult women in urban areas are overweight (Secretaría de Salud 2006).

Global environmental problems put additional pressure on urban centers. Increases in rainfall, temperature, and humidity are favoring the spread of diseases transmitted by mosquitoes over a wider range and higher altitudes (UNDP 2007). The rates of dengue fever, in particular, are increasing in poor urban settlements, where water is frequently trapped in cans, tires, and all sorts of containers, becoming breeding grounds for *Aedes aegypti*, the mosquito responsible for the transmission of this disease. Climate change, in fact, was considered responsible for 3.8 percent of dengue fever deaths worldwide in 2004, most of which occurred in societies with scarce resources and frail infrastructure (WHO 2009a).

Addressing the Health Needs of Women in the Urban Developing World

The increasingly complex health needs of women in the developing world can be addressed only through a comprehensive response built on four pillars: (1) a new generation of health-promotion and disease-prevention strategies; (2) universal access to a package of health-care services that is financed in a fair manner and addresses the triple burden of disease; (3) the adoption of innovations in the delivery of health-care services that make use of the various technological revolutions of our times; and (4) the endorsement and enforcement of human rights related to women's health. The remainder of this section discusses the use of these four pillars, taking into consideration the lessons of the PHC movement.

First Pillar: A New Generation of Health-Promotion and Disease-Prevention Strategies

To deal with the triple burden of disease faced by women in cities of the developing world, health systems need to renew public health interventions and expand their scope of action. Measures to control traditional health risks and prevent diseases should be strengthened. However, health systems also need to design and implement not just health policy, but *healthy* policies: to increase access to safe drinking water and sanitation, expand waste management services, improve public transportation and road safety, limit the consumption of tobacco and other drugs, prevent domestic violence, control the dissemination of unhealthy diets, increase physical activity, and control environmental pollution.

Some of the actions required to address health determinants may be implemented by health authorities. However, public health agencies cannot mandate by themselves the expansion of urban water pipelines or sewer systems for the urban poor, nor can they reorganize public transportation. Likewise, they have no authority to introduce sexual education contents in elementary school programs or implement judiciary reforms to protect victims of domestic violence.

The implementation of healthy policies requires coordination with other government agencies and sectors of society. The PHC movement has emphasized the need to act on the determinants of health. However, in developing countries PHC has been mostly involved with the direct provision of clinical and public health services. To generate additional improvements in the health conditions of women living in cities in developing regions and meet the emerging challenges, urban health systems must now assume other enabling functions, such as stewardship (Frenk 2009). Only strong ministries of health with solid regulatory and convening capacities will be able to prompt the design of the intersectoral policies that the urban health transition is demanding.

Public health measures related to women's health that need to be implemented in cities in developing nations include safe motherhood initiatives, sexual and reproductive interventions, preventive measures to address health risks related to emerging diseases, and investments to enhance urban epidemiologic security.

To improve maternal health it is necessary to expand access to prenatal and delivery care, thereby helping to foster healthy pregnancies and safe deliveries. This measure is critical given that there are still 350,000 maternal deaths annually worldwide (Hogan et al. 2010), 99 percent of which occur in developing countries. Urban women tend to have better access to medical services than women living in rural settlements, but maternal deaths are still a common event among poor women living in urban centers in developing regions.

Sexual and reproductive health has become a major concern among urban women in low- and middle-income countries. Efforts are needed to increase access to modern contraceptive methods and to methods that can prevent sexually transmitted diseases (STDs). Special attention in this regard should be given to teenagers, since the prevalence of unwanted pregnancies and unsafe abortions in this age group is very high in uneducated adolescents living in urban poverty. As mentioned earlier, young women are also becoming particularly vulnerable to HIV infection and other STDs. Human papillomavirus (HPV) infection, for example, is gaining importance, given its relationship to cervical cancer. This infection, which is highly transmissible, is more prevalent in developing countries than elsewhere. It is estimated that one out of five women in Africa is infected with HPV (Brocklehurst and Bartram 2010). An effective vaccine against this disease is now available. However, its cost limits its extended use in low- and middle-income countries.

Public health strategies to confront the increasingly prevalent ailments that transcend the field of reproductive health are also required. Salient among them are public health interventions to address cervical and breast cancer. Despite the magnitude of the problem, in developing nations there is an alarming lack of awareness about the increasing importance of noncommunicable diseases. More information directed to the general public should be disseminated, and better data to guide policy should be generated.

Access to screening procedures for the early detection of cervical and breast cancer should also be expanded. As mentioned previously, cervical cancer is one of the main causes of death in women in low-income countries, although effective and affordable treatments are now available. An interesting challenge would be to place cancer and other noncommunicable diseases in the global health agenda. The goal would be to expand the United Nations' Millennium Development Goals to include health targets related to noncommunicable diseases common in low- and middle-income countries, such as hypertension, diabetes, and certain cancers (Farmer et al. 2010).

Health promotion and preventive measures to control overweight in women should also be implemented, since being overweight is a major risk factor for three of the five main causes of death in women in low- and middle-income nations (ischemic heart disease, stroke, and diabetes).

Finally, public health investments to enhance human security are also needed, including epidemiologic surveillance and improved preparedness to respond to emergencies, natural disasters, and potential pandemics, to which urban concentrations are more prone and vulnerable. Pregnant women are especially susceptible to the human influenza A H1N1 virus, which clearly illustrates the differential impact that certain pandemic diseases can have on women's health.

Second Pillar: Universal Access to Health Care Services

In addition to health-promotion and disease-prevention strategies, urban health systems in developing nations need to mobilize additional financial resources to confront diseases and injuries that have already occurred. The Ministry of Health, the traditional steward of health systems, should approach the Ministry of Finance and the members of the Congress or similar administrative bodies and convince them of the need to increase the investment in health in order to meet the challenges of a population that is increasingly exposed to risks associated with costly, noncommunicable diseases. These additional resources, however, should be managed using financial arrangements that protect the population against catastrophic health expenditures. Protection against such expenditures is now considered one of the three main intrinsic objectives of health systems (Murray and Frenk 2000).

Catastrophic and impoverishing health expenditures are a common event in cities in developing nations, since the supply of health care tends to be dominated by private services, mostly financed out of pocket. Even in the Latin American region, where social security has had an expanding presence, only 20 percent of the population have access to public insurance (Fay 2005).

The best way to protect urban populations from "financial shocks" caused by injury, illness, or other health-related events is to collectively pool risks in some sort of public insurance program to meet health events without having to pay out of pocket. Innovations in the aggregation of risk should be considered, since access to traditional social security schemes is limited by the fact that a high proportion of the population in cities of developing countries are either self-employed or work in the informal sector of the economy.

Expanding women's access to health care beyond maternal care is a major challenge in cities of developing countries. Maternal deaths are still very common, especially in low-income countries, and should be addressed without hesitation. Health-care networks should be upgraded by improving the supply of equipment, medications, and safe blood, and health-care providers should be trained to assure timely diagnosis and treatment of obstetric emergencies. However, health systems in cities of the developing world also need to provide services for noncommunicable diseases. Cancer, in particular, is a challenge facing women in low- and middle-income countries that deserves more attention. Insofar as it is a STD, cervical cancer represents the unfinished agenda related to common infectious diseases. In contrast, breast cancer exemplifies the emerging challenges associated with the new lifestyles of women of developing countries. Meeting these challenges requires a two-pronged strategy: to improve early detection and to increase access to treatment, which is more effective when instituted at early stages of the disease.

Access to treatment of mental disorders, depression in particular, should also be expanded. The results of the WHO World Mental Health Surveys show that less than 15 percent of women with moderate to severe mental disorders in low-income and low-middle-income countries receive treatment, in contrast with almost 40 percent of women in high-income and upper-middle-income countries (Kessler and Ustun 2008).

Another major challenge is the quality of urban health services in developing regions. To increase the quality of care, health authorities can strengthen the regulation of individual and institutional providers through accreditation, certification, and other procedures.

Health systems in urban centers also have to introduce incentives for providers to reward high-quality care and responsiveness. Similarly, households can benefit from incentives tied to health-promoting behaviors, as shown by conditional cash-transfer (CCT) initiatives. These programs, implemented worldwide, have successfully met educational, nutritional, and health objectives in poor populations. In many countries, CCT programs have adopted a gender perspective in that the cash transfer is provided to women, who are thus empowered by their control over family resources.

Finally, urban public health systems can define packages of essential health services that make entitlements explicit. These packages are not only useful for planning and quality-assurance purposes; they also empower health-care users, who know exactly what they can demand.

Third Pillar: Innovations in the Delivery of Health-Care Services

The delivery of personal health-care services in cities of low- and middle-income countries has suffered from several problems, including the segmentation of populations, the poor responsiveness of health-care organizations to population needs, and the concentration of care in traditional health facilities (clinics, emergency units, and hospitals). The solution to most of these problems is integration: of populations through the creation of universal health-care systems; of health and healthy policies through the implementation of intersectoral strategies; of levels of care through the design of networks that guarantee the continuity of care; and of formal and informal health-care spaces through the extension of the supply of health care and health-promoting activities to a diversity of spheres—homes, schools, workplaces, and recreational areas—in order to move from health *centers* to healthy *spaces*.

The integrated model for the delivery of personal health services in urban settings should be based on networks that make intensive and extensive use of the instruments generated by the information and communication revolutions: databases, computers, and mobile phones. The use of cellular phones for health purposes is especially promising, since these phones are becoming the communication technology of choice even in very poor nations (Jordans 2009).

In the field of maternal health, mobile technology should be used to provide support during pregnancy. These systems can offer general health and health-care information to pregnant women, provide emergency-care tips and alerts, and supply post-delivery support. These same systems can also be used to offer information about emerging risks to which women are frequently exposed and remind women of the need for preventive care. Telephone hotlines can be implemented to provide support to victims of domestic violence and depressed women.

Fourth Pillar: Rights Revolution

To improve women's health, urban health systems have to make use of organizational and technical innovations—but they also require a firm ethical foundation. There is a need not only for ideas but also for ideals. More today than ever, the women's health movement must promote the ethic of universal rights, so that every girl and woman may have the same opportunity to achieve her full potential. It is in our ability to care for each other, in our determination not to leave anybody behind, in our vision of health as a right-related objective that we may find the building blocks for a better world.

The rights revolution of the twentieth century plays a key role in this regard. Rights have become the dominant language of public good worldwide, and health systems in urban centers in the developing world have to take advantage of this fact.

The first step in this direction is to endorse the idea of health care as a human right (Sen 2008). Such rights are, by definition, inherent to every person. The implications of a rights-based approach are clear: It is unethical to limit access to health services on the basis of the labor, ethnic, or legal status of any person. The human nature of the right to health care also implies that support for this claim can come from anywhere in the world. This opens an enormous field of action for international advocacy and global solidarity.

The second step in this direction is to create the necessary consensus to turn what is sometimes an abstract right into legislation in order to guarantee the effective exercise of the right to health care.

Finally, other rights related to the health of women also need to be supported and guaranteed, including reproductive rights, sexual rights, the right to be free from torture, and the right to a life free of violence (UNIFEM 2010a).

Overcoming the Obstacles to the Implementation of a Comprehensive Response to Women's Health Needs

The implementation of a comprehensive response to women's health needs in cities of developing nations based on the four pillars discussed herein can face diverse obstacles. In this section, some of these potential obstacles are discussed and examples of ways in which they can be successfully confronted are presented. Most of these examples stem from the recent Mexican health-care reform.

Intersectoral action in health is probably as old as modern public health. As mentioned in the first section of this chapter, the sanitary and the housing measures adopted in Western European cities in the nineteenth century yielded enormous health benefits. Despite this fact, low- and middle-income nations have not been able to develop a consistent tradition of intersectoral policies. Until very recently, most public health actions focused on common infections and reproductive events, and were developed within the strict frontiers of the health sector.

The changing nature of emerging health risks, associated with unhealthy lifestyles, is demanding regular collaborations of the health system with sectors such as education, finance, water and sanitation, transportation, and public security, and their international character is calling for closer relationships with sectors such as trade, foreign affairs, and even defense. Among the factors that can help strengthen the implementation of intersectoral actions in health are a supportive governance structure (legislation and institutions mandating the integration of public actions and strategies), a capable and accountable health sector, solid health research institutions, and strong civil society organizations working in the health arena (WHO 2010a).

One of the best examples of successful collaboration to meet health-related goals affecting women is in the area of tobacco control. To confront this major health risk, which is more prevalent in urban than rural settings, broad collaborations were established between research and policy institutions at both international and national levels, which eventually led to the design and promotion of the WHO Framework Convention on Tobacco Control. In some developing countries, national health authorities have been able to develop comprehensive tobacco control policies, which have included raising tobacco taxes, eliminating advertising and promotion, and creating smoke-free environments, thanks to the participation in the design and implementation of these policies of legislators and policymakers of the health and finance ministries, as well as academic institutions and nongovernmental organizations.

Several intersectoral policy initiatives have also been implemented in developing countries to address the emerging challenge of overweight and obesity, which has turned into a major pandemic. In Mexico, the Ministry of Health has worked closely with the Congress and the Ministry of Education to regulate the marketing of unhealthy food and implement school-based programs to promote healthy nutrition and physical activity (WcP Observer 2010).

Regarding pandemics, the response to the recent H1N1 influenza pandemic clearly shows the importance of broad collaboration between international and national health authorities at the global level, and among sectors at the local level. The timely and effective response to this threat was the result of the existence of global and national preparedness plans, the establishment of international epidemiologic networks, the enactment of transparent communication strategies, especially in those places first affected by the flu epidemic, the implementation of measures to control the dissemination of the disease, and the timely treatment of affected individuals. This broad response involved the participation at the local level not only of the health authorities but also of the ministries of finance, public security, foreign affairs, and defense, as well as the media.

The main obstacles to the expansion of social protection in health and to the expansion of the types of interventions available to women in cities of the developing world are the lack of resources and the scarcity of successful experiences that can be adapted to the conditions of low- and middle-income countries. The following initiatives demonstrate that these obstacles can be overcome.

Knowledge is one of the best instruments that urban authorities have at their disposal to mobilize additional resources for health. In their discussions with the local congress and the finance authorities, urban authorities can make use of global evidence showing that, in addition to its intrinsic value, a well-performing health system contributes to the overall welfare of society by relieving poverty, improving productivity, increasing educational abilities, developing human capital, protecting savings and assets, stimulating economic growth, and enhancing security.

The recent Mexican health-care reform is an interesting example of how evidence can be used to mobilize fresh resources and promote an initiative that is now providing social protection in health to all Mexican citizens, including the 50 million individuals, most of them poor, who lacked traditional social security (Frenk et al. 2006; Frenk, Gómez-Dantés, and Knaul 2009). Poor families in Mexico can now enroll in a new public insurance scheme known as *Seguro Popular*, which assures legislated access to a comprehensive package of health services.

Several international initiatives have also been successful in expanding the types of interventions offered by the health sector in cities of the developing world, especially those interventions addressing the emerging diseases affecting women in developing countries, such as cancer. For example, a major breakthrough was the approval of a $50 million grant from the Bill & Melinda Gates Foundation to create the Alliance for Cervical Cancer Prevention, whose mission is to work toward the prevention of cervical cancer in the developing world (Alliance for Cervical Cancer Prevention 2010). Similar efforts are being implemented in the breast cancer field. In 2002, the Fred Hutchinson Cancer Research

Center and Susan G. Komen for the Cure created the Breast Health Global Initiative, which in turn launched the "Guidelines for International Breast Health and Cancer Control" (Breast Health Global Initiative 2008). Recently, *Lancet* published a call to expand cancer care and control in countries of low and middle income (Farmer et al. 2010). At the local level, Colombia and Mexico, in the context of major health reforms, have demonstrated that universal access to the treatment of breast cancer is now possible in middle-income countries.

The main obstacle to the use of technological innovations in the delivery of health-care services in the developing world is access to these technologies. However, this is no longer a problem in the case of mobile phones, which are being increasingly used for health purposes. According to Vital Wave Consulting, there are 2.2 billion mobile phones in the developing world and by 2012 at least half of all individuals living in remote areas of the planet will have regular access to this technology (Vital Wave Consulting 2009).

In Peru, mobile phones are being used to send pregnant women advice on nutrition and potential problems during pregnancy (Pregnant women in Peru 2010). In South Africa, SMS (cellular phone text messaging) is used to promote education on AIDS (Project Masiluleke 2009). In Mexico, a program designed by the Carso Health Institute provides diabetic women with cell phones to monitor their blood sugar levels and adjust their drug intake (DiabeDiario 2009). Also drawing on the widespread use of cellular phones, call centers to support victims of sexual and domestic violence can now be found in urban centers all over the developing world.

Mobile phones are also being used for public health purposes. In China, mobile phones were used in an emergency reporting system for infectious diseases after the Sichuan earthquake (Yang et al. 2009). The influenza pandemic prompted the design of a mobile phone application that contains a questionnaire that helps identify if someone has the H1N1 virus (The HMS Mobile Swine Flu App 2009). In Peru, alerts of disease outbreaks are being sent through text messages, voice mail, and e-mail.

Finally, converting the attention to women's health needs in urban centers of developing countries into rights and entitlements is a particularly tough battle, since as the historian Lynn Hunt has written, "human rights are still easier to endorse than to enforce" (Hunt 2007: 208). However, several steps are being taken in this direction. There is a global movement for the recognition of health care as a human right. This movement is taking advantage of the fact that this right is enshrined in several binding international treaties and national constitutions (The Right to Health Care 2008).

Several initiatives have also been made to monitor the efforts of national health systems to eventually incorporate the right to health care into local legislations and turn this right into concrete entitlements (Backman et al. 2008).

The 1994 Cairo International Conference of Population and Development and the 1995 Beijing World Conference on Women greatly advanced the cause of reproductive rights, which have expanded considerably since then and permeated most of the local legislations in the developing world.

The movement against domestic violence has also rendered major achievements in the field of rights. For example, based on the findings of a national survey that showed a prevalence of domestic abuse of 21.6 percent among female users of health services, the Mexican Congress recently passed a law that punishes psychological, physical, and patrimonial violence against women and provides for the immediate arrest of the presumptive aggressor and the protection of the victim (Secretaría de Salud 2009).

Conclusion

The changing context of urban conglomerates in developing countries offers the opportunity to re-evaluate women's health needs. The increasing exposure of urban women in low- and middle-income countries to health risks associated with noncommunicable diseases demands the design of comprehensive approaches. To confront these novel challenges, health systems are being forced to design innovative public health strategies, increase social protection in health, expand the pool of interventions available in health-care units beyond maternal care, make use of the tools generated by new information and communications technologies, and take advantage of the global movement to recognize health care as a human right. Those local health systems willing to meet the challenges of the twenty-first century in this comprehensive way will improve not only the health of urban women, a desirable goal in itself, but also the well-being and security of their entire populations.

This chapter applies to the field of women's health some ideas presented in a previous work by Julio Frenk and Octavio Gómez-Dantés entitled "Urban Health Services and Health Systems Reform," in *Urban Health: Global Perspectives*, ed. D. Vlahov, J. I. Boufford, C. Pearson, and L. Norris. San Francisco, CA: Jossey-Bass, 2010: 221–36.

Chapter 2

Policy for a Better Future:
A Focus on Girls and Women

Ruth Levine

The world over, sound public policy requires a very specific type of vision—the vision to see into the future. Public policymakers need to anticipate how the actions they take today will make the people and institutions they serve either more vulnerable to both predictable and unknown future challenges or more resilient to those very same challenges. This is no easy task, in large measure because the pressures of the present—political, financial, and otherwise—often prevent attention to the middle distance and constrain the willingness to invest in the sorts of policies and programs that bring the greatest future benefits. But when long-term conditions and consequences are considered, we inevitably come to an understanding of the importance of appropriate, high-impact investments in the lives and livelihoods of the girls and young women of today.

Thinking about the future brings to mind an insightful metaphor held by the Aymara Indians of the Andean highlands. The Aymara refer to the future not as most other cultures do, which is as something in front of us that we look toward. Instead, they think of the future as being in back of them, hidden from sight; what they can see before their eyes is the past. So they have an image of walking backward into the future. That notion—which we might call 20/20 hindsight—is a fascinating challenge to our own notion that we face the future with a clear view of what is ahead. If we think more like the Aymara, then we realize how carefully we must walk: taking clues from what we can see based on past trends, but with the realization that there are vast uncertainties that we cannot see.

Those who are responsible throughout the world for major decisions about the laws, regulations, and use of public funds can make the best choices for the future by orienting their actions based on four major trends: changes in the size and age structure of populations (including population movement, particularly urbanization); changes in the type of distribution of health threats; environmental dynamics, especially climate change; and long-term economic trends. Unlike other important and headline-grabbing influences on national and global prospects, such as elections and the eruption of conflict, these four trends have remarkably predictable features, in some cases for decades into the future. Through them, we can look out twenty or even thirty years and have a good sense of how different the world will look. We can see the type of world for which the young people of today must be prepared.

At the same time, there are limits to inevitability. Within each of these trends we can identify a set of changes that are certain to occur, and then a range of scenarios that reflect uncertainty. So, for example, although we know that the average global temperature is rising, we are unsure about the pace and magnitude—variables that are a function, in part, of today's actions to control greenhouse gas emissions. Although we can play out demographic scenarios, social changes such as age at marriage and desired family size over the next decade influence the long-term prospects. In many cases, the potential variation and uncertainty hold clues to near-term policy actions that can influence what scenario plays out in reality.

In this chapter, I highlight what these large-scale trends tell us about what the world is likely to look like ten to fifty years hence. And I identify some of the ways in which a recognition of these trends should inform public policy, particularly with respect to policies that affect adolescent girls and women.

The Size and Structure of Populations

Let's look at the first trend, demographic change. Over the past forty years, almost all of the major developing regions of the world have witnessed a dramatic fall in the number of children born to each woman, along with significant improvements in life expectancy with the reduction of preventable childhood mortality, improved living conditions, and improvements in health among older adults. Those shifts, of course, came later to the developing countries than similar declines in fertility and mortality in the countries that now have relatively high average incomes. Given the population momentum—the echoes of high-fertility periods through subsequent cohorts—we can predict with confidence that between 2005 and 2030, most of the world's population growth will occur in the less-developed countries in Africa, Asia, and Latin America. Whereas Asia's share of the world's population will be at about 60 percent through 2050, Europe's share will shrink as a percentage of global population and Africa's will increase in relative terms (UNPD 2008).

An important transition in the age structure also will take place. Worldwide we currently have the largest cohort of adolescents, a real youth bulge of 12- to 24-year-olds estimated at 1.5 billion, representing a profound social challenge and perhaps opportunity.

Over the next decades, the average age of the population will rise, and we will see an increasingly dramatic divergence in average age between the countries that are now high income and those that are low and middle income. By about 2020, the average age will be right around 40 years in the developed world and about 20 years in least-developed countries (UNPD 2008).

Our shared demographic future has many implications for the world our children will inherit, and what their preparation should be. In particular, in most regions of the world, there has been—and will continue to be—a reorientation in women's roles from being primarily associated with reproduction to being increasingly associated with economic productivity. This implies the need for schooling that yields skills valued in the marketplace, as well as attention to the legal protections for women's income and assets. Moreover, it is likely (and has already been observed) that countries facing a rapidly aging population and their attendant health and other personal service needs will turn to the relatively young populations in the developing world for a major share of the workforce. Over time, immigration policies—particularly those that bring in service workers but do not provide a full share of citizen's rights—are likely to expand. Women's opportunities to migrate from poor to wealthy countries for jobs in the service sector will increase, as will the need for policymakers to ensure that laws are in place to assure them a full measure of human rights and employment protections.

Movement to Cities

If the change in raw population numbers and structure are relatively easy to predict based on the past, so is the future of cities—or at least that the future *is* cities. More than half the population in developing countries now live in urban areas. These are not only the so-called megacities, but also and importantly the secondary and tertiary cities.

By 2030, an estimated 5 billion people will live in cities, eight out of ten of them in developing countries (UNFPA 2007).

The rapid expansion of cities has tended to occur in an uncontrolled way, without attention to urban planning or sufficient investments in the water, electrical, or other infrastructure needed to support rapid population growth. Thus, we have seen the establishment of informal settlements on the outskirts of cities that are characterized by very poor shelter, limited public lighting, open sewage and trash heaps, very limited access to clean water, and high levels of crime and insecurity (Montgomery 2009).

With respect to the potential and the problems of urbanization, policies in low-income countries, as well as the interventions by international donors such as bilateral and multilateral agencies, have tended to be uninspired. For the most part, donor attention has focused not on cities but on rural areas, tending to promote economic opportunities and social service delivery in rural areas. This is in part because the conditions are systematically worse in rural areas than in cities and in part because of the motivation to reduce the pace of rural-to-urban migration.

Policymakers at the national and international level have difficulty confronting city problems, and the municipal governments and politicians upon whom the burden falls have in general not been equal to the task. In many cases, the informal settlements are outside of the legal jurisdictions of municipal authorities, and the poor residents have little political sway. In addition, it is not unusual for heads of state to be political opponents with the mayors of their country's largest cities, which may result in unfavorable budget outcomes for cities.

History has demonstrated that little can be done to stem human movement to cities. People are pulled to cities by the promise of job and school opportunities, as well as family and cultural factors. Virtually regardless of how harsh the conditions are, the attraction of cities persists. The policy challenge, then, is not how to restrict internal migration, but rather how to ensure that the public sector is able to manage the inflow as well as the natural growth of urban populations. A further challenge is to consider how to take advantage of the dynamic of urbanization to make for a more livable world in the future.

With regard to adolescent girls and women in urban areas, the key challenges largely have to do with security and health. In many developing countries, young girls migrate alone or with their families to urban settings where they are exposed to sexual violence as well as environmental risks, and where the social networks that might protect them from harm are more fragile (Temin and Levine 2009). They may be drawn into unregulated, invisible, and often unsafe domestic work, which in some settings is sheer servitude, or into the informal sector of small-scale shops and home-based assembly and other manufacturing.

Epidemiologic Change

A clear trend, and one that is likely to intensify, is the increase in the prevalence of chronic disease in developing countries. This is a dramatic phenomenon resulting from both our success in reducing the toll of infectious disease and the adoption of unhealthful behaviors.

The figures are startling. Already heart and respiratory disease affecting adults top the causes of death in the developing world, and by 2030 chronic diseases such as diabetes, cancer, and chronic obstructive pulmonary disease (chronic bronchitis and emphysema) are predicted to be far more significant causes of mortality than diarrhea, malaria, and tuberculosis in most low-income countries. Between 1990 and 2020, we anticipate a 120 to 140 percent increase in developing countries in mortality due to cardiovascular disease. Diabetes already extracts a high toll—in Tanzania, more than 10 percent of those 35 years and older in urban areas have this disease. Globally, an estimated 171 million people were affected by diabetes in 2000; by 2030, that figure is anticipated to grow to 366 million, with 86 percent in developing countries (Wild et al. 2004).

The near- and long-term consequences of the rise in chronic diseases are profound, at both family and social levels. In India, a very large share of family income may be devoted to health care when a family member is affected by diabetes (Ramachandran et al. 2007), and the same is likely true in many other developing countries. In many countries where studies have been conducted, close to one fifth of public spending on health is used for caring for people with diabetes (Adeyi, Smith, and Robles 2007).

Public policymakers are facing the need to both prevent and manage the challenge of chronic disease, which in many countries represents a more significant problem than the infectious diseases that international donors tend to see as their focus. Preventive strategies are numerous, ranging from ensuring that urban infrastructure permits and even encourages physical activity, to instituting taxes to limit the consumption of tobacco products, to exploring the use of polypills for population-level prevention of cardiovascular disease. There is, on the prevention agenda, a particular role for attention to adolescent girls, because it is during adolescence that many of the dietary and other "lifestyle" habits are established.

Climate Change

A fourth trend that shapes our collective future is environmental change of many sorts, and particularly climate change. With climate change, as we have seen, come changes in agricultural production, with the most negative consequences likely to affect many of the poorest regions; extreme weather and sea level rise, which particularly threaten countries with fragile infrastructures and island nations; and shifts in the geographic reach of infectious diseases, particularly insect- and animal-borne diseases.

Policies that foster adaptation to the likely environmental changes include major infrastructure investments to protect vulnerable populations. However, recent research has shed light on the potential for classic development interventions, and particularly investments in the education of girls, to both increase the resilience of societies to predictable environmental challenges and to mitigate the environmental changes themselves (Blankespoor et al. 2010).

Economic Shifts

While our shared economic future is less predictable than changes in population size, structure, and distribution, or environmental dynamics, we can draw upon clues from the recent past to make educated guesses about the global economy in the future.

We are likely to continue to see fast and potentially dramatic economic growth in Asia, particularly in the South Asian giant India, and in China. In high-income countries, economic growth rates are expected to be at about 2 percent over the foreseeable future; in low-income countries, we can expect up to 7 percent growth on average. By 2050 the total gross domestic product of China is predicted to surpass that of the United States, although the per capita income will remain much lower.

To some extent, the growth in large developing countries will continue to be export driven, responding to the demand for goods and services from high-income countries, particularly the United States. However, increasingly, the economic growth in large low- and middle-income countries will be driven by expansion of the domestic economy.

Several implications link directly to the prospects for girls and women. First, with increased aggregate income come new and increasing opportunities for public investments in infrastructure, research and development, and the social sectors, including health and education. The tendency is for decisions about those investments to be made in response to demands from powerful constituents and/or to be seen as "gender neutral." However, progressive public policymakers, realizing the disproportionate benefits that come with investments in the well-being of girls and women, will take advantage of the opportunity to increase infrastructure investments that reduce the time burden of women, who tend to be responsible for many domestic tasks, including obtaining water for family use. Second, the expansion of economic opportunities demands that women are seen as economic actors and that investments are made in the education options that will adequately prepare women to participate in a global labor market.

The Millennium Development Babies

This summary of major trends that are shaping the future of both developing and developed worlds—demographic (including urbanization), epidemiologic, environmental, and economic—is intended to motivate us to ask some basic questions: Are we ready for these changes, and are we adequately preparing our children? Is the public policy of today creating societies that will be more resilient to the challenges ahead? Are we making the most of the actions we are taking today—the level and type of investments in education, immigration, security, or other policies—to orient the "megatrends" toward the brightest possible future?

The trends shape what we will see over the next forty years, through 2050. This is, in fact, the productive adult period of the Millennium Development babies—those who were entering the world around the year 2000, when more than 190 leaders were signing the Millennium Development Goals. Those children are 10 years old today, at the very beginning of their adolescence.

Motivating the type of large-scale and consistent priority that public policymakers in developing countries, as well as their development partners, should give to the needs of girls and women requires looking at the demographic, economic, and other trends that are shaping our future and seeing both the gender-specific implications of those trends and how the decisions we make today can help to ensure that the future is as bright as possible.

This chapter was prepared while the author was employed by the Center for Global Development in Washington, D.C. The views expressed do not necessarily represent those of the U.S. Agency for International Development or the U.S. government.

Chapter 3

Girls' Health and Educational Needs in Urban Environments

Varina Tjon-A-Ten, Brad Kerner, Shweta Shukla, and Anne Hochwalt

The majority of the world's population now live in urban areas. More than one-third (37 percent) of the urban population in developing regions live in slum conditions and struggle with the associated problems of inadequate public services, inadequate social infrastructure, and a lack of education (United Nations 2006, 2008c). According to a United Nations survey, children's attendance at primary school is higher in urban areas than in rural areas (84 percent attendance vs. 75 percent attendance), yet children from the poorest households, regardless of where they live, have the lowest attendance (65 percent) (United Nations 2008c). Additionally, girls account for 55 percent of the out-of-school population (United Nations 2008c). Worldwide, for every 100 boys out of school there are 122 girls out of school (World Bank 2009). In developing countries, one out of five girls does not complete sixth grade and only 43 percent of secondary-school-age girls are in school (UNICEF 2007). These numbers prevail despite important accomplishments of the United Nations Millennium Development Goals focusing on universal primary education (Goal 2) and gender equality (Goal 3).

The importance of ensuring that girls not only enter school, but stay enrolled when they reach puberty is an enduring issue, having been of concern in many societies for more than a century. The novelist Jane Austen wrote: "Give a girl an education and introduce her properly into the world, and ten to one but she has the means of settling well, without further expense to anybody" (Austen 1814). A decade ago, former United Nations Secretary Kofi Annan called out: "The first step is for societies to recognize that educating girls is not an option; it is a necessity" (Annan 2000).

Improving school attendance for girls can be life changing, especially in developing countries. Educated girls have a positive impact on gender equity, child and maternal health, reduction of birth and mortality rates, and reduction of poverty (Tembon and Fort 2008; Winter and Macina 1999). Keeping girls in school not only enhances their families' lives and well-being but also contributes to national economic growth (Dollar and Gatti 1999; King and Mason 2001). For example, when a girl in the developing world receives seven or more years of education, she marries four years later, has fewer children, and sees child and maternal mortality decline (Summers 1994). In Africa, children of mothers who receive five years of primary education are 40 percent more likely to live beyond age 5 (Summers 1994). Furthermore, an extra year of primary school can increase a girl's eventual earnings by 10 to 20 percent, and an extra year of secondary school can increase wages by as much as 15 to 25 percent (Psacharopoulos and Patrinos 2002). Finally, when women and girls earn income, they reinvest 90 percent of it in their families, compared with only 30 to 40 percent for men (U.S. Department of State 2010).

Yet it is not just families that benefit from improved female education; nations also experience economic gains. A recent World Bank study of 100 countries revealed that every 1 percent increase in the proportion of women with secondary education boosted a country's annual per capita income growth rate by 0.3 percentage points (PLAN 2008). It also showed the staggering costs of failing to educate girls to the same standard as boys. Sixty-five low-income, middle-income, and transition countries that did not offer girls the same secondary school opportunities as boys missed out on an annual economic growth of an estimated $92 billion (PLAN 2008). Countries in South and West Asia and sub-Saharan Africa have the worst record on educating girls to the secondary level, costing the sub-Saharan region alone more than $5.2 billion a year due to gender disparity in schools (Dollar and Gatti 1999; PLAN 2008).

Barriers to Girls' School Attendance

Many factors interrupt girls' school attendance and participation. For example, in western and central Africa, drought, food shortages, child labor, HIV/AIDS, and poverty contribute to low school enrollment and high dropout rates that prove to be particularly devastating for girls (United Nations 2008c). In many countries, the lack of birth registration and the lack of control to enforce compliance make providing and enforcing compulsory education (where it exists) very difficult (Melchiorre 2004). Cultural biases, traditions that support educating only boys and keeping girls at home to work, fear of sexual harassment or abuse by teachers or other students, and fear of impregnation are additional factors interrupting girls' school attendance (United Nations 2008c; Kirk and Sommer 2006; Lawson 2008; Sommer 2009b).

Although not definitively proven, many health and education specialists believe that the onset of menstruation affects a girl's attendance or participation in school (FAWE Uganda 2004; Gathoni 2009; GWE-PRA 2001; UNICEF 2005; Stromquist 2007; IRIN 2010b; Kirk and Sommer 2006; Sommer 2009a; Kariuki 2003; Mati 2003; DeJaeghere 2004). In developing countries, there are often no major differences in attendance at the preschool or early primary school levels between boys and girls. But in the higher primary grades and secondary school, the number of girls in school declines almost by half (Herz et al. 1991). Reasons cited as contributing to the dropout and absenteeism rates include the absence of adequate safe, clean, and private latrines and clean water supplies, inadequate access to sanitary products, and girls' ignorance of practical information on managing menses.[1]

The onset of menstruation points to an important issue that may lie with women. Women prefer not to talk about menstruation, and if they do, they do not address the issue directly, choosing to use nonspecific expressions ("not feeling well" or have "stomach cramps") or euphemisms ("red flags hanging" or "monthly celebrations") (Tjon-A-Ten 2009). It is critical that women start an open dialogue—with women and men—about all aspects of female sexual and reproductive health, including menstruation and menstrual hygiene. Support must be given to men and women in developing countries who want an upfront approach to talk about sexuality within the framework of education without losing track of deeply embedded and persistent cultural traditions and customs.

What happens when the priorities and needs of girls are driving forces, for example, in school design and school infrastructure? What happens when girls are given accurate information about puberty and menstruation? What happens when girls are provided with sanitary pads, and as a result do not feel embarrassed or anxious about staining their clothes with blood and being teased by boys? There is conclusive evidence that girls' attendance in school is increased through improved sanitation (Bharadwaj and Patkar 2004). A recently published Oxford study (Bradshaw 2010) shows that free sanitary pad distribution to girls has a positive impact on school attendance. Further research and programs suggest that simple, carefully crafted solutions to support girls' menstrual health needs may have positive results, while the work of nongovernmental (e.g., Save the Children in Ethiopia) and governmental (e.g., Rajasthan [India] Ministry of Health) partnerships with private companies (e.g., Procter & Gamble) may have broad reapplication to girls living in cities and provide some answers to these questions. The remainder of this chapter reviews examples of these initiatives and draws lessons from the experiences.

Addressing Menstruation and Education: The Girls' Puberty Book Project in Tanzania

An in-depth research study on girls' experiences of menstruation and education conducted in 2006–2007 in rural and urban northern Tanzania determined that poor sexual and reproductive health education, coupled with the onset of menstruation and puberty, was interrupting girls' school participation. The research included observation, in-depth interviewing, review of curriculum and relevant policy documents, and, most important, conducting participatory activities with adolescent girls. This research method used in rural (Rombo District) and urban (Moshi) Tanzania with 120 girls not only led to a greater understanding of the needs of young girls but sparked the idea for the development of a "girls' puberty book," which was subsequently written by the researchers (and Tanzanian girls) in partnership with local collaborators (Sommer 2009b).

In Tanzania, much secrecy surrounds the topic of menstruation. Traditionally the paternal aunties, the grandmothers, and the older women convey puberty guidance to girls. However, as families become separated due to urban migration and the impact of HIV/AIDS, there is less extended family guidance being passed along to girls. And, just as parents in the United States may be uncomfortable talking about menstruation, parents in Tanzania often refrain from talking about this issue with their daughters. Therefore, in exploring this sensitive topic, the researchers found that capturing girls' voices and recommendations was fundamental to knowing how to solve the challenges they were facing.[2]

A primary focus of the fieldwork was three participatory activities conducted with groups of girls. The first asked girls to write "menstrual stories" in Swahili. Writing anonymously, they each submitted a page about the first time they experienced their menstrual periods, describing how they felt, how they managed their first menstrual flows, and whom they talked to or sought advice from (if they talked to anyone). Girls were also asked to include their advice for younger girls who had yet to experience their first menstrual periods. More than 100 girls wrote their stories, and most reported that they had talked to no one at the onset of menstruation. In a second activity, girls submitted their (anonymous) puberty questions for which they had no source of information. In a third activity, groups of girls designed a puberty curriculum to be passed along to the Ministry of Education. When analyzed, the three activities revealed the gap between what girls felt they knew and the guidance they wished to receive.

Based on this information, the research team concluded that a prior idea—developing a colorful and informative "girls' puberty book," including girls' own stories, to inform and empower girls and to help parents and teachers open a dialogue about puberty topics—would be a useful remedy to address this gap in girls' knowledge about puberty and menstrual management. They envisioned a book that would be distributed at no cost across Tanzania through various nongovernmental organizations (NGOs) working with prepubescent girls. The Nike Foundation provided support through a seed grant to develop and publish an initial 16,000 copies of the book and to pilot an effort to build support and identify sources to further sustain the book's publication in Tanzania.

The research team believed that this approach would overcome at least two difficulties in the girls' educational environment. First, teachers in many schools are predominantly male and for gender and cultural reasons are not an appropriate source of support for pubescent girls with menstrual-related questions. Second, teachers in most schools are overloaded with a full curriculum and do not have adequate reference materials for teaching girls about menstrual onset. For both reasons, developing a book that was not dependent on schoolteacher interaction for girls' knowledge and empowerment seemed critical.

The thirty-four-page book with colorful illustrations, pictured in Figure 3.1, written at a 10- to 14-year-old reading level, has three sections. The first section contains very basic puberty guidance—it intentionally does not address issues of safe sex, HIV, or family planning—and was adapted from a puberty curriculum that the government of Tanzania was already developing for use in schools. The second section reproduces five menstrual stories culled from the research. The third section outlines a number of educational activities related to menstrual management and associated puberty changes. They include a true/false section to counter some of the myths about menstruation, a question-and-answer section based on the anonymous puberty questions girls submitted, and a menstrual calendar to teach girls how to track their periods.

The book aims to reach girls at a window of opportunity in early adolescence, before other pressures, such as sexual relations, confront them. It targets the changes of early puberty rather than taking on topics such as practicing safe sex. During preparation of the book, the authors asked parents, teachers, and other adults to review the manu-

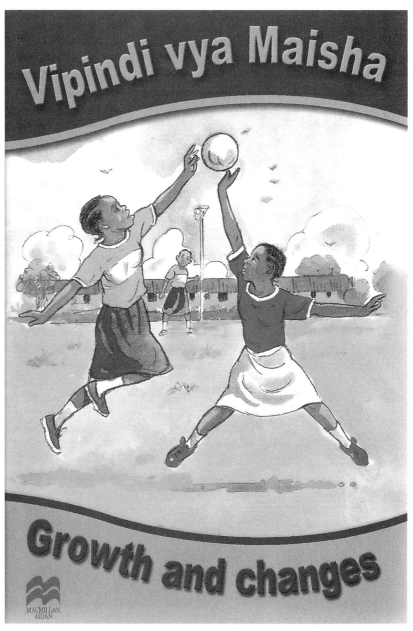

Figure 3.1. The cover of *Vipindi vya Maisha* (Growth and Changes). (Photo courtesy of Marni Sommer.)

script, and the book was field tested with 11- and 12-year-old girls (the middle of the target age group).

With an initial print run of 16,000, the book (called *Vipindi vya Maisha*, or Growth and Changes) was distributed through numerous NGOs, including Family Health International, the International Youth Foundation, and Care International (Figure 3.2). To broaden support for the book, the authors presented a copy to the permanent secretary of the Ministry of Education, who loved it and sent it to the Ministry of Education's curriculum committee for review and incorporation into primary school curriculum. The committee gave the book conditional approval in November 2009, with final approval received in August 2010. The local United Nations units, UNFPA (the United Nations Population Fund) and UNICEF (the United Nations Children's Fund), also supported it, financing the publication and dissemination of more than 100,000 copies. In August 2010, Vodacom, a large mobile phone company, decided to fund an additional 50,000 to 100,000 copies of the book.

Three things are critical to repeating this book's success in other countries: First, such a book must be socially and culturally appropriate to the context in which it will be distributed. Second, participatory

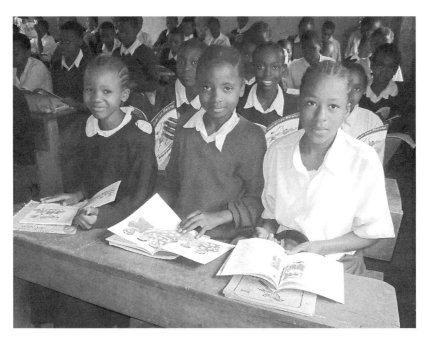

Figure 3.2. Tanzanian school girls reading the *Vipindi vya Maisha* puberty education book in class. (Photo courtesy of Marni Sommer.)

research activities are essential to gathering the material for the book. Third, having the approval of parents and adults and reviews of young girls who will use the book is critical. Distributing 100,000 copies of such a book across a country is achievable only when the book is developed from within and for the society in which it will be distributed.

The Effect of Menstruation on Girls' School Experience: Save the Children's Program in Ethiopia

Save the Children is a leading independent organization for children in need, with programs in 120 countries, including the United States. It aims to inspire breakthroughs in the way the world treats children and to achieve immediate and lasting change in children's lives by improving their health, education, and economic opportunities (Save the Children 2009b).

Save the Children has an active Adolescent Sexual and Reproductive Health (ASRH) program that focuses on creating access to reproductive health information and services, working with parents to communicate better with their teen children, training health providers to meet the needs of young people, involving youth in improving the services offered at the health facilities, and involving young people in peer-to-peer outreach on HIV prevention. Save the Children places a special emphasis on reaching younger adolescents, promoting comprehensive sexuality education—which includes a focus on puberty and body literacy—while connecting these youth with caring adults.

As in Tanzania, a considerable number of girls in Ethiopia navigate puberty without proper information about the physical changes they can expect, without support from family members, without schools that have a "girl-friendly" water and sanitation infrastructure, and without information on feminine hygiene products. Ethiopian adolescents have limited access to sexual and reproductive sexual health information and services, and the sociocultural context perpetuates an environment in which these issues remain taboo to discuss with parents (Save the Children 2009a). Within this context, Save the Children has been working in Ethiopia since 1998 to improve adolescents' sexual and reproductive health with comprehensive, multifaceted programs that work from an ecological model, reaching adolescents as well as their parents, teachers, and communities.

Ethiopia has a population of 85 million (Central Intelligence Agency, *World Factbook 2010*), of which 29 million are young people (ages 10 to 24) (Population Reference Bureau 2008), with 17 percent of the population living in cities (Central Intelligence Agency, *World Factbook 2010*).

Boys in Ethiopia complete an average of eight years of their primary and tertiary education, while girls complete only an average of seven years (Central Intelligence Agency, *World Factbook 2007*). As a developing country, Ethiopia is faced with reproductive health challenges particularly among younger adolescents and out-of-school youth, including early marriage and sexual debut coupled with limited access to high-quality, youth-friendly reproductive health information and services.

Due to teachers' hesitancy, in-school youth in Ethiopia do not receive practical sexuality education, and very young adolescents (10 to 14 years old) are completely overlooked. Moreover, girls in Ethiopia live with many challenges, including gender inequity, early marriage, early and unwanted pregnancy, unsafe abortion, and sexual abuse. Although many strides have been made in the past decade by the government of Ethiopia with the creation of a National Adolescent and Youth Reproductive Health Strategy, it has taken time for these policies to be realized and implemented at the community and health-facility level (Ethiopian Ministry of Health 2007). Many donors, international NGOs, and local community-based organizations have been concerned with adolescent sexual and reproductive health and have been filling the service-provision gap for adolescents.

More recently, Save the Children began to pay particular attention to the needs of girls in their early adolescence who were making the critical transition from primary to junior secondary school, because of the declining school attendance and high dropout rate of girls during this transition. Save the Children had programs to improve the quality of education within primary schools, but it had not looked at sexual and reproductive health factors, such as puberty and menstruation among girls, and how they could be contributing factors to girls' educational attainment.

Before designing the ASRH program, Save the Children conducted qualitative research with forty-nine girls, forty-seven parents, and fifty-two teachers to obtain nuanced and in-depth information that would help in the design and implement a context-specific, culturally appropriate program that addressed the impact of puberty on girls' educational experiences. The findings from this research, summarized in the following list, cannot be generalized to all girls in Ethiopia but do represent the experiences of girls within the program areas who later helped in the design of the program.

- Information on reproductive health—particularly on puberty, feminine hygiene, and menstruation—is very limited. Few girls reported receiving some information on reproductive health and puberty from science and biology classes.

- Girls learned about feminine hygiene from peers and sometimes from elder sisters and mothers. Many experienced their first period on their own without prior information about the onset and nature of menstruation.
- Many girls were surprised or panicked by their first menstruation.
- Some girls described not wanting to go to school when menstruating because they felt they could not fully participate in school activities.
- Girls, teachers, and parents all agreed that girls' menstruation and related issues have an effect on school performance and attendance.
- Most of the girls use cotton or cloth from old dresses as sanitary protection materials and complain about their lack of comfort and inadequate protection quality. Only a few described having used sanitary pads.
- Most girls, particularly those in rural areas, had never seen sanitary pads, although most had heard about them. Almost all girls were enthusiastic about learning about these alternative menstrual blood management products.
- While participants said they looked forward to the opportunity to use sanitary pads, they also expressed concern about sustained usage due to cost.
- Girls stated that school latrines have limited privacy and poor hygienic conditions. Teachers and girls also confirmed that there are no hand-washing facilities at the schools.

Based on these results, Save the Children developed a four-part program. First, it created community dialogues and community spaces where mothers, teachers, community leaders, and girls could come together to talk about puberty and menstruation and begin breaking down taboos that prevented discussion of these issues. These important dialogues helped create communities that truly cared for adolescent girls and helped parents recognize the importance of talking about subjects their parents never addressed with them. The conversations helped families and teachers begin to understand the challenges that adolescent girls face in school when they are menstruating, and together the families and teachers are finding ways to make communities and schools more girl friendly.

Second, Save the Children developed a school-based sexuality education program to teach adolescent girls about puberty, menstruation, and menstrual hygiene. They linked this effort to a larger curriculum for very young adolescents in which girls also learned about the risks of early marriage and preventing pregnancy, coupled with other life skill-building exercises, to help them negotiate a healthy adolescence. Save the Children trained teachers and girls' peer leaders to roll out this life-skills curriculum as extracurricular learning opportunities.

Third, Save the Children collaborated with communities to improve the water and sanitation infrastructure within schools. Save the Children feels, as a basic human right for children, that every school should have a safe and clean bathroom. For girls, this becomes a profound need when managing their menses. Unfortunately, too many schools in Ethiopia have no bathrooms, or pit latrines. Girls describe such an environment as being unsafe and undignified, and one that inhibits learning. When working in a school that has no latrines, Save the Children consults with girls on what a girl-friendly latrine would look like and uses this information to craft plans and involve communities in the building of new latrines. The new latrines built for girls are separate from boys' latrines and have doors that lock from the inside as well as a place to dispose of menstrual hygiene materials.

Fourth, Save the Children exposed girls to all the menstrual hygiene products available to them—both traditional and commercial products. Girls in the program have been provided with a three-month supply of sanitary napkins to help them understand that alternative, more absorptive methods exist and to encourage them to expose their sisters and mothers to these same products. By understanding what products are available and seeing how they work, girls may help their parents understand the impact these products will have on girls' learning experiences. This exposure also provides girls with negotiation power within their families, influencing parents to prioritize monthly funds for the purchase of sanitary napkins, thus helping the girls attend school without fear of menstrual leaks and boys' ridicule.

As the program got off the ground, Save the Children undertook a KAP—Knowledge, Attitude, and Practices—survey involving nearly 800 girls from Addis Ababa, Limu, Agaro, Dendi, and Ginchi districts to assess the level of girls' knowledge of their menstrual cycle and their attitudes about going to school during their menses, and to ascertain how much school they missed due to menstruation-related issues (Table 3.1). Save the Children disaggregated the results by residential location to understand the unique challenges faced by urban and rural subpopulations. Overall, the data suggest that the Ethiopian girls in urban schools were generally more knowledgeable about and less affected by the onset and management of their periods than their rural counterparts. Nonetheless, the data showed major areas for improvement among both communities.

In terms of knowledge indicators, more urban girls than rural girls rated themselves as having very good or excellent knowledge about their menstrual cycle (27 percent for urban girls and 18 percent for rural girls), but both groups had low levels. Further, when the survey delved into spe-

Table 3.1. Save the Children's Knowledge, Attitude, and Practices (KAP) Survey Results

	Rural Girls	Urban Girls
Knowledge		
I have knowledge of my menstrual cycle. (Percentage of girls who answered "very good" or "excellent" on a 5-point scale of poor, fair, good, very good, or excellent)	18%	27%
I have knowledge of the biological and physiological changes that occur during puberty. (Percentage of girls responding "false" on a true-false scale)	26%	26%
I have knowledge of the fertile period during the menstrual cycle. (Percentage of girls responding "in the middle of my cycle" from a selection that included during, right after, in the middle, just before, or throughout my period, or others, or don't know)	6%	6%
I know where to find materials to manage menstruation. (Percentage of girls responding "true" on a true-false scale)	50%	62%
Attitudes		
I prefer to stay home and not go out during menstruation. (Percentage of girls who answered "strongly agree" or "agree" on a 5-point scale of strongly agree, agree, neither agree nor disagree, disagree, or strongly disagree)	49%	33%
I feel I cannot go to school when menstruating. (Percentage of girls who answered "strongly agree" or "agree" on a 5-point scale of strongly agree, agree, neither agree nor disagree, disagree, or strongly disagree)	61%	34%
I feel less confident during my period. (Percentage of girls who answered "strongly agree" or "agree" on a 5-point scale of strongly agree, agree, neither agree nor disagree, disagree, or strongly disagree)	56%	32%
I am afraid of my next period. (Percentage of girls who answered "strongly agree" or "agree" on a 5-point scale of strongly agree, agree, neither agree nor disagree, disagree, or strongly disagree)	44%	24%
I missed 1 or more days of school in the last 3 months because of problems related to menstruation. (Percentage of girls responding 1–3 days up to more than 5 weeks on a scale that also included none and don't know)	45%	10%

Source: Save the Children's Protecting Futures program in Ethiopia, funded by Procter & Gamble. Data from the baseline report from January 5, 2009 (with data collected in October 2008), prepared by Brad Kerner, Adolescent Reproductive Health Sr. Specialist, Save the Children Federation, Inc., April 2010.

cifics around girls' knowledge of the signs of puberty and the fertile period of the month, there was no difference between urban and rural girls. Only 26 percent of all respondents (urban and rural) were familiar with the signs of puberty, and only 6 percent actually knew the time of the month when they were most fertile. These findings are not surprising, and it is clear why all girls had low actual knowledge levels of puberty, menstruation, and fertility: Although urban girls have more exposure to media and information sources about puberty—which may lead this group to believe they have good knowledge of their menstrual cycles and changes during puberty—education and intergenerational dialogue on this topic are lacking. School curricula do not include these topics, teachers are inexperienced in puberty education, and only small numbers of parents talk to their girls about these issues due to cultural taboos.

The research also revealed parental misinformation and lack of intergenerational communication about puberty and menstruation. One mother said: "One day my daughter came from school and she was bleeding. I lost my temper, and I repeatedly asked her what she committed in the school. I suspected she had sex. So I punished her. My neighbor, a teacher, told me this is her first menstruation. I didn't want to hear her. I know when a young girl bleeds, it is what we have all passed through [i.e., sexual activity]."

When the girls were asked if they knew where to find products within their communities to manage menstrual blood, the percentage of urban girls who knew where to locate products was higher than the percentage of rural girls (62 percent of urban girls vs. 51 percent of rural girls). This, as well, is not surprising, since urban girls pass pharmacies and shops on their way home from school.

To examine attitudinal data, the survey asked girls if they preferred to stay home and not go out during their period. Among urban girls, 33 percent reported they preferred to stay home, whereas 49 percent of rural girls preferred to stay at home during their period. Girls were also asked if they felt less confident during their period. Fewer urban girls than rural girls reported feeling less self-confident (32 percent vs. 56 percent)—and the number of urban girls stating they were afraid for when their next period would arrive was also much lower than the number for rural girls (24 percent vs. 44 percent).

Clearly, rural girls have lower self-confidence, are much more likely to stay home from school when menstruating, and fear having periods. The girls' survey responses indicate the likely explanation for this: When asked why they miss school during their periods, rural girls (73 percent) and urban girls (45 percent) stated they missed school due to fear of being ridiculed, mostly by boys, if they soiled their clothes (Figure 3.3). The research also indicates why girls fear being harassed by boys. One 14-year-old girl shared that boys draw red crosses on the girls' notebooks when they believe certain girls are menstruating, saying "red terror" has arrived.

To examine girls' school absenteeism while menstruating, the survey asked if the girls missed school during the last three months due to menstruation or issues related to menstruation. There was a huge difference between urban and rural girls—only 10 percent of the urban girls missed one or more days of school, compared with 45 percent of rural girls. Further, the data showed that while no urban girls missed more than four days in the last three months for this reason, 14 percent of rural girls did so.

Many lessons learned during the program have helped shape future iterations of girl-focused programming. The following are some of the key lessons from the initial Ethiopian program.

1. Utilize a whole-school approach: Instead of focusing only on the key grades when girls start to drop out, a whole-school approach

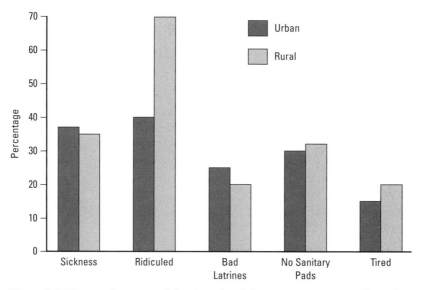

Figure 3.3. Reported reasons girls miss school. In a recent survey conducted by Save the Children, girls were asked if they knew the reasons why most girls miss classes during their menstruation. The top three reasons cited by both urban and rural girls included (a) fear of being ridiculed if they had their dresses soiled by blood; (b) a general feeling of sickness; and (c) the lack of sanitary materials.

Source: Save the Children's Protecting Futures program in Ethiopia, funded by Procter & Gamble. Data from the baseline report from January 5, 2009 (with data collected in October 2008), prepared by Brad Kerner, Adolescent Reproductive Health Sr. Specialist, Save the Children Federation, Inc., April 2010.

is needed that targets all girls with age-appropriate sexual and reproductive health information, as well as all teachers—especially male teachers—so they can all be more sensitive to girls' menstrual management needs in school.

2. Improve hygiene: Start with products girls are currently using and teach them how to improve their hygiene practices.
3. Introduce sanitary pads (if available): It is acceptable to introduce pads to girls, even provide them with a one- to three-month supply, so they can have the knowledge of how these methods are used.
4. Integrate learning into full, life-skills education: A thirty-minute educational session on menstrual management is not enough—integrate this learning into longer life-skills education.
5. Do not forget the boys: Boys are interested in learning about puberty and menstrual cycles, and can develop empathy when properly engaged.
6. Create caring communities: Too many parents are unable to talk to girls about puberty and menstruation, yet adolescent girls signal that they want to receive this information from their parents.
7. Engage and build: The order of the intervention components works best when communities are engaged first, then girl-friendly latrines are built, then girls are educated.

Through all of these program components, Save the Children is working to build communities that truly care for the well-being of adolescent girls. Creating a dialogue between girls, parents, and teachers to help break down taboos is the starting point. Success is achieved when communities recognize that girls should not miss school simply because they are girls and menstruate, and start to demand and construct learning environments that are girl friendly. When girls' school attendance begins to increase, then these Save the Children programs have been successful.

Telling the Story: Cultural Biases and Taboos Limit Girls' Education in Rajasthan

India is a land of stories. The following is a compilation of a number of stories that—like those of Tanzania and Ethiopia—capture the nature of barriers to girls' education. Although this tale is set in a rural area, it has relevance (with some adjustments) for understanding the experiences of urban girls. The protagonist is a 15-year-old girl, Banwari. Banwari comes from the state of Rajasthan, one of the least-developed and largest states in India, and one that has a reputation for gender inequality and patriarchy.

Banwari is the oldest of six siblings, and she has grown up believing that she needs to take on more and more household chores. For example, she walks barefoot to the nearest well, which is four hours away, to fetch water for her entire family. Banwari's father decided to enroll her in a nearby government school that does not cost him any money. Banwari loved being in school with other girls. But all this changed one day when she started menstruating.

When she started bleeding, she did not understand what was going on. She sat in a corner, totally mortified. Finally, when her mother noticed that her yellow kurta was stained red, she quickly took a piece of an old sari, made a bag from it, and stuffed it with some sand and cotton, just as she did for her own menstruation. She gave it to her daughter and said, "Banwari, get some rest and make sure you don't enter the kitchen or visit the temple because you're impure."

This began a monthly ritual for Banwari. The cloth bag did not stop the leaking, the staining, or even the subsequent infections. In school, there was not enough water to wash the cloth or a private place to change it. Banwari's parents decided that she was better off not going to school. "We don't want the men in the village to know that our girl is now grown up," said her father. And her mother silently agreed.

Banwari could be any of the 80 million rural girls and women in India. It is a country in which, for every 100 boys, only 83 girls ever see the inside of a school. And the statistic gets worse: As girls approach adolescence, the number drops to 76 girls for every 100 boys (Government of India 2010).

As mentioned earlier in this chapter, there are several reasons why girls' school attendance begins to drop off at the secondary level, including poverty, the pressure to marry early, and the lack of basic amenities, such as toilets, in schools. But the most important factors interrupting girls' school attendance are the onset of puberty and girls' lack of knowledge about what is happening in their bodies and lack of access to quality sanitary protection.

Recognizing these challenges, Procter & Gamble initiated a program called Protecting Futures in seventeen underdeveloped markets in Africa and India. Focusing on keeping girls in school, the program provides puberty education and access to quality sanitary protection to vulnerable girls.

Providing puberty education and affordable sanitary napkins is critical to making sure girls stay in school and do not lag behind boys when it comes to education. In 2008, Procter & Gamble partnered with the Ministry of Health in the state of Rajasthan on a pilot project called Parivartan, which covered three districts and 360,000 menstruating women, roughly half of whom were adolescent.

Initial fieldwork with village doctors uncovered that women often used materials such as sand, coconut husk, hay, and grass—practically anything that absorbs—for sanitary protection. Reasons for adopting these subhygienic practices were affordability, lack of awareness that sanitary napkins exist, and accessibility. Cultural taboos prevent women from purchasing menstrual products from retail shops operated by men, the dominant format of retail in India.

In partnership with the National Rural Health Mission, part of the Ministry of Health in India, accredited social health activists (ASHAs) provided girls with puberty education and products (at subsidized rates) inside the private confines of homes. ASHAs are women who go to homes and talk about health issues, dispense medicines and contraceptives, and provide pregnancy counseling.

Response has been encouraging. An independent survey conducted by the Nielsen Company (AC Nielsen 2010) revealed that as many as 60 percent of those surveyed were aware of the program, 40 percent had purchased the product, and of those who did purchase the product, 85 percent converted to sanitary pads from traditional methods.

But back to the story of Banwari. What has happened to her, and how have changes produced by the program affected her life? Banwari had reconciled to a life of staying at home until one afternoon an ASHA knocked at her door. She wondered, "Why is this lady who talks about contraceptives and pregnancy coming to my home?"

The ASHA had a pack of sanitary napkins. She opened one, showed it to Banwari, and explained how it was better than traditional means for better and longer protection, and to prevent staining. Banwari's mother shooed her away saying that they didn't care for these "newfangled ideas," and she'd rather spend the money on food for her family. Banwari discreetly signaled to the ASHA and asked her to wait outside her house. She spoke with the nurse, bought her first pack of sanitary napkins, and hid them from her parents.

The ASHA continued to visit Banwari's home regularly and educated both mother and daughter on the benefits of sanitary napkins versus traditional methods. Eventually, Banwari did not have to hide her napkins. She went back to school, and when asked what she dreams of, she said she wants to become an English-speaking tour guide in Jaipur.

Conclusions

As these cases illustrate, girls in developing countries must progress but cannot do so until they receive education and guidance on the changes happening in their bodies and on the pragmatics of how to manage their menses. Without this, they will continue to be unable to participate fully and actively in society. Leaders must take responsibility and face the pressing challenge of addressing the issues of puberty, menstrual hygiene, and menstrual management as one means of opening up female educational opportunities. The burden of the lack of sanitary hygiene protection, as a result of which girls and young women cannot participate in school when menstruating, can be lifted when girls and young women have decision-making power with regard to menstrual hygiene and management.

However, breaking the vicious circle of illiteracy and incompetence so more girls can successfully contribute in the development of their countries does not imply a quick technical fix, such as providing girls and women with sanitary napkins. It means changing perceptions, developing new health initiatives, reallocating resources within existing educational and health programs, and refocusing. It requires undertaking a broad range of projects including adopting a life-cycle approach to the education of young girls that includes teaching about puberty, menstruation, and fertility; supporting entrepreneurs who want to start or have already started small businesses to produce sanitary hygiene products from local materials; and giving increased attention to water and sanitation issues, especially in urban settings, as they relate to the overall well-being of girls when they begin to menstruate. All of these actions are critical to supporting vulnerable girls' menstrual health needs, helping young women stay in school, and promoting their empowerment.

Chapter 4

Making Cities Safe for Women and Girls: Integrating a Gender Perspective into Urban Health and Planning

Claudia Garcia-Moreno and Manupreet Chawla

The expansion of cities stems from the natural demographic growth of urban populations as well as from migration from rural to urban areas. People come to cities in search of better jobs, higher incomes, and more conveniently accessible services. Over the past twenty years, in many developing countries young women between the ages of 18 and 24 years have flocked to cities in search of work. As a result, young adult females outnumber young adult males in many Latin American and Asian cities (ECLAC 2008; United Nations 2009). The health of this subpopulation is affected by the risks and opportunities of urban and urbanizing environments (Montgomery 2009).

Many rapidly growing cities lack planning and, as a result, have areas of inadequate housing and of insufficient water, sanitation, transportation, and other facilities. African, Asian, and Latin American cities in particular have experienced significant growth in such slums and informal settlements over the past two decades (WHO 2010e). Women head about one third of households in these poor urban areas (UNFPA 2009).

Such conditions have enormous health implications, significantly raising the risk that women will experience sexual, reproductive and mental health problems, intimate partner violence, sexual and other forms of gender-based violence, and traffic-related injuries or death. Although urban populations enjoy better health on average than do rural dwellers, urban populations are socially and economically diverse, and many of the urban poor experience health risks comparable to those affecting rural villagers (Montgomery 2009). Therefore, health policies for urban areas should be based on disaggregated data instead of on a city's total average measures of health (Montgomery 2009).

Women's specific needs and concerns must be considered when devising programs and policies to improve living conditions and health services in urban communities; currently, however, policymakers and urban planners often fail to do this. Uneven access to maternal health services among the urban population exemplifies the failure to adequately address all urban women's needs: Although access to maternal health services is generally better in urban areas than in rural areas, access to health care in poor urban environments is usually comparable to that in rural areas (WHO 1996).

A 1998–2000 Demographic Health Survey for India compared the health of urban and rural populations by poverty level; Figures 4.1 and 4.2 illustrate the study's results. Figure 4.1 depicts differences among subpopulations of urban and rural residents in terms of how many received at least one prenatal-care visit. A higher percentage of urban women received prenatal care than did rural women; however, large differences exist within each group relative to standards of living. The graph shows that only 69.7 percent of very poor urban women in India received any prenatal care between 1998 and 2000, a percentage compa-

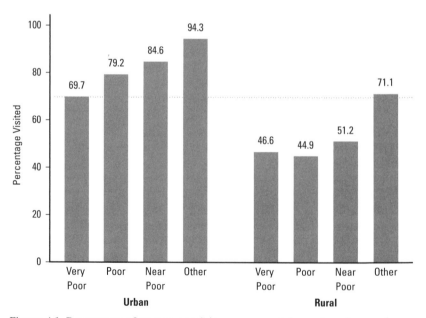

Figure 4.1. Percentage of women receiving any prenatal care in urban and rural India (1998–2000).

Source: Montgomery 2009.

rable to that of rural women living in the upper half of rural living standards (Montgomery 2009).

This study also shows that poor urban women are approximately as likely to have a physician or a nurse-midwife present during childbirth as are upper-income rural women (see Figure 4.2). By this measure of health, large differences exist between very poor and better-off urban women.

Health and Safety Risks Women and Girls Face

A safe and healthy city is one in which women are guaranteed all of their rights. It ensures their health and well-being by improving access to services and promoting, among other things, the elimination of gender-based violence while at the same time promoting equal opportunities for women in terms of access to economic resources, political participation, education, and employment (UNIFEM 2010b). In a safe and healthy city, women and girls are not discriminated against and can enjoy public spaces and public life without fear of being assaulted;

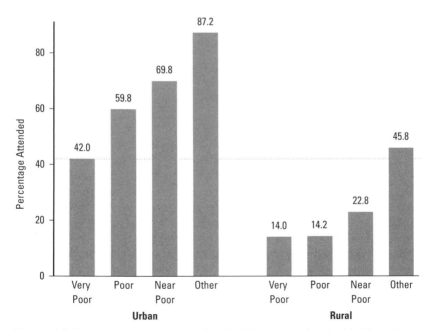

Figure 4.2. Percentage attendance of a physician or a trained midwife at time of delivery in urban and rural India (1998–2000).

Source: Montgomery 2009.

they can access water and sanitation without putting themselves at risk of violence or infectious diseases; they can access schools, health care, and other services; and they can enjoy streets that are safe for pedestrians (among whom women are a majority). Making cities safe and healthy for women and girls means ensuring their access to basic services (e.g., health, education, and legal services) and preventing violence against them.

Low social status, discrimination, and the lack of basic human rights compromise the health of women in many societies. In many countries, women may not be able to leave the house, obtain contraception, or obtain other health services without permission from a third party. In other situations of poverty and limited employment opportunities, young women may resort to sex work, which—along with a lack of knowledge and effective use of modern contraceptives—increases their risk of unintended pregnancy and unsafe abortions, sexually transmitted infections, and other health problems. As these examples show, women's health is directly linked to their empowerment and to gender equality (goal 3 of the Millennium Development Goals). Therefore, policies and programs that improve women's capabilities, increase their opportunities for education, economic and political participation, and guarantee their safety must be in place to complement initiatives and programs aimed at improving their health (Grown, Gupta, and Pande 2005).

In urban settings, women face harassment in schools, parks, and streets, particularly when they are using public transportation; they may risk rape and other types of sexual assault, as well as other forms of street violence. Women modify their behaviors and their use of public spaces in response to such omnipresent violence and fear of violence, especially when they are in neighborhoods with underprivileged populations. A study conducted in Montreal, Canada, in 2000 showed that 60 percent of women—compared to 17 percent of men—reported that they were afraid of walking alone in their own neighborhoods at night (Michaud 2003). Because they appear fearful, women are more likely to be perceived as weak, helpless, and vulnerable and so are more likely to be victims of violence (Falú 2007). In a study in Cali, Colombia, fear of violence in public—along with low educational levels and the existence of family violence—was shown to be significantly associated with poor mental health among adolescents (Prince et al. 2007). Further, girls were found to be three times more likely than boys to show signs of depression and anxiety (Prince et al. 2007).

Poor mental health is also more prevalent among urban women than among urban men and is more common in poor urban neighborhoods than in other urban neighborhoods (Almeida-Filho et al. 2004). Poor mental health among women can indirectly affect the health of children and other family members by affecting a woman's capacity to provide care. Poor mental health among men can also affect a community's health; for example, the lack of employment opportunities in urban areas can adversely affect the mental well-being of men in urban communities, which can lead them to misuse alcohol and to use violence, including toward their partners (Parkar, Fernandes, and Weiss 2003). Therefore, poor mental health in urban communities has a direct effect on the overall health—both mental and physical—of a community and, particularly, on the health of its women and children. Poor mental health can also lead to violence, which in turn can further deteriorate mental health.

A 2005 World Health Organization (WHO) multi-country study examining the prevalence of intimate partner violence against women in both rural and urban settings found that in countries with both a predominantly rural and an urban site (Bangladesh, Brazil, Peru, Thailand, and the United Republic of Tanzania), the prevalence of partner physical or sexual violence, or both, was higher in the urban sites in all countries except the United Republic of Tanzania (WHO 2005). The study also found a statistically significant association between exposure to violence and poor health (Ellsberg et al. 2008). In all of the urban sites, women who had been abused were significantly more likely to have had thoughts of suicide or to have made actual attempts at suicide, compared to women who had not experienced any partner violence (Figure 4.3).

Violence against women violates their basic human rights and negatively affects their health in many ways. Beyond direct physical injury, violence against women increases the risk of other health problems such as depression, sexually transmitted infections, chronic back pain, drug and alcohol abuse, unintended pregnancies, and adverse pregnancy outcomes (Campbell 2002; Garcia-Moreno and Stoeckl 2009). Violence has also been shown to be associated with HIV. In Tanzania, women testing positive for HIV at a voluntary testing and counseling center were two to six times more likely to have experienced violence in an intimate relationship than those who tested negative for HIV (Maman et al. 2000). Additionally, violence against women increases the risk of gynecological disorders including chronic pelvic pain, irregular vaginal bleeding, vaginal discharge, pelvic inflammatory disease, and sexual dysfunction (Heise, Ellsberg, and Gottenmoeller 1999). Because gender inequality is deeply rooted in the attitudes of many community members, health-care workers should team up with social activists, urban planners, women's organizations, and religious and other leaders in encouraging safe health practices (Falconer et al. 2009).

Issues relating to violence against women often are not taken into account in designing urban policies and planning urban environments.

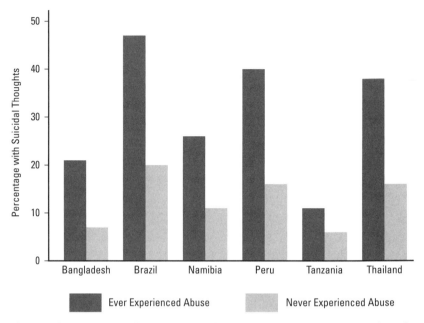

Figure 4.3. Percentage of ever-partnered urban women reporting thoughts of suicide relative to their exposure to physical or sexual violence, or both, by an intimate partner.
Source: WHO 2005.

Even programs that specifically target urban violence fail to address the issues surrounding women's specific exposures to violence. If the goal of improving women's health is to be achieved, the highest level of political commitment at both national and international levels will be needed not just to provide services but to design and institute policies and allocate the resources necessary for gender equality and the empowerment of women (Grown, Gupta, and Pande 2005).

Challenges to Making Cities Safe for Women and Girls

In addition to violence and crime, social, economic, cultural, and family issues contribute to the insecurity and fear women and girls face (UNIFEM 2010b). Poverty and inequality increase the risk of experiencing violence. A woman in a poor urban slum is more likely than women elsewhere in the city to have to cross unsafe parts of town, walk through badly lit streets, and wait for transportation in unsafe places. Poverty and inequality also isolate women, and may prevent them from forming and utilizing social support networks when violence occurs.

Poor housing conditions in slums disproportionately affect women's health. A lack of adequate ventilation in slum housing, coupled with the use of solid fuels and open fires for cooking, lighting, and heating results in indoor air pollution. This puts women at high risk for acute respiratory infections and chronic obstructive pulmonary disease (Montgomery 2009). In addition, in some countries fire-related deaths account for a high number of deaths among young women, some due to cooking accidents and some possibly related to family violence. Since women are often targets of both street and home-based robbery, poor housing conditions can further predispose them to being victims of assault.

Poor water and sanitation systems in urban slums are another challenge. More than 170 million urban residents have no access to even the simplest forms of latrine, which forces them to defecate in the open (WHO 2010e). As a result, women and girls often delay going outside to relieve themselves and only do so at night, which makes them more vulnerable to violence and adds to their insecurity in public spaces. In India, the National Slum Dwellers Federation and Mahila Milan installed community toilets managed by local women and accessible on a pay-and-use system, an example of gender-based planning that greatly improved safety and cleanliness (Grown, Gupta, and Pande 2005).

Although 90 percent of households in urban areas have some access to improved drinking water sources, oftentimes the water source is not on the premises (WHO 2010e). When drinking water is unavailable near the house, women or girls are usually responsible for fetching it. Carrying heavy water containers over long distances can increase the risk for head, neck, and back injuries and can also put women and girls at increased risk of violence and robbery, all of which can be avoided by installing drinking water sources closer to homes (Grown, Gupta, and Pande 2005).

Finding Solutions

Confronting the challenges and obstacles to making cities safer for women and girls and to improving their health requires a multisectoral approach. Governmental and nongovernmental partners must be involved, and different levels and types of services must be addressed. Water and sanitation, emergency services, police, security personnel, health providers, health policymakers, women's organizations, youth groups, and more must all be part of the solution.

The first step should be to develop an understanding of how men and women experience living and working in the city differently, paying close attention to how these differences affect access to and utilization of services, including health care. In other words, a gender perspective should be integrated into urban planning and design. Women must have a voice in this process, as they are the experts on how safe and unsafe public spaces feel (UNIFEM 2010b) and on the challenges they encounter in seeking better health for themselves and their families. To make programs that address women's safety in cities sustainable, the voices of diverse groups of women must be heard when developing and proposing policies and solutions.

Planners should acknowledge that not all groups of women have the same experience; therefore, information from women of different ages, backgrounds, and ethnicities must be gathered (UNIFEM 2010b). Even when designed to benefit both men and women equally, a gender analysis of policies understands how each action, program, and policy will affect men and women differently. Such a perspective also creates the understanding that urban planning is not neutral but reflects the power relations that determine the differences in the way men and women live their lives (Michaud and Chappaz 2001). Participation in decision-making also empowers women and girls by enabling them to take control over their own health and security instead of being dependent on male decision-makers (Michaud 2003). In a study of slum areas in Karachi, Pakistan, the researchers found that in the face of acute pregnancy and delivery complications, an emphasis on first locating male decision-makers to obtain their consent to provide hospital care to women caused critical delays in the women's care (Fikree et al. 1994).

Proposals for and implementation of gender-responsive initiatives reflect society's changing gender roles, with women increasingly making their own health decisions and working outside of the home. Some examples of public policies that include a gender perspective follow.

A Gender Perspective on Public Transportation

Public transportation policies are an important element in urban planning and can have a significant impact on health issues in general and on death and injury levels specifically. Women's voices should hold significant weight in shaping public transportation policy—particularly in the design of programs to improve safety. Women and men tend to use public transportation differently: Unlike men, women do not simply travel from home to work, or from point A to point B; they tend to perform multiple, diverse tasks throughout the day, which requires them to make many stops in a crisscross or zigzag pattern across the city (Peters 2002 in UNIFEM 2010b). Using public transportation to reach multiple destinations may involve paying multiple fares, thereby increasing the cost for women (Kunieda and Gauthier 2003). Programs geared toward making cities safer for women must incorporate women's perspectives and needs if they are to ensure both the safety and the affordability of public transportation for women.

Often, women travel at nonpeak hours, when transportation services are less available (Peters 2002; World Bank 2006). For example, women who sell in the markets will often travel during the early hours of the morning. This may increase their vulnerability as a result of inadequate lighting and the presence of fewer people on the streets at those hours.

In addition to the focus on motorized transportation, attention and support should be given to the safety of pedestrians and bicyclists; walking and biking, in addition to providing transportation, have multiple health benefits. However, injuries and deaths from traffic accidents, including pedestrian and biking accidents, are one of the leading causes of death and disability among adolescents and young adults in urban settings (WHO 2007b). A detailed analysis of pedestrian injuries in Mexico City found poverty, insufficient traffic signals and road lighting, being female, and time pressures on urban parents that limit their close supervision of children to be among the risk factors for pedestrian traffic accidents (Híjar, Trostle, and Bronfman 2003; Bartlett 2002). Public health planners in developing countries should utilize media campaigns to promote the use of safety interventions, such as helmets by bicyclists and motorcyclists. Emphasis should also be placed on the need to clear dangerous roadside objects, maintain existing roads, institute speed limits, and avoid routing high-speed traffic near dense settlements, busy markets, schools, and children's playgrounds (Montgomery 2009).

Enabling women to use intermediate forms of transportation, such as bicycles in some settings, has been very powerful in terms of both access to services and empowerment (UNIFEM 2010b). Coordinating mass transit systems with dedicated bicycle or pedestrian paths offers benefits on multiple levels by encouraging healthy lifestyles, providing safe and effective access to health-care services and food sources, and promoting integration across cities (WHO 2010e).

Another concern is harassment—also known as "eve teasing"—of women in buses and trains. In many countries, this problem significantly affects a woman's travel behavior (Kunieda and Gauthier 2003). While economic power imbalances and sociocultural constraints often result in greater dependence of women on public transit, public transit may not meet their needs, especially for travel free of harassment. Specifically, women may experience violence and sexual harassment while waiting at bus or train stops, while traveling to these stops along unsafe routes, and while traveling on public transit. Furthermore, many women carry things as they travel, including merchandise and children, making them even more vulnerable to harassment (Peters 1998).

As described in Safe Cities (UNIFEM 2010b), in India, the Blank Noise project, an Internet blog/forum, enables women and girls to share their personal experiences of sexual harassment while using the city's public transit services (Blank Noise Blog 2009). Blog posts characterize the type and extent of harassment faced by women in public transit, which range from whistling to staring, talking to breasts, passing comments, accidental touching, flashing, stalking, tickling, masturbating, spitting, honking, and unsolicited photography. Based on women's suggestions, strategies to curtail harassment of women in transit have been proposed and implemented in some cities; these include increasing the number of security personnel, avoiding overcrowding by increasing the number of buses, and offering women-only taxis or buses (Haniff-Cleofas and Khedr 2005b).

Other efforts to address harassment during travel include different versions of "women-only" programs for subways, buses, trains, and taxis that have been implemented, for example, in Mexico City, Tokyo, Osaka, New Delhi, Lebanon, and Rio de Janeiro (Loukaitou-Sideris et al. 2009). However, it is important to note that such programs—although they create awareness—perpetuate gender norms and behaviors that discriminate against women and so should be in place only temporarily. Rather than segregating women and girls, the goal should be to create cities where women can travel and enjoy the city independently and at any time of day.

Efforts to address the problem of sexual harassment of women and girls while using public transportation should include training transport staff on the effects of violence and insecurity on women, their health, and their use of transport. This is also an opportunity to provide broader training to transportation staff on gender discrimination and on relevant policies and laws that may be in place but that are not being implemented (UNIFEM 2010b). At such a training in New Delhi, India, the 3,500 bus drivers who met proposed solutions that included stopping the bus until the perpetrator gets off and taking detours to drop women closer to their destinations at night (Jagori 2007). By allowing passengers to walk shorter distances to their destinations, the latter strategy can also benefit the elderly and the disabled.

Safe, affordable, and reliable public transportation is important to a community's overall health. When such public transportation is more accessible, women and girls can avail themselves of health-care services more easily (Global Campaign for Education 2004). Since life-threatening problems during pregnancy, delivery, and the postpartum period can occur unexpectedly, fast access to emergency care is crucial in preventing maternal mortality (Montgomery 2009). Indeed, access to reliable and safe transportation is an important element in obtaining emergency medical help in a timely manner.

In addition to initiatives for providing safe and harassment-free transportation services, other initiatives aimed at improving the public environment for women and girls have also been proposed. To promote the good use of spaces, women in Nairobi, Kenya, have adopted a creative initiative called "Adopt-a-Light Limited," with the goal of ensuring that women can travel city streets without experiencing any form of violence. This program—which has the motto "Advertising with a Purpose"—encourages businesses to adopt and maintain streetlights in exchange for the use of those streetlights for advertising (Kunieda and Gauthier 2003). The program has successfully installed 185 streetlights along the major highways and in the slums of Nairobi.

Planning a city's public spaces in a gender-responsive manner, with active participation by women, can ensure a safe, healthy, and sustainable environment that women and girls of all ages can enjoy (UNIFEM 2010b).

Hearing the Voices of Women

Women in Cities International (WICI) works to increase women's safety by identifying and disseminating information and solutions that promote women's equal access to public space. Using community dialogues, the organization establishes an understanding of the factors that lead to gender exclusion. Through focus groups and women's safety audits, WICI helps women identify safety problems and devise solutions. The organization also promotes partnerships between women and their local governments (WICI 2006).

The safety audit tool has proven useful in promoting women's participation in urban planning. First developed in Toronto, Canada, in 1989 by the Metropolitan Action Committee on Violence Against Women and Children (METRAC), the tool has been modified for use in communities all over the world and has helped change physical environments to make public spaces safer for women and girls. In addition, the tool has helped make local policies and programs more gender sensitive in their promotion of safety, has increased the confidence and skills of the women participating in the audits, and has increased awareness of the issue of women's safety (Lambrick and Travers 2008).

The tool encourages women to become experts on their own environments, enabling them to formulate local and context-specific solutions to safety problems (UNIFEM 2010b). During a women's safety audit, a group of women together assess the site of interest, usually a known unsafe public space (e.g., a shopping center, a pathway between residences, a water site) and identify what factors make it unsafe, such as its isolated location, negative graffiti messages, and lack of lighting (Rodigou et al. 2008). Based on the assessment, the women propose solutions and recommendations to the local government and other community members, empowering themselves in the process to lead community processes (Metropolitan Action Committee 2002; UN-HABITAT 2008a). Such checklists have been utilized in countries as diverse as Tanzania and France to bring people together to identify problems and propose solutions (Mtani 2002; Lieber 2002).

The safety audit, which has been internationally recognized as a best practice tool, is not the only assessment tool available; various other surveys and exercises have also been used by planners to determine how women and girls feel in the spaces they use (Dean 2002). In London, for example, the "Fearometer" exercise is used to identify triggers that make women afraid in public spaces. In this exercise, women rate factors on a scale that measures their perception of safety: The scale runs from "safe" at one end to "afraid" at the other. Then, they recommend ways to improve their environments and discourage neighborhood crime (Royal Town Planning Institute 2007).

Different approaches have been taken to conducting women's safety audits. In India, a women's non-governmental organization has involved women and girls in identifying and marking characteristics of unsafe public spaces in cities on maps (Jagori 2007). In the United Kingdom, the Somali Women's Neighborhood Health and Safety Group has held one-on-one interviews with community members to gather information on unsafe spaces (Cavanaugh 1998). Other approaches—such as creating scale models of spaces and observing activities (Cavanaugh 1998), surveying the public (Evans and Dame 1999), taking photographs (WISE 2005), and making presentations to the public using storyboards (Phaure 2004)—have also been used to target different groups of women.

Such initiatives can foster partnerships between local governments and women's organizations. For example, the United Nations Development Fund for Women (UNIFEM) has started a program in Latin America in which the organization is funding a baseline assessment of the different forms of violence experienced by women and the locations where such acts are perpetrated. Here, too, the end goal is to encourage women in the community to participate in developing action proposals to make public spaces safe and to create partnerships (UNIFEM 2010b).

Qualitative data from women regarding their personal experiences of violence and their fear of using public spaces can also be very useful when planning and designing cities with spaces that are safe and easily accessible by women. By prioritizing the safety of women and girls, planners can design the public environment with good lighting, directional signs, fast and easy access to emergency equipment and phones, and spaces that are clear, open, and easy to navigate.

Generating Public Awareness

Interest in, and advocacy to improve, the safety and health of women and girls in urban areas is relatively new and needs to be sustained. Knowledge and understanding of the issues involved should continue to be developed; and the efficiency and effectiveness of assessment tools and programs should also be tested through research and evaluation. Raising public awareness about women's particular needs and concerns is another critical step; through this process, women and their communities can be empowered to make recommendations and take action. UNIFEM has launched an initiative to generate awareness of gender inequalities and of the mandate to eliminate violence against women using public events, poster campaigns, documentaries, and newspaper articles and other media outlets in different countries in Latin America (UNIFEM 2003). However, awareness alone is not enough; it needs to be accompanied by policy changes, and at times legal changes, and political and financial support for programs and interventions.

In Argentina, a local women's organization teamed up with the UNIFEM regional program Cities Without Violence Against Women, Safe Cities for All to launch an urban artwork competition. With the goal of raising awareness of women's equal rights to enjoy the city and its public spaces, program leaders made an effort to involve community members from all sectors. The winner's artistic creation was displayed in a public park for two months, where it continued to disseminate information in an engaging, interesting, and attractive manner.

In Chile, a women's shelter started a campaign to take back the street, organizing a march to generate awareness of violence prevention. This initiative has transformed into a permanent campaign, and by means of demonstrations and discussion of cases of violence, it continues to attract community attention (Valdés 2008).

Media campaigns can quickly reach a large audience using television advertisements, newspapers, Internet, and radio. In Colombia, emotionally charged advertisements depicting images relating to violence against women and displaying current, local statistics on the issue are broadcast. In some countries, blogs and public forums have successfully created online communities where all participants can feel comfortable, safe, and respected (Blank Noise Blog 2009). These Web sites provide women and girls the opportunity to post pictures of locations where they were sexually harassed, to tell their stories, and to lobby for change.

Documentaries, too, can shed light on issues that contribute to violence against women in cities and bring attention to the programs and resources in place to make communities safer for women. By showing such documentaries to target audiences—on local television stations, in schools, and in other public arenas—awareness among multiple audiences can be generated (UNIFEM 2010b).

Need for Mobilizing Entire Communities

Not just women but *all* members of a community need to acknowledge the importance of the safety and health of urban women and girls as an issue deserving action and support. A community itself is ultimately responsible for—and influenced by—threats to the safety and human rights of its citizens, and when multiple sectors of the community recognize this, action and support to end violence against women will come more easily. Female leaders representing different age groups, economic levels, ethnicities, and interests can establish networks with other community members. The WHO recently launched a campaign—"A Thousand Cities, A Thousand Lives"—to encourage cities around the world to adopt a multisectoral approach to promoting urban health (WHO 2010f). The campaign will portray community members campaigning for urban health: hopefully female leaders will be well represented so that women's voices and perspectives will be incorporated into proposals and programs targeting urban health.

Community meetings must take into account the needs of women and girls and be planned and organized in a way that encourages their participation. The meetings must offer a safe and positive space where personal experiences and ideas can be voiced in an open, nonjudgmental way (UNIFEM 2010b). Further, the meeting places should be easily accessible by public transportation, language translation and child care should be provided, and the meetings should be held at times that do not conflict with work or school hours (Cowichan Women Against Violence Society 2002). Participation in learning and training activities and in group discussions may be intimidating for women who are not used to public speaking or working in groups, so the goal should be to facilitate an environment where women can comfortably share their experiences and propose solutions.

Mobilizing a community to address issues relating to gender equality and violence against women should be a holistic process involving all groups that can then effectively mobilize their individual constituencies (Michau 2007). This includes boys and men, so youth and men's groups, in addition to women's organizations, should be targeted.

The male leaders in a community—including government officials, elders, business owners, and sports coaches, among others—can prove effective in influencing youth and men, particularly in challenging their attitudes and behaviors regarding gender equality and gender-based violence (Michau 2007). Initiatives involving boys and young men can help build equal relations between boys and girls and women and men, increase respect for women's autonomy, and provide a platform for learning nonviolent conflict resolution. Such initiatives also provide opportunities to initiate discussions on deconstructing traditional norms of masculinity, particularly those that perpetuate violence and discrimination, and promote the need for men's increased involvement in family affairs and child care (UN-HABITAT 2004a).

Awareness-raising and capacity-building campaigns should promote an understanding of the magnitude and consequences of different forms of violence inflicted on women and girls. Campaigns should inform public officials and service providers—including those involved in urban planning and policymaking—so that they are able to respond in a supportive, nonjudgmental way. Police and community security workers should also be targeted by these campaigns, as studies have shown that women are often reluctant to go to the police (UN-HABITAT 2002). If police are well trained and understand the issues related to violence against women, they can play an important role in both family and community safety.

Training sessions where new ideas and concepts are introduced can take many forms. In Jamaica, a project by the Sistren Theatre Collective utilizes theater to mobilize the community to take action to prevent violence against women; in particular, it targets young men at risk of perpetrating violence. This program promotes behavior change by teaching techniques using active audience participation and culturally appropriate communication strategies (Sistren Theatre Collective 2009). Similarly, storytelling and group discussions are other informal means of introducing new concepts and of encouraging audience members to reflect on their daily experiences, obstacles they face, and environmental issues in the context of violence, fear, and gender inequality.

Recruiting role models whom participants respect and with whom they relate can also help deliver messages (Michau and Naker 2003). Various examples exist, using male sports figures and coaches, singers, and politicians. In Canada, for example, an aboriginal fellowship center organized a weeklong workshop to help women cope with their experiences of abuse and violence. Elders who shared the participants' struggles and challenges conducted the sessions. This experience was powerful for both the leaders and the audience; it was particularly empowering for the participants, as they could see the leaders living healthy and productive lives, which served as a source of inspiration and support (Ministry of Community Services 2005).

UNIFEM offers a training module—developed for use by government officials, civil society, and women's organizations—that provides information on how to raise awareness and offer training to improve the safety of cities for women. Topics such as women's human rights, causes of violence in cities, the public's attitudes toward violence, and the limitations of past approaches to women's safety are highlighted (Centro de Intercambio 2005).

Planning and Design of Programs

Community members who recognize the need to improve health and safety in cities for women and girls can actively participate in the design of proposals and solutions. Proposed solutions and interventions must take into account the resources currently available in the city, gaps in the present infrastructure, existing policies, and other groups working on similar matters. Programs and interventions should build on what exists and be designed to be sustainable (Greed 2007).

Much can be accomplished through the creation of networks and partnerships that can pool together resources and work toward a common goal. The various actors working to create safe cities for women and girls—such as the media, municipal urban planning departments, governments, and nongovernmental organizations, particularly women's organizations—must work together if they are to make a significant impact.

Multisectoral partnerships need coordination and a clear definition of roles and responsibilities. This takes time and leadership. Since time is also needed to change community attitudes concerning women and girls and their safety, a program designed to make cities safe for women will usually be most effective if it operates over a long period of time (Whitzman 2007). To ensure a program's sustainability, coordinators must plan and act carefully, and sound technical and financial resources must be found.

To make a long-term impact, short-term pilot projects are not enough; sustained, scaled-up programs are necessary. These require planning, prioritizing, and assessing budgetary requirements properly. Monitoring and evaluating all initiatives, particularly at the initial stages, are critical in order to assess and improve as the work moves along, build and share evidence of good practices and lessons learned, and establish a body of knowledge that will enable more and better actions in the future.

To conclude, making cities healthier and safer for women and girls ultimately contributes to making cities better for everybody (UNIFEM 2010b). A city that promotes and protects its citizens' rights, including those of women; that implements actions to address violence against women; that ensures access to basic amenities such as water, sanitation, education, and health care; and that designs the environment to allow women to circulate freely and without fear is a city committed to the health and well-being of its citizens. This commitment can greatly improve not only women's health but everyone's health.

This chapter was developed from a presentation made by C. Garcia-Moreno at the Penn-ICOWHI Eighteenth International Congress, Cities and Women's Health: Global Perspectives. It is based in part on the Safe Cities Module of the Virtual Knowledge Centre to End Violence Against Women and Girls launched by UNIFEM in 2010. The Safe Cities Module was developed by Women in Cities International and Red Mujer y Habitat. The views expressed in this chapter are those of the authors and do not represent policy of the World Health Organization.

PART II

Urbanization, Space, and Geography

Chapter 5

Design of Healthy Cities for Women

Eugenie L. Birch

Cities are places where women can live healthy or unhealthy lives. By definition, cities are large, are densely settled, and support heterogeneous populations. When properly designed, they provide clean water, efficient transportation, universal education, health services, personal and property protection, and solid and sanitary waste disposal. And in a perfect world, all their residents occupy affordable, durable, structurally sound housing that meets minimum standards with regard to the provision of light, air, sufficient living space, and basic services (e.g., water, electricity, heat). Their residents also reside in neighborhoods that accommodate or are proximate to jobs, community services, recreation, and fresh food. Finally, in a perfect world, cities support design practices that go well beyond the basic service provision just described to promote living habits that contribute actively to excellent health.

In the developing world (or Global South), these practices may encompass implementing innovative water, waste disposal, and transportation systems, participating in mapping exercises to document new slum settlements and their populations for the purposes of service delivery, or supporting self-help or other cooperative ventures to develop standard housing and other efforts to modernize or fully integrate new neighborhoods into fast-growing cities. In contrast, in the developed world (or Global North), design practices attend to addressing the needs of areas of concentrated poverty but also include crafting land use and building codes that promote active living, such as New York City's recent passage of a requirement that all new multifamily residential buildings have bike-storage rooms; employing competitive rating standards, such as the Leadership in Energy and Environmental Design for Neighborhood Development (LEED-ND) rating system, developed to produce districts that "protect and enhance health"; and implementing citywide sustainability plans that incorporate women's health-inducing elements, such as those of New York City, London, and Singapore (US DHHS 2009a).

Although no city in the world meets all of the standards outlined at the start of this chapter, some are inching toward them. Cities in the developed world are often at a distinct advantage because they are in regions that are already highly urbanized and relatively prosperous and have manageable rates of urbanization and comparatively small city sizes, whereas those in the developing world are in generally less highly urbanized, economically poor regions, confronting runaway rates of urbanization, and have average city sizes that are much larger than those of the Global North—all factors making the provision of basic services, much less advanced design ideas, difficult (Spence, Annez, and Buckley 2009). Nonetheless, the cities of the Global South have the advantage of being able to avoid the settlement-pattern mistakes of the Global North if they so choose and/or can rally the resources to do so. More important, for both types of regions there are common design specifications for cities, neighborhoods, and homes that promote better female health regardless of the level of development. To explore these ideas, this chapter establishes the physical/social and economic foundation for pro-female-health design by outlining worldwide urban settlement patterns and the associated issues. It then reviews common design specifications for cities, neighborhoods, and homes and discusses their application in different developmental contexts.

Worldwide Urban Settlement Patterns and Associated Issues

As is well known, the world population crossed the "majority-urban" line in 2008; but not so well known are many other factors that characterize the urban environment in which women live and have important ramifications for their health. These factors include the distribution of the urban population between the developed and developing worlds; the location and population levels of different-sized cities; the relative rates of urbanization; current and future demographic profiles; the relationship between level of urbanization and economic development; and the nature of women's labor force participation in today's global, primarily urban economy.

Location of Urban Populations, Rates of Urbanization, and Service Provision

Of the 6.8 billion people in the world, 82 percent (5.6 billion) live in the developing world and half (3.5 billion) are city dwellers. Of the urbanites, 74 percent (2.5 billion) live in the developing world, up from 54 percent (0.8 billion) in 1975. Demographers anticipate the urban population to experience an 85 percent increase by 2050 (rising to 6.3 billion, or two thirds of the world population), primarily in the developing world (United Nations 2008b, 2010b) (Table 5.1).

Half of all urbanites live in cities with populations under 500,000 (Table 5.2), and a third (or 1.6 billion) live in cities with populations under 100,000. The remaining half live in 960 cities, of which megacities (10 million population or more) constitute 2 percent of the total number and hold 9 percent of the population; large cities (5 to 10 million population) constitute 3 percent of the total number and 7 percent of the population; medium cities (1 to 5 million population) constitute 41 percent of the total and 22 percent of the population; and small cities (500,000 to 1 million population) constitute 54 percent of the total and 10 percent of the population (Table 5.3). Basically, 95 percent of cities with over 500,000 people have fewer than 5 million people, sizes that are large enough to accommodate designs to promote women's health (United Nations 2008b, 2010b).

But even more important than the basic data are regional variations (see Tables 5.1–5.3). Three quarters of all urbanites (2.5 billion people) live in the developing world. And in the past generation, Asia surpassed Europe and North America as being the most dominant urban region. It holds more than 50 percent of the world's urban population (about 1.7 billion people), 49 percent of those living in the smallest cit-

Table 5.1. Urban Population by Region 1975–2050

Place	Population (in billions)				Share of Population			
	1975	2010	2025	2050	1975	2010	2025	2050
World	1.5	3.4	4.5	6.3	100%	100%	100%	100%
Developed world	0.7	0.9	1.0	1.0	47%	27%	22%	16%
Developing world	0.8	2.5	3.5	5.3	54%	74%	78%	84%
Asia	0.6	1.7	2.4	3.4	38%	50%	53%	54%
Africa	0.1	0.4	0.7	1.2	7%	12%	15%	19%
Latin America/ Caribbean	0.2	0.5	0.6	0.6	13%	14%	12%	10%
Europe/ North America	0.6	0.8	0.9	1.0	41%	24%	20%	16%

Sources: United Nations. 2008. *World Urbanization Prospects: The 2007 Revision.* New York: United Nations Department of Economic and Social Affairs; United Nations. 2010. *World Urbanization Prospects: The 2009 Revision.* New York: United Nations Department of Economic and Social Affairs.

Table 5.2. Share of Urban Population by Region and Size of City 2010

	World (number)	Asia	Africa	Latin America/ Carib- bean	Europe/ North America
Megacity: 10 million people	324,000,000	66%	7%	20%	13%
Large city: 5–10 million people	245,000,000	56%	6%	12%	23%
Medium city: 1–5 million people	77,000,000	54%	13%	14%	23%
Smaller city: 0.5–1 million people	350,000,000	48%	12%	12%	23%
Smallest cities: <500,000 people	1,777,500,000	49%	13%	13%	26%

Sources: United Nations. 2008. *World Urbanization Prospects: The 2007 Revision.* New York: United Nations Department of Economic and Social Affairs; United Nations. 2010. *World Urbanization Prospects: The 2009 Revision.* New York: United Nations Department of Economic and Social Affairs.

Table 5.3. Share of Cities by Region and Size of City 2010

	World (number of cities)	Asia	Africa	Latin America/ Carib- bean	Europe/ North America
Megacity: 10 million people	21	55%	10%	20%	15%
Large city: 5–10 million people	33	58%	6%	12%	24%
Medium city: 1–5 million people	388	53%	12%	13%	22%
Smaller city: 0.5–1 million people	518	50%	13%	12%	25%
Smallest cities: <500,000 people	n.a.	n.a.	n.a.	n.a.	n.a.

n.a. = data not available.

Sources: United Nations. 2008. *World Urbanization Prospects: The 2007 Revision.* New York: United Nations Department of Economic and Social Affairs; United Nations. 2010. *World Urbanization Prospects: The 2009 Revision.* New York: United Nations Department of Economic and Social Affairs.

ies (under 500,000 population), and 53 percent of those living in the 960 larger cities. It contains 51 percent of all cities with over 500,000 population, and of these it contains 55 percent of all megacities (and 66 percent of all the people [177 million] living in them[1]). In contrast, Europe and North America, with only 24 percent of the world's urban population, dominate in the small- and medium-sized city category, having 46 percent of the population in such cities and 47 percent of the total number of cities in that category. Notably, Europe and North America contain only 15 percent of all megacities and 13 percent of the megacity population (United Nations 2008b, 2010b).

Urbanization rates are also highly variable, a factor that sets important constraints on designing healthy cities for women because rapidly urbanizing places can barely keep up with the onslaught of newcomers, regardless of whether they are rural migrants or newborns. As may be expected, two regions stand out for their low percentages of urban population but high annual rates of urbanization: Asia (42 percent urban) and Africa (40 percent urban). For Asia the annual urbanization rate has been 1.6 percent for the past 34 years, for Africa the rate has been 2.6 percent, and both areas anticipate high, albeit slower, rates in the years up to 2025: 0.9 percent for Asia and 2 percent for Africa. In contrast, figures for North America (82 percent urban) and Europe (73 percent urban) reveal slow urbanization rates. Since 1975 the urbanization rates have been 1.1 percent for North America and 0.2 percent for Europe, and in the next fifteen years the rates are anticipated to be lower (North America, 0.8 percent; Europe, –0.3 percent). Latin America is an outlier—it is highly urbanized (79 percent) and has and will have annual urbanization rates comparable to Asia and Africa (1.7 percent in the past and 0.9 percent in the future) (United Nations 2008b, 2010b).

These data, along with the population numbers, give an indication of the scale of urban conditions worldwide and offer an appreciation of where the locus of attention should reside and where room for innovation may exist. Rockefeller University demographer Joel E. Cohen captures these issues dramatically with a summary comment: "Poor countries will have to build the equivalent of a city of more than 1 million each week for 40 years" (Cohen 2011: 27).

Underlying these data are two key points: First, of the total urban population, 35 percent (1.2 billion) are poor and live in slums; and second, the majority of the urban poor (1.1 billion) are in the Global South, a figure that amounts to 43 percent of all urban dwellers in the developing world (United Nations 2008b). The remainder (60 million) live in the developed regions and represent 6 percent of all their city dwellers (Commission on Social Determinants of Health 2008: 61). About

60 to 70 percent (700 million or more) of slum dwellers are women and girls. The slums in which they live are overcrowded, unserviced or underserviced (absence of clean water, sewer, schools, and health clinics), and lack durable, structurally sound housing, security of tenure, and efficient transportation (Garau and Sclar 2005). In the developing world, slum or informal settlements are prominent urban features located either in interstices of inner cities or on peripheral, often vulnerable land in crowded, poorly planned neighborhoods. Their prominence can be seen, for example, in Nairobi, where 60 percent of the population live in informal settlements or slums, and in Mumbai, where 55 percent of the population live in slums. In Mumbai, these settlements dominate the city. In the developed world, slums are deteriorated neighborhoods in inner cities and inner ring suburbs, located among abandoned factories, brownfields, and other rundown environments (Jargowsky 2003).

Anticipated urban growth will likely generate demand to house more than half a billion people in next decade alone (Garau and Sclar 2005: 9). Indications of current settlement patterns in the rapidly expanding cities of the Global South show that the highest rates of growth are occurring in peripheral, sprawling informal settlements (Birch and Wachter 2011).

The smaller, but still significant, numbers of people who live in concentrated poverty in the developed world face health problems similar to those seen in the slums of the Global South. In the United States, for example, 8 million people live in 2,500 neighborhoods where 40 percent of the population is below the poverty line. Seventy-five percent of these neighborhoods are in central cities, including Chicago, Houston, Los Angeles, and New York, and this population is unevenly distributed nationally, with the South having 40 percent, the Northeast having 23 percent, the West 21 percent, and the Midwest 17 percent of the total (Jargowsky 2003).

Living conditions in both the informal settlements of the developing world and the neighborhoods of concentrated poverty in the developed world pose serious threats to women's health and well-being. The sprawling-growth phenomenon of both places has the potential to affect the ranking of women's health issues, placing unintended violence (e.g., traffic accidents) and nutrition-related problems (e.g., obesity) at a higher level than in earlier years (Lopez et al. 2006; Campbell and Campbell 2007). Yet, the most important ills, chronic and infectious diseases, still remain. (See Chapter 1.)

Worldwide statistics for poor women show worse than national averages for key health indicators (maternal mortality, incidence of infectious and chronic diseases, especially HIV/AIDS, obesity) and such accompanying characteristics as low levels of education, nutrition, physical fitness, and personal safety. Women in both the developing and developed world share comparable levels of poor health. However, as Table 5.4 demonstrates, global life expectancy data provide a view of regional disparities (overall women in the developed countries can expect to live 50 percent longer than those in the poorest countries— they are more urbanized and less poor). These disparities point to the urgency of attending to the least-developed countries in the Global South because of the scale of the problem in those places (United Nations 2008b: 86–89; UN-HABITAT 2010a).

Looking at environmental quality, specifically data on drinking water and sanitation, which are among the most critical elements for good health, can help illustrate the scale of women's health issues in the developing world. The World Health Organization (WHO) reports that only 35 percent of the population in developing countries have inadequate sanitary facilities[2] and 6 percent have substandard drinking water[3] (WHO 2010b: 52) (Table 5.5). But WHO's assessment masks the fact that disaggregated data reveal much higher rates for populations that live in informal settlements. The Population Research Bureau has found that only 42 percent of poor city dwellers in the developing world have piped water (Montgomery 2009: 8). An additional burden ensues: Securing water falls to women and girls, who represent 72 percent of those collecting water from standpipes or other delivery points (WHO 2010b: 29). These and other domestic conditions, such as early marriage and poverty, also prevent girls from attending school.

Recent special issues of *The Economist* (For Want of a Drink 2010) and *National Geographic* (Water, Our Thirsty World 2010) pinpoint some cities with water/sanitation problems. In Addis Ababa and Lagos, for

Table 5.4. Women's Life Expectancy by Region (in years)

World	68.6
Developed world	79.8
Less developed world	66.2
Least developed world	53.2
Africa	50.4
Asia	70.7
Latin America/Caribbean	76.0
Europe	78.4
North America	80.8

Source: United Nations. 2008. *State of the World's Population 2007.* New York: United Nations Department of Economic and Social Affairs.

Table 5.5. Water and Sanitation Levels in Urban Areas 2008

		Water		
			Clearly Substandard	Problematic
		Other		
	Piped into	Improved	Unimproved	Total
Place	Dwelling	(*a*)	(*b*)	(*a* + *b*)
World	79%	17%	4%	21%
Developed world	98%	2%	0%	2%
Developing world	73%	21%	6%	27%
Southeast Asia	52%	40%	8%	48%
East Asia	96%	2%	2%	4%
West Asia	93%	3%	4%	7%

		Sanitation			
			Clearly Substandard		Problematic
			Open	Unim-	
		Shared	Defecation	proved	Total
Place	Improved	(*a*)	(*b*)	(*c*)	(*a* + *b* + *c*)
World	76%	15%	5%	4%	24%
Developed world	96%	n.a.	0%	4%	4%
Developing world	68%	8%	7%	20%	35%
Southeast Asia	79%	10%	8%	3%	21%
East Asia	61%	30%	6%	3%	39%
West Asia	94%	6%	0%	0%	6%

n.a. = data not available.

Source: World Health Organization. 2010. *Progress in Sanitation and Drinking Water: 2010 Update.* Geneva: World Health Organization.

example, "a quarter to a half of the population have no access to decent sanitation and not many more will have access to piped water. No Indian city has a 24-hour domestic water supply" (For Want of a Drink 2010: 4). Demographer Joel Cohen captured the situation dramatically when he stated that half the infrastructure needed to accommodate urban population growth will be built in the next forty years (Cohen 2011: 30). Other analysts have pointed out that the cost of outfitting existing slums in the next ten years alone could reach $300 billion (Garau and Sclar 2005: 143).

Women living under these physical conditions are clearly in a survival mode attempting to secure the basic services necessary to maintain good health. Designing cities for women's health in the developing world requires attention to these issues, but also requires attention to other phenomena. For example, discriminatory human rights customs or law resulting in major disparities in female autonomy in health-care decisions, access to health care and education, and other areas must also be taken into account. When the United Nations Development Fund for Women reports that "more than one in four women does not have a final say in decisions related to her own health" (Goetz 2008), then designers need to think not only about providing basic services but also about choosing sites for health-care facilities that adapt to current social situations.

In the developed world's neighborhoods of concentrated poverty, environmentally related ills are important but are of a different sort. The lack of affordable housing, physical deterioration of the units (and the neighborhoods), crowding, crime, and associated drug use, and limited access to fresh food dominate. Like their counterparts in the developing world, households in these areas suffer from other poverty-induced characteristics: high levels of joblessness, high levels of female-headed families, high school-dropout rates, poor nutrition and/or lack of access to fresh food, limited safe recreation, and so forth. Here the health issues are more related to life expectancy and quality of life than to survival.

Demographic Profiles

Adding to the characteristics of the global urban environment are the current and future demographic profiles. As of 2000, the old outnumber the young. By 2050, one person in three in the developed countries and one in five in the developing countries will be over 60 (Cohen 2002: 84, 2011: 26). By 2050, 80 percent of the elderly will live in the developing world, will number more than one billion, and will constitute 25 percent of the area's total urban population (WHO 2007a: 4) (Table 5.6).

Notably, in the most elderly category (80+ years), women outnumber men today and will also do so in the future. This phenomenon is accompanied by projected changes in the birth rate that will lower the proportion of children under 4 years old. (The developed and developing countries again show differences—in the developed countries young children will drop from 6 percent in 2000 to 5 percent in 2050, while in the developing countries the change will be more dramatic—from 11 percent in 2000 to 7 percent in 2050.) The result will be an expected major shift in the dependency ratio (the percentage of elderly and young children supported by the working population); in the developed countries, the dependency ratio will increase from 48 percent

Table 5.6. Aging Urban Population 2009–2050 (in millions)

Place	Total Elderly 2009	Urban Elderly 2009	Total Elderly 2050	Urban Elderly 2050
World	0.787	0.393	2.0	1.4
Developed world	0.264	0.193	0.363	0.4
Developing world	0.516	0.2	1.7	1.0

Source: Author's estimates based on World Health Organization, *Global Age-Friendly Cities: A Guide* (Geneva: WHO, 2007), and United Nations, *World Urbanization Prospects: The 2009 Revision* (New York: United Nations Department of Economic and Social Affairs, 2010).

in 2000 to 69 percent by 2050, and in the developing countries, it will decrease from 60 percent in 2000 to 53 percent in 2050 (Cohen 2002: 84, 2011: 30–31).

These data have important implications for the design of cities, neighborhoods, and homes. Of particular importance will be enabling elderly women to have active lives and age in place by providing access to health services and assuring personal safety. Additionally, caregiving to the young and the elderly and the changes in the dependency ratio point to two other considerations. First, recent research demonstrates that the more educated a woman is, the more responsive she is to public health campaigns for herself and for those to whom she gives care (Harpham 2009). This finding about education supports the likely success of crafting multisector designs to promote better health—providing both basic services such as clean water and transportation *and* such community facilities as schools and health clinics. Second, with high levels of dependent people (young and elderly), women's participation in the labor force will be more important than ever, and city designs need to take women's multiple roles into account.

Level of Economic Growth and Female Labor Force Participation

An analysis of world gross domestic product (GDP) demonstrates a strong relationship between high levels of urbanization and economic prosperity, important considerations in the selection and use of specific design practices. For example, in 2006, the United States was 81 percent urban and had a GDP per capita of $38,000 (in 2000 dollars), whereas in 2004, China was only 39 percent urban and had a GDP per capita of $5,300 (in 2000 U.S. dollars) (Spence, Annez, and Buckley 2009: 4–5). Further, 97 percent of the world's GDP comes from industry and services, a factor that favors urbanization, as both industry and services benefit from agglomeration, the clustering of enterprises that promotes economies of scale and other efficiencies (Sattherwaite 2008: 38).

These official data hide an important element: the strength of the informal economy in various places.[4] Estimates of the average financial contributions of the informal sector to regional economies range from a low of 13 percent in North America and Australia/New Zealand to a high of 42 percent in Africa (Schneider 2002: 4–19) (Table 5.7). The informal economy is an important component of the global workforce (paid workers), which now numbers 3 billion, 60 percent of whom are in the informal sector.[5] Female workers (numbering 1.2 billion) constitute 40 percent of the workforce, and 60 percent (720,000) are in the informal sector.

But more to the point, for women, the informal sector is a partial lifesaver. Often barred in developing countries from entering the formal labor market by cultural convention, family obligations, poor education and skills, and lack of capital, women working in the nonagricultural informal sector are able to earn some income (Chen et al. 2005: 6). In addition, coverage of Nobel Prize-winning microfinance programs by international journalists has outlined the potential of this sector to improve women's health (Kristof and WuDunn 2010). However, the bottom line is that this work is low wage and has no legal (job security, freedom from harassment) or health protection. Some informal sector jobs, like rag-picking (sorting through garbage to find cloth and other items for resale), dominated by women, can be hazardous to the worker's health (Alliance of Indian Wastepickers 2010). Other common informal sector jobs are in the world's 3,500 economic protection zones

Table 5.7. The Informal Economy: Percent Gross Domestic Product (GDP) and Jobs

	Percent Contribution to GDP	Percent Contribution to Urban Labor Force
Africa	42	48
Asia	26	33
Central and Latin America	41	45
Transitional Europe	38	n.a.
Western Europe	18	16
North America, Australia, New Zealand	13	n.a.

n.a. = data not available.

Source: Schneider, F. 2002. Size and Measurement of the Informal Economy in 110 Countries Around the World (paper presented at Workshop of Australian National Tax Centre, ANU, Canberra, Australia, July 17).

(areas with tax relief and few or no government regulations), where women form 70 to 90 percent of the employees (Wick 2010). However, as products of globalization, these jobs are footloose subject to wage competition. In sum, these data strengthen the rationale for insisting that designs for healthy places for women include safe workplaces either near or in the home or in areas serviced by inexpensive, efficient transportation from the home.

So why is this contextual discussion important? First, it reveals an important fact, the nature and scale of women's health issues will vary in different regions, in different-sized cities, and in different economies. The developing world, especially Asia and Africa, by virtue of the scale and speed of urbanization in these areas, commands immediate attention. Addressing traditional environmental conditions is essential, but due to emerging sprawling peripheral urban growth, new concerns such as traffic-induced injuries are also important. Second, and more important, the contextual discussion provides evidence that gendered health concerns cross the wide divide between the developed and developing countries. This finding supports the articulation, adoption, and adaptation of principles for urban planning and design that address women's health needs and have worldwide application.

Common Design Specifications for Healthy Cities, Neighborhoods, and Homes for Women

Places designed to promote better health are critically important for women who live in either informal settlements of the developing world or areas of concentrated poverty in the developed world. But what would such cities look like? The answer to this question requires scrutinizing the basic building blocks of a city and of a neighborhood and its contents and infrastructure. It also focuses on universal principles that specify general arrangements but assume that their execution demands extensive community participation and governmental/nongovernmental and private sector coordination to work out place-specific details (Garau and Sclar 2005; WHO 2007a; Commission on Social Determinants of Health 2008).

Neighborhoods and Their Contents

Ideally, neighborhoods are mixed-use places where people can live, work, and play within a walkable circumference. Neighborhoods range in population from a few thousand people to tens of thousands, depending on the ability of the land to carry the required structures and services. Ideal neighborhoods can accommodate women of all ages and, unlike many places today, have features that enable elderly women to have active lives (WHO 2007a).

Located on appropriate land, ideal neighborhoods are resilient, invulnerable to natural disasters (e.g., floods, earthquakes) and man-made disasters (e.g., brownfields), and on land not needed for agricultural or other uses that support city life. They are legally secure, that is, on land where municipal authorities have established and documented ownership and permitted development.

Neighborhood contents in these communities include structures protected from the elements and such hazards as fire. These structures include (1) housing that is affordable, of sufficient size, structurally sound, and constructed of durable materials; (2) space for retail and other commercial activities; and (3) space for community use including schools, health clinics, government service centers, and places of worship. Individual structure designs incorporate features that promote healthy living for women across the age span. These features include mixing the types of buildings to accommodate different uses, such as small entrepreneurial businesses or residential-care facilities integrated with family housing. Other features include building entrances near transit stops/stations or along transit corridors, signage about the kinds and distances to transit stations, bike routes and pedestrian ways, facilities for storing and parking bicycles, replacement of elevators with stairways either throughout a building or, in taller buildings, on alternating floors, yet also offering accessibility through ramps or other means to the elderly.

Ideal neighborhoods have open space within a ten-minute walk of housing. Open-space programming accommodates activities that are culturally and age appropriate. For example, elderly women may require quieter spaces provided with benches (yet in full view of others and having interesting views), while girls need safe places for active sports or walking. Another design device is the reuse of obsolete facilities, such as viaducts or unused railways, for open space to transform potentially dangerous places and structures that could harbor criminal or other threatening activities to safe public realms. Wherever possible, neighborhood open space networks should connect to regional ones.

Finally, ideal neighborhoods have a range of retail and community facilities. These include full-service grocery stores and places for farmers' markets located near housing or work, community gardens where space allows, and community centers with health clinics and other services accessible to women and girls that are also near homes or places of work (Figure 5.1).

These universal principles have different applications in the developing and developed world. For example, in the developing world where

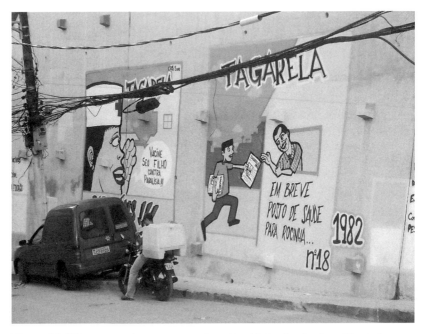

Figure 5.1. Women receive messages about health in the favela of Rocinha in Rio de Janeiro through a public art/poster vehicle. (Photo courtesy of Gregory Scruggs.)

informal settlements are the norm for many women, various strategies have emerged for supplying healthy housing and neighborhoods. These include sites and services arrangements where a public or nongovernmental organization secures land, lays it out with streets sufficiently wide to allow light and air to circulate and to accommodate service and transit vehicles (see infrastructure section later in this chapter), and allocates parcels to households (sometimes with an already poured cement slab) for family members to construct their dwellings. Or in already built-up slums, public or nongovernmental organizations undertake upgrading activities that include providing water, sewage, and power, improving streets, regularizing or legalizing land tenure, selective clearance of buildings, and adding such community facilities as schools and clinics. Women's groups, especially those associated with the Huairou Commission, the global coalition of women's community development groups founded in 1996 and including such associations as Kenya-based GROOTS (Grassroots Organizations Operating Together in Sisterhood), Germany-based MINE (Mothers Centers International Network for Empowerment), and U.S.-based National Council of Neighborhood Women, have fought for these services for their neighborhoods, primarily in disadvantaged communities of the Global South and North. In addition, they have secured physical spaces, community centers, for their work. Depending on the neighborhood needs, they use these multi-service places for health clinics, training workshops, and daycare (Yonder and Tamaki 2010; Purushothaman et al. 2010).

These features contribute to healthier living for all slum dwellers but aid women and girls disproportionately. For example, the provision of water relieves women and girls of the daily burden of securing the family's water supply; supporting a women's center offers services of benefit to the whole population but at the same time validates women's roles as leaders by strengthening their group identity, offering visibility, and formalizing their positions in the community (Yonder and Tamaki 2010: 1).

In the developed world, neighborhood revitalization processes do not have to address the basic service and layout provisions described previously, but they do include improving the physical conditions of deteriorated and obsolete housing and providing easily accessible community services and open space. In some instances, public and nongovernmental organizations sponsor wholesale clearance and reconstruction of neighborhoods according to the standards listed earlier. Examples from the United States include the HOPE VI program, which has rebuilt rundown public housing projects in many cities, and Richmond, Virginia's Neighborhoods in Bloom program of targeted investment in selected neighborhoods for capital improvements (e.g., street improvements, lighting), rehabilitation of dilapidated housing, construction of infill housing, and code enforcement, coupled with loans for extinguishing violations. Again, these improvements are not gender specific, but due to the high incidence of female-headed households and children in these types of neighborhoods, the improvements result in healthier neighborhoods for women and girls. Within the gender-specific interventions is the provision of women-managed community centers offering space for education, health care, and temporary housing (Yonder and Tamaki 2010: 83).

Infrastructure

Infrastructure is expensive and thus forces a preference for high-density neighborhoods, those featuring attached, clustered, or multifamily housing, that justify and support capital investments in hard infrastructure (e.g., transportation, water/sanitation) and soft infrastructure (e.g., schools, health clinics). An essential feature is a comprehensive transportation network that knits a city's neighborhoods together and affords opportunities for taking advantage of regional employment and/or such large-scale citywide facilities as hospitals, large-scale cultural and sports venues, specialty stores, and other facilities that require a large population base for support. Such a system offers modal choice and has interconnected streets, pedestrian ways, and bike paths. Designs incorporating minimal dead-end ways (or cul-de-sacs) and small blocks often meet this goal; this specification encourages but does not require grid layouts. Some cities, including New York, have determined standards for maximum size of blocks (200 feet by 300 feet in New York City) (*Active Design Guidelines* 2010: 37). Such standards are not universal but are dependent on many factors, including climate, land availability, and cultural customs.

The transportation network should provide for trips of different durations and lengths and should allow for different modes—pedestrian, mass transit, vehicular. Thus, its components (streets, sidewalks, underground facilities such as pedestrian tunnels, metros, bike paths) need to be wide enough to take care of many kinds of vehicular and foot traffic but not so wide as to discourage walking, and they should be well lit so as to provide for safety at all times of day. Addressing questions of street width takes design imagination. Safety requirements (e.g., access by fire engines) and surface mass transit (e.g., bus rapid transit [BRT]) standards call for wide streets (e.g., the U.S. standard for fire engines is 20 feet plus parking with a 100- to 150-foot turning radius; the BRT lane requirement is 20 to 80 feet), but such roadways are not conducive to pedestrian or bike traffic. Resolving this conflict includes carving "refuge" islands in the center of right of ways and providing underground passageways, signals with countdowns, and buffered pedestrian and bike paths (*Active Design Guidelines* 2010: 41).

Sidewalks merit much attention. First and foremost, they are necessary, not optional, features. In both the developing and developed countries, a tendency to favor vehicles over pedestrians has led to the construction of neighborhood-piercing limited-access highways and other road-building schemes where sidewalks and their ongoing maintenance are totally absent. Rectifying this lack of attention to pedestrians is of highest importance to women and girls, who often do not have other mobility resources. Second, sidewalks should be built wide enough to accommodate sufficient traffic (e.g., the New York City standard is that sidewalks accommodate twelve people per minute per yard (*Active Design Guidelines* 2010: 41). Third, sidewalks should be well appointed: Ideally, they should be well lit with continuous, well-drained, smooth surfaces; accessible to the disabled, elderly, and baby carriages; supplied with drinking fountains and seating; and buffered from vehicular traffic and bicycle traffic. Bike paths have the same requirements as sidewalks with the added demand for space for bike storage at home and at all destinations (work, retail, recreation).

A well-designed transportation network encourages more people to be on the street, a phenomenon that has many positive health outcomes. First, these arrangements foster personal safety. A well-known fact of urban life is that the more "eyes" that are on the street, the less crime will occur (Jacobs 1961). So offering sidewalks, bike paths, mass transit, as well as venues to go to—stores, schools, jobs, and so forth—brings people, especially women, into the public realm. Second, the presence of sidewalks, bike paths, and mass transit encourages more physical activity and gives people reasons for walking to easy-to-reach community services, transit stations, stores, and open space. (In the United States an acceptable walking distance is a half or quarter mile, depending on the type of venue. A child can walk a half mile to school; a mother might want to walk only a quarter mile to a grocery store.) Many manuals that explain and set out the standards for such designs exist (American Planning Association 2006; Hack et al. 2009). With obesity reaching epidemic proportions in cities worldwide and urban women being most prone to the condition, providing opportunities for physical activity like walking is a critical design imperative. Third, once people are on the street, public and private decision-makers have reasons to make the ways more attractive. The presence of people provides a rationale through either the ballot box or the pocketbook for these decision-makers to offer attractive landscapes (trees, flowers, public art) and streetscapes that avoid blank walls (e.g., shop windows), curb cuts, and other impediments to the pleasant pedestrian experience. User-friendly public spaces create a virtuous circle that reinforces and enhances the original use.

In addition to a comprehensive transportation network, a second infrastructural element is green infrastructure, a system of open spaces of varying sizes and other such design features as rain barrels and green roofs and walls, woven into the system in appropriate places. Green infrastructure provides drainage for storm water, offers opportunities for rainwater collection and storage, serves recreational uses—playgrounds with permeable surfaces accomplish this end—and supplies the "real estate" for water and sewer pipes where they are nonexistent (Birch and Wachter 2008). Retrofitting these features in an informal settlement in the developing world or an area of concentrated poverty in the developed world is quite possible but may require selective clearance of buildings. However, knitting green infrastructure into cities in the developed and developing world is occurring with increasing frequency, especially in places that use its features to enhance inadequate sewers and public space amenities. Exemplary work in this regard has occurred in Philadelphia, São Paolo, and elsewhere.

Last but not least is the infrastructure pertaining to community services (e.g., schools and health clinics). The key here is to provide decentralized, neighborhood-based facilities accessible safely and conveniently to women of all ages.

Exemplary Design Guidance and Projects

In recent years, public policymakers and their advisors have devoted considerable thought to designing healthy cities, neighborhoods, and homes. Some of this thinking is directly attributable to the presence of the Millennium Development Goals outlined by the United Nations in 2000 that set worldwide poverty reduction objectives to be achieved by 2015. Although these goals are not specifically focused on urban places or on women, their achievement would improve the urban environments and women's lives and health. Each of the eight goals has a direct or indirect urban planning and design implication and has triggered special studies to monitor progress, which in turn have stimulated additional research to establish standards and publicize best practices.

An example of such a study is the World Health Organization's Commission on Social Determinants of Health, whose final report devotes many pages to urban life and states that while infectious diseases still dominate, "urbanization itself is reshaping population health problems" to include obesity, violence and crime, traffic accidents, and neuropsychiatric disorders that urban planning and design guided by the principles discussed in the previous section of this chapter can help alleviate (WHO 2008a: 62, 66). Other examples are WHO's *Global Age-Friendly Cities: A Guide* (WHO 2007a), the United Nations' Millennium Project's Task Force on Improving the Lives of Slum Dwellers (United Nations 2005), and the U.S. Green Building Council's LEED-ND codes that also support the general principles of land use and transportation outlined in this chapter (Plouffe and Kalache 2010).

Individual cities have become involved as well. Between 2009 and 2010, New York City published its *Active Design Guidelines*, adjusted its zoning and building codes to require such things as bike-storage facilities in new residential and commercial buildings, laid out miles of dedicated bike paths, and converted critical streets like Broadway in Manhattan's Theater District to open space. Long-term projects include a massive rehabilitation of abandoned and deteriorated housing that took place between 1980 and 2000, the construction of sewage pollution control plants and a new water tunnel, and heavy investment in mass transit.

In the developing world, many cities have adopted a number of the principles relating to transportation choices including Curitiba, Brazil (noted for its BRT), and Bogotá, Colombia (noted for substituting a

BRT and bike system for a costly subway). Since 1993, Medellín, Colombia, evolved its Integral Urban Project, a multisector slum-upgrading program that has received worldwide attention for its originality (e.g., using cable cars to transport 40,000 people daily in one formerly inaccessible neighborhood; carving out space in multipurpose community centers and parks around stations) and effectiveness (including extensive community participation and government agency coordination) (Blanco and Kobayashi 2009) (see Chapter 10). Further, women in Mumbai slums have organized with the help of professional women to secure basic services such as water, sanitation, and better housing (see Chapter 6).

UN-HABITAT's 100 Cities Initiative, a Web-based information portal announced in April 2010 as part of UN-HABITAT's World Urban Campaign, gives further publicity to ongoing individual city efforts that directly and indirectly promote better women's health. Available in beta form at www.100citiesinitiative.org, it details projects in several cities. Philadelphia is one example; the Web site highlights its water and sanitation improvement plans, community gardens, and fresh food initiatives, all efforts that have the potential to improve women's health in the city's neighborhoods of concentrated poverty.

Conclusion

As Neal Peirce wrote in *Century of the City: No Time to Lose,* "notwithstanding the staggering challenges that 21st century cities face, great fonts of knowledge, skills and both local and global networks do exist and are poised to be tapped. If the world's cities seize these opportunities, they will have more than a fighting chance of succeeding; ignore them and blind forces . . . may set this urban century on a destructive course" (Peirce and Johnson with Peters 2008: 53). This statement applies forcefully to the situation related to cities and women's health. Public and private decision-makers, scholars, professionals, and citizens realize that challenges are massive and known, as the contextual discussion of this chapter exhibited. The scale and speed of urbanization, the demographic shifts, particularly related to aging, and the shape of the global economy have specific implications for the health of women and that of their families. Further, the knowledge among the fields needed to meet the anticipated challenges exists. This chapter focused on the general design principles that will assist in bettering the physical urban environment, ones that can be boiled down into a few simple ideas—mixed land use, good transportation, plentiful open space, affordable, durable housing, recognition of the needs of women across their age span, and so forth. These ideas are only one part of the story. Improving women's health demands collaborative work among a variety of professionals, extensive consultation, education at all levels, and most important a belief in the power of linking research and practice in the field of urban planning and design to research and practice in the field of women's health.

Chapter 6

Are Women Victims, or Are They Warriors?

Sheela Patel

The health hazards posed by living in a slum are by now well documented: From quality of housing to access to clean water, the urban poor are highly vulnerable to a number of health problems, many of which affect women disproportionately. Women and their survival strategies form the foundation of how poor communities subsist in cities, yet most programs do not truly address their needs or make use of their resources. Most urban health interventions simply provide short-term fixes and do not build women's capabilities to deal with the ongoing issues with which they struggle on a daily basis. If a woman is given a prescription for medicine to alleviate her cough yet continues to spend much of her day in a tiny shack inhaling fumes from her cooking stove and from the vehicles speeding past outside, she will continue to have respiratory trouble. If she is instructed on how to cook healthy meals for her family yet cannot afford to buy enough food, her children will continue to suffer from malnourishment. If she is educated about the importance of sanitation but has no access to clean water, her family will continue to contract gastrointestinal disease.

Simply seeking to "manage poverty"—to make the existing system work better for marginalized people—may help a few in the short term. Yet transformation of the lives of the poor is a marathon rather than a 100-meter dash. To truly improve health outcomes for poor communities in urban areas, and particularly for poor women, development and health professionals must work with communities to address the underlying issues of habitat and environment that play a major role in well-being.

Despite all the challenges facing them, women are not simply waiting for help to arrive. Rather, women in urban communities across India and dozens of other countries are already taking steps to address the problems presented by their habitats. They are saving money for new and improved houses, negotiating with officials for access to water and electricity, and even building their own community toilet blocks. Though women are often treated as victims, they are warriors. It is simply a question of lighting their fire.

The Alliance: SPARC, Mahila Milan, and NSDF

The Society for Promotion of Area Resource Centres (SPARC) is a nongovernmental organization (NGO) that was established in Mumbai in 1984 by a group of professionals who sought to explore new ways of working with the urban poor. SPARC's initial work in Mumbai was with pavement dwellers and focused specifically on women. SPARC supported pavement women in forming a network of neighborhood collectives called Mahila Milan—Hindi for "women together." These collectives provided a means for women to build their confidence while addressing tangible problems in their lives.

In 1986, the National Slum Dwellers Federation (NSDF), which at that time was a federation of slum community leaders from eight cities in India, sought an alliance with these newly emerging neighborhood collectives in Mumbai. The NSDF was addressing issues of eviction and seeking to build and develop a sense of identity for slum and pavement dwellers in the city. The NSDF explored a strategy to provide access to city services and resources by pavement dwellers.

SPARC's role has been mainly one of assistance to NSDF and Mahila Milan in building their leadership by providing organizational outreach, facilitating the exploration of new strategies and activities, and opening spaces for the organizations of the poor to begin dialogue (and hopefully partnerships) with various levels of government to address issues of poverty. NSDF and Mahila Milan have developed leaders who undertake these activities on an ongoing basis. As the poor have established their needs and priorities, SPARC has sought to support the poor in their transformation from passive beneficiaries and supplicants to active participants in changing their own life situations, acting as a bridge between the formal and informal world in the dialogue on development priorities.

NSDF and Mahila Milan groups meet regularly and participate in frequent exchange visits with groups in other cities, states, and even countries to learn about one another's strategies and approaches. When a local federation devises new solutions to address a problem, it shares them with the rest of the alliance. This strategy builds confidence by showing local groups that change is possible and helps the poor use processes developed in other cities to demand similar changes in their own city. It also builds a critical mass of the urban poor who support each other while striving to collectively bring change to their settlements. Real change takes time, requiring patience, persistence, and long-term strategic thinking; the support of the alliance helps local groups maintain morale and motivation throughout the process. These activities and their impact on the lives of the urban poor are discussed in greater detail later in this chapter.

Urbanization in India

To the international community, the narrative of the past decade in India is one of phenomenal economic growth and a vast increase in opportunity—the India of global trade and information technology outsourcing. Less frequently noted is a correspondingly massive growth in India's urban population and the vast increase in the numbers of urban poor, visible in the vast slums that characterize most Indian cities and the terrible conditions in which millions work and live (Figure 6.1). The economic strides India has made in the past few years are real

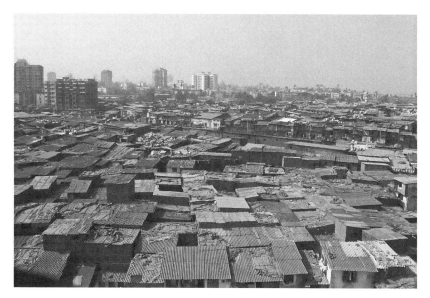

Figure 6.1. Dharavi slum in Mumbai. (Photo courtesy of the Society for Promotion of Area Resource Centres [SPARC], the federations, and friends of SPARC.)

and significant, yet if India does not rise to the challenges presented by rapid urban growth, it will struggle for years to come to translate economic gain into improved quality of life for its people. Simply put, if government officials cannot deal with the migration that they are seeing in their cities today, what will they do ten years from now?

If we are to truly tackle the challenge of creating healthy cities, then we must address the urban poor's lack of sanitation, adequate housing, and basic services. The practice of blaming the urban poor for their situation and their cities' troubles has emerged from a perception among planners and governments that urbanization, particularly when it means the migration of the poor into cities, is an unhealthy trend. In India, this attitude has resulted in the allocation of development funds to unsuccessful attempts to reverse the flow of people from rural to urban areas, while neglecting urban investment for fear of "encouraging the poor" to come to the city.

Though government officials in India have begun to recognize and take steps toward addressing the plight of the urban poor in recent years, the desires of private developers still take priority in most cities' urban policies. The textile mills of Mumbai, for example, though long empty, have largely been sold to private developers rather than brought back in to the public space as part of an urban renewal strategy. Meanwhile, nearly 60 percent of the city's population live in slums, many of which lack basic services and facilities.

Such myopia regarding urban development is not confined to India. Countries around the world face similar challenges as development and urbanization proceed at a breakneck pace.

Women in India

Although India guarantees its citizens a number of fundamental rights, including the right to equality, women continue to be second-class citizens in many regions and in many aspects of life. Despite laws requiring equal pay for equal work, men outearn women by anywhere from 50 to 90 percent. Though child marriages were outlawed in 1929, 40 percent of all child marriages in the world still take place in India (UNICEF 2008). Likewise, although dowries were prohibited in 1961, the practice is still widespread in many regions. Perhaps most troubling of all, the United Nations Development Programme estimates that an estimated 42 million Indian women—the highest number in the Asia-Pacific region—are "missing" due to sex-selective abortion, infanticide, and discriminatory treatment in access to nutrition, health care, and other basic needs (UNDP 2010).

A great deal of research thus far has focused on the plight of women in rural and northern areas of India, where gender imbalances are higher and economic prospects bleaker. Relatively little research has been done on health outcomes for women living in cities, who represent a rapidly growing percentage of the Indian—and world—population. The impacts of the urban environment on women are only beginning to be understood, but it is clear that they are significant and important.

Women are often dismissed, along with children and the elderly, as vulnerable and helpless victims in need of external assistance or intervention. Yet in the alliance's experience working with women in slums across India, nothing could be farther from the truth. By working together, women can assert their strength in powerful ways.

Urban Development and Women's Health

Until communities and households have access to safe water, sanitation, and basic amenities, the impact of poor people's environments overwhelms any effects of habits and practices, medicines, or nutrition. From overly crowded living spaces to lack of access to clean water, life in the slums presents a number of threats to residents' health.

Slum populations exhibit higher rates than the general population of nearly all major illnesses. At any given time, an estimated 4 to 8 percent of the slum population in India is suffering from a short-term illness, with an additional 3 to 6 percent suffering from chronic disease (Karn, Shikura, and Harada 2003). Incidence of disease and other health problems in urban areas are negatively correlated with water consumption, housing quality, family income, and literacy: As each of these indicators goes up, disease rates go down. Most discussions of women's health are confined to issues of family planning and reproductive health. Yet it is becoming clear that a number of health issues affect women differently, and often more severely, than men.

Health issues are often treated as technical problems to be fixed with technocratic solutions. Yet health cannot be divorced from the politics of power and decision-making. Addressing urban women's health issues is not a simple matter of fixing the health system, utilizing new health technologies, or improving health service delivery; it requires fundamental changes to the politics that produce the framework of inclusion and exclusion. Real, lasting improvement to women's health requires a different approach to decision-making, one that brings the urban poor, and women in particular, into the process.

The following pages provide an overview of the health issues with which poor urban women struggle, and a glimpse at the ways in which they are working to overcome the systemic problems that produce poor health outcomes.

Migration

In India, a city's economic growth spurs population growth, as those living in rural areas leave their villages to escape grinding poverty, hoping to make their fortunes in the big city. Though the real city is a far cry from the glamorous Bombay of Bollywood films, for most it is still better than home—for all the dirt and noise, even children can earn more as trash pickers in the city than entire families can earn in rural villages. In the city, nearly everyone can find a way to get two square meals a day. Consequently, a vast informal sector of unskilled workers—day laborers, rickshaw wallahs, street food vendors, maids—has sprung up in many cities to serve the burgeoning middle and upper classes.

Men come to the city from the villages to work, and they sleep on the pavements or rent rooms with dozens of others. It is only when women come to join their husbands and start families that huts begin to spring up on the pavements and in the slums (Figure 6.2). Yet municipalities often persist in portraying slum and pavement dwellers as dangerous, dirty criminals rather than acknowledging that the vast majority are simply families who have nowhere else to go. For many years, the state persisted in demolishing slum and pavement dwellers' huts, unwilling to acknowledge any responsibility to help the poorest, most marginalized people in the city. As urban areas grow by leaps and bounds, however, it is becoming increasingly clear that the existing infrastructure, housing, and service provision are woefully inadequate.

Sanitation and Waste Disposal

Sanitation and drainage have been recognized as important factors in urban health for over a century. The first investment in a comprehensive drainage system in Mumbai (then Bombay) was the result of an intervention by French and Egyptian representatives at a conference on cholera in 1867. Bombay, referred to as a "cholera nest," was seen as a threat to public health worldwide; subsequently, quarantine restrictions were imposed by the Egyptian Board of Health on ships carrying pilgrims departing from Bombay. Arthur Crawford, the then municipal commissioner of Bombay, argued that to maintain the city's role as an important port within the British Empire and to overcome the fear of exporting cholera, financial assistance was required to improve the city's sanitation (Dossal 1991; Harrison 1994).

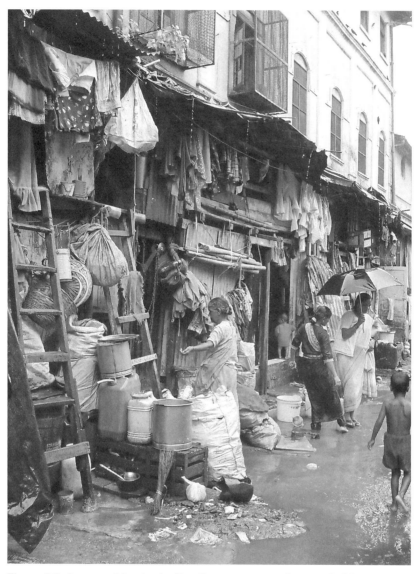

Figure 6.2. A waste picker in the Byculla pavement settlements in Mumbai segregates material to sell. This 4-foot-wide dwelling is about 65 square feet, which explains why water cans and clothing are stored on the dwelling's exterior. The ladder leads to a mezzanine level where younger children sleep. (Photo courtesy of the Society for Promotion of Area Resource Centres [SPARC], the federations, and friends of SPARC.)

In the twenty-first century, the city still struggles to meet its sanitation needs. When city authorities sought a loan from the World Bank to expand its sewer systems and improve waste treatment, for example, it neglected the fact that over 50 percent of Mumbai's population live in slums and informal settlements with limited access to toilets. Consequently, a huge amount of the city's fecal waste would not even go into the sewers planned to treat its waste: Although some formal buildings may have toilets connected to the city's sewer system, much of the waste in slums is disposed of, untreated, in storm drains that often flow directly into a canal, river, lake, or the sea, posing a health threat to the broader city.

Therefore, the priority from the point of view of informal settlements is the provision of toilets rather than the development of the city's sewer systems. The Brihanmumbai Municipal Corporation (BMC) responded to this problem by offering to provide minimum sanitation for 1 million people who did not have access to sanitation infrastructure—about a fifth of the total number lacking adequate sanitation facilities. Yet the provision of universal minimum sanitation has yet to be addressed systematically.

The lack of toilets presents a particularly severe problem for women. Concerns about modesty and harassment lead many to eat and drink less in order to minimize defecation, resulting in malnourishment, or to suppress defecation and urination till the cover of night, causing damage to internal organs in extreme cases. Although more girls are going to school, more are also leaving school at an early age, especially with the onset of puberty, due to the lack of toilet facilities at or near schools, as discussed further in Chapter 3.

Water

Water consumption among slum dwellers is extremely low—estimated to be between 26 and 33 liters per capita per day in Mumbai, far less than the citywide average of 135 liters per day (Karn, Shikura, and Harada 2003). This fact is worrisome in and of itself, suggesting that slum dwellers do not have enough water with which to drink or wash. Yet not only do slum households consume less water, but the water they drink from their taps is often contaminated: Though most large cities in the developing world treat their water supply, contaminated tap water is a frequent problem. Families who can afford to purchase water filtration systems do so, but families living in the slums must use the unfiltered tap water and hope for the best. The World Bank estimates that 21 percent of communicable diseases in India are related to unsafe water (Reuters 2010); in urban slums, water-related diseases are, unsurprisingly, a major problem. The annual incidence rates of diarrhea, typhoid, and malaria are estimated as 614, 68, and 126 cases per thousand people, respectively—much higher rates than are found in the country overall.

Furthermore, children are more likely to become ill from water-related diseases than adults are, and are at increased risk of death from waterborne illnesses, particularly diarrhea—the leading cause of death for children under 5. Since women are children's primary caregivers, more childhood disease translates into an increased burden for women, as well as an increased risk of their becoming ill themselves.

Malaria, usually associated with poor rural areas, is a growing problem in India's cities, particularly in slum areas. Pools of water at construction sites, in trash heaps, and in cisterns, where it is stored due to inadequate piped water supply, create breeding grounds for the mosquitoes that spread the disease. Urban incidences of malaria have gone from being a negligible problem in the 1950s to approximately 15 percent of malaria cases in India today. Improved water provision, drainage, and trash collection would reduce the number of breeding sites for malarial mosquitoes and help eradicate the disease in urban areas.

Water issues are particularly significant for women, who spend most of their time in the home carrying out domestic tasks, many of which—particularly cooking and cleaning—require the use of water. Furthermore, the tasks of water collection and waste management are traditionally women's responsibility, so when water and sanitation services are not available or functional, the impact is heaviest upon women.

Household and Public Space

Tuberculosis has long been common in urban areas where large numbers of people live in close quarters. Unsurprisingly, then, as India urbanizes, tuberculosis cases are on the rise. Poor nutrition and sanitation make people more susceptible to the disease, and cramped living conditions contribute to its spread. The median floor area of homes in slum areas in India is approximately 10 square meters (approximately 2.2 square meters per capita), while pavement dwellers' households have an average floor area of 8 square meters (Karn, Shikura, and Harada 2003). Such close quarters contribute to the spread of disease and the spread of tuberculosis, in particular: The tuberculosis rate is 7 to 18 cases per thousand people in Mumbai as compared to just 3.3 cases per thousand people in India overall. India currently accounts for one fifth of all tuberculosis cases globally, with an estimated 330,000 Indians dying of tuberculosis each year. Improvements in urban sanitation and living conditions would help reduce these numbers as more people flock to cities and end up in slums.

Women, who spend more time in the home than other family members, are most affected by cramped living conditions. They also bear the brunt of household-specific environmental hazards, from inhaling smoke and chemicals from the stoves and fires kept in cramped houses to breathing harmful fumes from burning trash.

Common space is extremely important in the daily life of slum dwellers: Since the private space inside homes is often limited, common areas outside provide space to carry out such tasks as washing and bathing as well as to socialize and interact. This space is especially important for women and children, who are largely confined to a small area near their homes, making the availability and quality of common space critical to the well-being of women and children living in slums. In many slum areas, however, the constant parade of motor vehicles poses a safety threat, and exhaust fumes contribute to respiratory problems. Further, inadequate trash collection allows huge piles of household waste to accumulate in streets and alleyways, providing a breeding ground for germs and mosquitoes alike.

Reproductive Health and HIV/AIDS

Though women living in urban areas are often assumed to have access to reproductive health services at city hospitals and clinics, this is not usually the case for women living in the slums and on the pavements. One study conducted by the India Institute of Public Health found that women who lived in slums had significantly less access to reproductive health services, from contraception to skilled birth assistants, than women who did not live in slums (Hazarika 2010).

Urban development and migration have also contributed to rising HIV/AIDS rates among Indian women. Heavy urban concentrations, migratory patterns, extreme poverty, and insufficient health infrastructure have been linked time and time again to the spread of HIV (Zulu, Dodoo, and Ezeh 2004). Poor women who migrate to the city and find themselves without work or income may be forced to resort to sex work to earn a living, which puts them at extremely high risk of contracting HIV.

Consequently, UN-HABITAT 2010b states that women living in urban slums are at greater risk of contracting HIV/AIDS than those in rural areas (UN-HABITAT 2010b). Furthermore, for those who are HIV positive, the high risk of disease in slum areas presents a serious threat to their compromised immune systems. Health interventions targeting people with HIV/AIDS may be futile if the individuals being treated go home to slums with no clean water and no sanitation system.

Addressing Habitat-Linked Health Issues

UN-HABITAT's recent *State of the World's Cities 2010–2011* report cites provision of basic services and development in slum settlements, security of tenure to poor families in slums, and involvement of the poor in decision-making and community development efforts as three important components of efforts to eliminate slums. A discussion of strategies for involving women in improving their communities follows.

Working with Women

Many health professionals, however committed they may be to women, see women primarily as beneficiaries and consumers of professionals' information and health solutions. Under the guise of helping women, health professionals all too often simply tell women what they must do. And yet the information that professionals offer is often grossly ill-suited to the reality of women's situations. Health workers talk to poor women who have no access to clean water about hygiene and washing hands, or train women in providing nutritious meals to their children when the family hardly has enough money to buy enough food each day.

Health workers must think carefully about how to communicate insights and knowledge to women in a way that is relevant to their lives. Many of the outcomes health professionals hope to achieve are not possible within the existing health system. Rather, it is necessary to change the politics underlying the framework of who is included and who is excluded in development outcomes—a task that requires a different way of bringing people and women into the process.

Surveys

The power of knowledge is one of the most important tools poor urban communities have. In many cities, little to no accurate information about slum dwellers—their numbers, their length of tenure, their livelihoods, their living conditions—exists. The assumptions made about the urban poor are consequently prejudiced and inaccurate. The urban poor are not drug addicts, thieves, or freeloaders, but hard-working families down on their luck with no place to go. They are employed as maids, cooks, trash pickers, and laborers. They are not "freeloading" on the city—rather, they often pay above market rate for basic services like water and electricity. Perhaps most important, slum and pavement dwellers can afford to survive in the city on the low wages they are earning only *because* they are living on the pavements and have low housing costs. Cities cannot clear the streets of pavement dwellers without losing the low-wage workers on which their economies are built unless they are willing to help provide low-cost housing.

Therefore, forcing city authorities to face the facts of urbanization is often the first step in achieving the goals of safe and healthy living conditions for the urban poor. The simple act of asserting these facts can be immensely powerful. Conducting a census of a slum or pavement settlement is a way for communities to communicate with those in power using the "official" language of numbers and statistics. Furthermore, by collecting information themselves, the urban poor learn about their neighbors, their communities, and their collective strength, all while bringing rich background information and context to the raw numbers.

Negotiation

Even short-term interventions are usually more effective when undertaken by communities rather than imposed by outsiders. Furthermore, the process of working together to solve health problems within a community can help build trust among women that can serve as the foundation for collective work to address their underlying problems.

Although they have no professional health training, the women of Mahila Milan collectively took on that role in their weekly meetings, which focused on sharing knowledge and experiences. In a community atmosphere, women were able to explore stories and experiences related to health that they might not have felt comfortable sharing in an atmosphere dominated by professionals. This trusting, comfortable environment allowed women to admit their health problems and seek help from health professionals. Women from the collectives therefore became partners with the health and social work professionals in closing the communication gap between their groups.

For example, for many years when the pavement women of Byculla took family members to the hospital for medical care, they were often told that they would have to provide blood or expensive medication before the patient could be admitted—items the women could not afford. Yet as one Mahila Milan leader, Samina, explained, things changed when these women joined Mahila Milan and decided to go to the doctor as a group. "Now Mahila Milan goes together if anybody needs to go to the hospital," she said. "If they are told to go and get the blood or go and get the medicine, we call not one doctor but five doctors, and we ask them, 'Who's this hospital meant for? This hospital is meant for the very poor, and the poor don't have the money to get blood, and they don't have the money to get medicine. Otherwise, say it is a rich people's hospital. But you know that rich people don't come here—they go to their own hospital and they do their own treatment.' After explaining this to the doctors, the doctors help us get blood or they give us some blood and we pay for some of it. They also explained to us that there are government sources where you can get cheaper or free medicine." The support of the group gives the women the courage to assert their needs and constraints to those who had previously intimidated them.

After SPARC had been working with the women of the Byculla pavements for about six months, the pavement women came to the SPARC staff and told them, "Now we groups of women can get our services. We can go and heckle the doctor in the hospital and make sure we get some help. We can deal with the education system; we can learn some of these tricks. But what we can't do is work towards getting a secure home for the next generation of children. We don't want our grandchildren to be living in the same spaces that we are." It was clear that although women had learned to use their collective power to make the existing system work for them, they were running up against the limits of the system itself. True change to their lives would require change to their housing, shelter, and infrastructure—to the very politics of land and space.

Toward that end, a critically important factor in women's health and well-being is their ability to negotiate with powerful institutions. Poor people do not have the luxury of making demands based on abstract principles and sticking to them. They must negotiate and dialogue with their tormentors if they hope to see changes in their lives. As they are denied access to many traditional avenues of power and authority, poor women are often forced to plead with those in power for aid or assistance. To escape the position of eternal supplicant, they must be strategic. By utilizing the power of association, women have learned to collectively negotiate with academics, government officials, and representatives of international development agencies. This process of dialogue and negotiation is critical not only for poor women who seek straightforward medical care, but also for those who seek to improve their fundamental living conditions by upgrading their homes or building a new community toilet.

Involvement of the Poor in Planning Processes

A contributing factor in India's difficulty in dealing with the growth of cities is a preponderance of archaic planning laws that provide only for the needs of the formal economy, despite the fact that huge segments of the urban population, particularly the poor, work in the informal sector. The wealthy live in the central city, while the poor who provide the services upon which they depend are pushed farther and farther into the city's outskirts, where services and infrastructure are scarcer. As a result, often the only way most poor people can get a piece of land in an area amenable to their livelihood is to encroach it, and the only way they can access amenities and services is to purchase them from a middleman, many of whom steal resources from the municipality.

Furthermore, even when the city does attempt to provide services to the poor, it often fails to take their actual needs and priorities into account. Because housing strategies are supply driven and centrally managed, they rarely reach the poor. Likewise, housing and toilet designs themselves are often ill suited to the needs of the poor, and particularly to the specific needs of poor women. Professional planners, architects, and engineers have failed to involve the poor, especially women, in the process of designing and building their own homes. Instead, city governments pull out the same old standard designs—expensive, difficult to maintain, and mostly doomed to failure. Despite their uninspiring track record, these standard models are duplicated again and again. Fresh, workable ideas for community improvements are badly needed. Yet they can emerge only from the perspectives of those who understand the communities in question—that is, the poor themselves. It is from the process of community experimentation that new standards emerge.

SPARC has therefore taken it upon itself to support slum and pavement communities in putting forth their own designs for structures and services. In preparation for the first SPARC housing exhibition, held at the Byculla Area Resource Centre in 1986, the Mahila Milan women acquired a mature understanding of matters relating to housing, from the costs of building materials to the process of construction. The women worked with engineers to construct life-sized model houses out of cardboard, cloth, and wood, and showed the engineers how big the kitchen should be and where to put the drain. With these houses they conveyed to the municipality and to architects which features were most important to them and what they could afford. For example, the women designed houses with lofts, permitting privacy for more than one generation to live together while keeping costs low. They also opted for community toilet blocks rather than individual household toilets, maximizing household space while improving hygiene by keeping toilets far from spaces used for cooking, eating, and sleeping. In this way, women are able to play an active role in creating spaces that are healthy and functional for them and their families.

Another design innovation was the idea of community toilet blocks built with communal spaces around or above the toilet itself. In densely populated slums, where there is little public space for people to gather, creating such a space in or above a community toilet is often an attractive proposition. The creation of such communal spaces also begins to transform the manner in which people relate to the structure, as they have an incentive to keep the toilets clean and functional. Some communities have also built caretaker's rooms atop the toilet blocks, providing an incentive for caretakers to do their jobs while providing a secure place for the person undertaking that job.

Furthermore, women are not only negotiating for changes to their housing, but learning to do the construction itself to upgrade their homes. Community toilet-building programs help the poor, particularly women, develop marketable skills and experiment with new solutions. Once women have learned to build toilets for their own communities, they are able to find work as contractors, helping other communities build toilets while bringing in a steady income.

Savings

When people hear "microfinance," they tend to think of microcredit—the small loans provided by NGOs and banks. Microsavings are much less widely known, yet they are actually more important to the poorest of the poor. Recent studies of microfinance show stronger effects for microsavings programs than for the more prevalent microcredit (Dupas and Robinson 2009). Research also suggests that although microfinance has an impact on people's lives, for most, it does not seem to provide a pathway out of poverty. The true value in microfinance may lie in what SPARC and Mahila Milan have been doing for years: helping the poor get through periods of financial instability and manage cash flow problems.

Mahila Milan's savings and credit programs build trust within a community. Women leaders visit every home in their community every evening to collect small amounts of money—typically no more than the change left over from a household's grocery purchases (Figure 6.3). For very, very poor households, even this small amount is a very important starting point in putting savings aside. Communities use these small savings to create a structure by which they learn to lend to each other, and in most cases, this lending is very humble: a few rupees to buy groceries when money is low or to buy a bus pass to go find a job. Yet larger loans are also available for emergencies—when a family member is sick or injured and needs to go to the hospital, for example. Over time, women increase their savings as much as they are able to, and many start saving for larger goals such as new housing.

Since every home is visited every day, members of the community know how others are doing and are there to support one another. If a woman

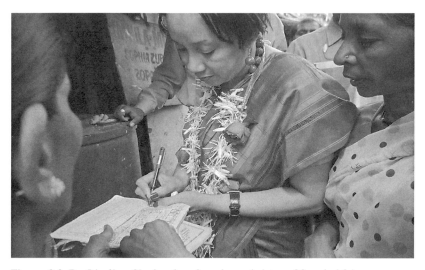

Figure 6.3. Dr. Lindiwe Sisulu, then housing minister of South Africa, accompanying the Mahila Milan on their daily savings round. Dr. Sisulu had visited India in 2005 to inaugurate Milan Nagar, a precedent-setting housing project constructed by Mahila Milan to house the pavement dwellers of Byculla, Mumbai. (Photo courtesy of Society for Promotion of Area Resource Centres [SPARC], the federations, and friends of SPARC.)

is facing violence in the house, the group knows it. If there's an illness in the family, the group knows it. In this way, the women support one another and their families through whatever crisis they are going through. Women get to know and trust one another—a critical step in building their ability to negotiate with the city for improvements in their lives.

From the savings process, the women also learn financial literacy. Since most women living in slums and on pavements are illiterate, they learn best through transactions. This process allows people control over their financial situations, the security of knowing that emergencies will not result in economic devastation, and the luxury of planning for the future.

Community Exchanges

Community exchange programs, in which members of poor communities visit each other's settlements to learn about each other's conditions, problems, and shared experiences, rest on a very simple concept: The poor learn best from the poor. Community exchanges, in contrast to development processes that rely on experts as "agents of change," actively involve slum residents and help them in transforming their own lives.

Exchanges are an important first step in breaking the isolation and helplessness that poverty brings to urban poor communities. Once communities see themselves as part of a larger group and an interdependent process, they can explore solutions to problems they face together. They can also learn from each other's successes.

Though these exchanges often begin at the local level, with visits between members of settlements within the same city, they are immensely valuable on a global scale as well. The poor are able to see that not only people within their settlement, city, or country are facing the same problems, but people around the world are grappling with the same situations and learning to overcome them. Through international networks like Shack/Slum Dwellers International, solutions to urban problems developed in India can be transferred to South Africa and Brazil, and vice versa. Many locals make a powerful global.

Conclusion

As this chapter has related, such partnerships among professional women and slum-dwelling women as SPARC, Mahila Milan, and the National Slum Dwellers Federation exemplify the kinds of productive synergies that result in better-designed neighborhoods and cities that have enhanced physical arrangements and social services. While far from perfect, progress is being made that will result in tangible improvement in female health. Equally tangible are new political roles for women, ones that will enable them to continue to address current needs and attack future concerns.

Chapter 7

Women with Disabilities and Cities

Rosaly Correa-de-Araujo

Ensuring that men and women across the life span and across diverse population groups live meaningful lives and enjoy the full economic growth and social benefits of communities worldwide is a critical humanitarian goal. In pursuing this goal, paying attention to the needs of women with disabilities, especially those living in cities, is of particular importance.

The World Health Organization (WHO) estimates that 10 percent of women worldwide are disabled, with a total of 300 million of these women and girls suffering from a mental and/or physical disability (Kern 1997: 244). According to a World Bank report, every minute, more than 30 women are seriously injured or disabled during labor. Regardless of the severity of their injuries and disablement, the 15 to 50 million women suffering from these injuries and disablements do not receive the necessary care or attention they deserve (World Bank 2010).

Generally, women report more incidents of disability than men and are at an increased risk of becoming disabled throughout their lives due to limited access to health care, poor conditions at work, and gender-based violence. Women with disabilities face stigma and exclusions and are more likely to get sick, be poor, and suffer from social isolation than either men with disabilities or women without disabilities. Women with mental disabilities are particularly vulnerable. For example, depressive disorders account for approximately 42 percent of the disability from mental or neuropsychiatric disorders among women compared to 29 percent among men (WHO 2010g). However, the broad range of mental health threats to which women are disproportionately susceptible—such as gender discrimination, violence, poverty, armed conflict, dislocation, and other forms of social deprivation—are still poorly understood (WHO 2010g). Women and girls with disabilities remain particularly vulnerable to specific types of abuse (e.g., being beaten at home, raped, and forcibly sterilized).

Women with disabilities are at a higher risk of acquiring HIV/AIDS due to lack of awareness and access to information and programs. Folk belief that individuals with sexually transmitted diseases, including HIV/AIDS, can rid themselves of the infection if they have intercourse with a virgin poses a particular risk for girls who have disabilities. These girls are seen as sexually inactive and, therefore, as easy targets.

In most industrialized countries, especially in urban areas, the challenge for women with disabilities is to achieve equality of opportunity; they seek access to the same opportunities available to women who do not have disabilities. In urban areas of industrialized countries, women with disabilities often have easier access to health care and rehabilitation services; some have access to education and vocational training opportunities as well. Many hold jobs and/or are married and have families. For these women in the industrialized countries of Asia, Europe, and North America, priorities are to increase access to jobs and self-employment; combat discrimination in the workplace; increase the availability of the attendant care necessary to enable many women with disabilities to work; change negative public perceptions and attitudes toward persons with disabilities; and provide easier access to public and private buildings, transportation, and various forms of communication.

In most developing countries, especially in rural areas, girls and women generally hold the largest share of the burden of poverty, both physically and economically. For women with disabilities, the situation is even worse, as they are even poorer, are often totally dependent on others for survival, usually have a dismal future, and have less access to food, health care, and education than other family members. In these countries, women are expected to perform all daily household work (e.g., cooking, fetching water and wood for fuel, going to the market, doing washing and laundry, minding younger children, gardening, cleaning the house and yard). However, girls and women with disabilities are often seen as not helpful and so are not expected or encouraged to help with these household tasks, even when physically or mentally capable; as a result, these women and girls are precluded from engaging in a number of activities that could help them develop skills and abilities for employment. They are rarely involved in the decision-making process, either within the family or within their communities. Decisions concerning girls and women with disabilities are generally made for them without any consultation. Furthermore, women with disabilities rarely have opportunities to get married, although many have children. In developing countries, women with disabilities are often victims of HIV/AIDS and other sexually transmitted diseases due to a lack of knowledge about these diseases and about ways to prevent them. Higher rates of HIV/AIDS are generally associated with the poverty under which these women live. In addition, cultural, legal, and institutional barriers persist, making these women and girls victims of discrimination (Depouy 1988). In certain countries, legal barriers preclude women with disabilities from the right to marry and form a family. For those with mental disabilities, marriage may not be allowed, based on the assumption that disabled people cannot fully understand the nature of the responsibilities associated with marriage. Examples of countries in which such laws prevail include Tanzania, Cambodia, and China (USAID 2010). Women and girls with disabilities also are at risk of being trafficked and forced into prostitution. Reports indicate that prostitution houses in Thailand specifically seek out deaf female children and adolescents because they are less likely to exhibit distress or find their way back home. Similarly, in Taiwan, children with mild developmental disabilities are six times greater than the general population to be prostituted (USAID 2010).

The goal of enabling women with disabilities worldwide to live meaningful lives and enjoy the full benefits of membership in a community is ambitious. It will require joint international efforts and local partnerships among urban planners, governments, and consumers. These groups must work toward the general goal of achieving gender equality and empowering women to embrace opportunities and contribute to sustainable urbanization while also focusing on the specific factors pertaining to women with disabilities. These factors include environmental constraints that limit people's activities in daily work, school, and community life. Because environmental barriers can have a significant negative impact on people's activities, access to affordable and accessible housing and transportation, to safe and healthy environments that protect women with disabilities from violence, abuse, and illness, and to quality and culturally competent health and support services is essential.

Several international efforts have addressed women's issues and, increasingly, are drawing attention to the special concerns of women with disabilities. Landmark events in this field include the 1979 Convention on the Elimination of All Forms of Discrimination Against Women (CEDAW),[1] the 1994 International Conference on Population and Development,[2] and the 1995 Fourth World Conference on Women.[3] The recommendations and consensuses that resulted from these conventions frame the contemporary discussion of women's health as grounded in gender equality and women's empowerment.

The United Nations reinforced these accomplishments in the 2000 Millennium Development Goals.[4] Women with disabilities constitute 10 percent of the world's population, and 20 percent of poor people worldwide are disabled—yet neither the Millennium Development Goals nor the policies, guidelines, programs, and efforts accompanying these goals specifically reference disability. Nevertheless, the eight Millennium Development Goals, listed in Table 7.1, are very relevant to women with disabilities, as they foster collaborative action to reduce poverty, improve health, and address educational and environmental concerns with a focus on the world's most pressing issues. Still, data gaps related to monitoring, evaluation, and application of the goals in relation to disability exist and should be repaired in order to mainstream disability in policies, processes, and mechanisms.

The World Health Organization's Community-Based Rehabilitation Initiative has the potential to significantly contribute to achieving the Millennium Development Goals in a way that benefits people with disabilities. It also can help bring the protection of the United Nations Convention on the Rights of Persons with Disabilities to communities. Currently implemented in over ninety countries, WHO's Community-Based Rehabilitation Initiative is a development strategy that provides rehabilitation, reduces poverty, equalizes opportunities, and promotes the inclusion of persons with disabilities in their communities. The initiative takes a multisectoral approach, coordinating the efforts of people with disabilities, their families, organizations, communities, and governmental and nongovernmental organizations (NGOs). Table 7.1 identifies potential strategies under WHO's Community-Based Rehabilitation Initiative that can significantly benefit persons with disabilities by contributing to the achievement of the Millennium Development Goals. As described by the World Health Organization, these strategies derive from the following facts:

- Poverty is both a cause and a consequence of disability. Eradication of extreme poverty and hunger can be achieved through livelihood and employment promotions under the community-based rehabilitation approach. (Goal 1)
- Children with disabilities (particularly girls) are the most marginalized and least likely to go to school. The correlation between low educational outcomes and having a disability is often stronger than the correlation between low educational outcome and gender, rural residence, or poverty. (Goal 2)
- Discrimination against women with disabilities, based on both gender and disability, increases the risk of violence and abuse. Women who care for family members with disabilities may themselves face significant hardships particularly where there are limited support services in the community. (Goal 3)

Table 7.1. Persons with Disabilities, Millennium Development Goals, and the World Health Organization's Community-Based Rehabilitation Initiative

Millennium Development Goals	WHO's Community-Based Rehabilitation Strategies Supporting the Millennium Development Goals and Persons with Disabilities
1. Eradicate extreme poverty and hunger	Identifying and overcoming barriers preventing social participation Exploring potential employment opportunities for people with disabilities in their communities Providing or ensuring access to skills training for income-generating activities and employment
2. Achieve universal primary education	Informing families with disabled children that they have a right to education Providing recommendations and practical assistance to make school environments physically accessible and to make teaching flexible and child-centered Referring children to specialized services to enable inclusion in primary education (e.g., referral for assistive devices)
3. Promote gender equality and empower women	Promoting equal access and participation for women with disabilities in all community development initiatives Supporting girls with disabilities to access educational opportunities Supporting the development of self-help groups for women with children with disabilities
4. Reduce child mortality	Ensuring early identification of children with impairments and referring children to specialized medical and rehabilitation services where necessary Providing disability awareness training to primary health-care staff to ensure children with disabilities are able to access general health care Providing basic home-based therapy interventions to promote child development
5. Improve maternal health	Raising awareness within communities that people with disabilities have sexual and reproductive health needs Supporting women with disabilities to access maternal health services in their communities Ensuring that traditional birth attendant training programs focus on disability

Table 7.1. Continued

Millennium Development Goals	WHO's Community-Based Rehabilitation Strategies Supporting the Millennium Development Goals and Persons with Disabilities
6. Combat HIV/AIDS, malaria, and other diseases	Reducing the stigma surrounding sexuality and persons with disabilities Promoting the provision of health information in accessible formats Developing tailored prevention programs for persons with disabilities where mainstream programs are inappropriate or ineffective
7. Ensure environmental sustainability	Ensuring communities involve persons with disabilities when designing safe water and sanitation facilities Making recommendations and modifications to ensure access to existing facilities Ensuring that disaster response training within communities considers the needs of persons with disabilities and appropriate strategies are in place
8. Develop a global partnership for development	Partnering and working with all sectors to achieve positive outcomes for people with disabilities

Sources: Millennium Development Goals. 2000. http://www.unmilleniumproject.org/goals/index.htm; WHO. 2000h. *Millennium Development Goals. Disability and Rehabilitation Team (DAR). Achieving the Millennium Development Goals for People with Disabilities.* http://www.who.int/disabilities/media/events/idpdinfo031209/en/index1.html.

- Worldwide, approximately 200 million children have disabilities. These children are more likely to die from life-threatening medical conditions, lack of access to health services, and neglect. Community-based rehabilitation programs can control these causes and reduce child mortality. (Goal 4)
- Morbidity and disability often result from pregnancy and childbirth complications. Also, women with disabilities can become mothers themselves and often need particular consideration while pregnant or when bringing up children. Community-based rehabilitation strategies can improve maternal health outcomes. (Goal 5)
- Infectious diseases are disabling. HIV, for example, can cause blindness, neuropathy, and dementia. Persons with disabilities are routinely excluded from HIV and AIDS policies and programs

due to widespread reluctance to regard this population as sexual beings. Community-based rehabilitation programs can contribute to combating HIV/AIDS, malaria, and other diseases. (Goal 6)
• Environmental risks and natural disasters cause illnesses and disability. Many people with disabilities live in communities with poor sanitation, including limited access to quality water. In addition, they are often excluded from disaster preparedness and management activities. (Goal 7)

Community-based rehabilitation relies on a partnership approach that involves all development sectors. Three global alliances work to achieve positive outcomes for people with disabilities: the Asia-Pacific Network, the Africa Network, and the American and Caribbean Network. Currently, WHO, the International Labour Organization (ILO); the United Nations Education, Scientific, and Cultural Organization (UNESCO); and the International Disability and Development Consortium are developing guidelines for implementing community-based rehabilitation programs. These guidelines will ensure that persons with disabilities have the same rights and opportunities to benefit from the Millennium Development Goals as do others in their communities.

Many countries have legislation pertaining to people with disabilities. For example, in the United States, important federal laws and statutes protect individuals with disabilities from discrimination in employment and the job application process, including the Americans with Disabilities Act, the Rehabilitation Act, the Workforce Investment Act, the Vietnam Era Veterans' Readjustment Assistance Act, and the Civil Service Reform Act. These laws and statutes share the fundamental goal of removing barriers to employment faced by individuals with disabilities; their limits differ depending on such factors as whether employers are in the public or private sector, the number of employees in an organization, and whether the organization holds federal contracts or subcontracts (U.S. Department of Labor 2005).

Gender discrimination is specifically addressed under Title VII of the Civil Rights Act of 1964, which makes it unlawful for an employer to hire or discharge any individual, or otherwise to discriminate against any individual, with respect to his or her compensation, terms, conditions, or privileges of employment, because of an individual's race, color, religion, sex, or national origin. This covers hiring, firing, promotions, and all workplace conduct. Gender discrimination is also addressed under Title IX of the Education Amendment of 1972, which prohibits sex discrimination in any educational program or activity at any educational institution that is a recipient of federal funds. In addition, Title IX prohibits all forms of sex discrimination in federally funded educational institutions, whether private or public, and covers, for example, issues related to sexual harassment, discrimination in admissions and counseling, and discrimination against married or pregnant students.

Estimate of Worldwide Population of People with Disabilities

There are numerous challenges to estimating the number of people with disabilities around the world. The definition of disability is complex and differs from region to region, from country to country, and within countries, depending on the purpose of each classification system or the definition needed to support disability claims. This variability in definitions of disability affects the resulting estimates. In addition, the collection of disability data is not standardized, which leads to inconsistency. Numerous surveys currently available include self-reported disability information, which may be inconsistent but may also be underreported, since these populations are subjected to stigma and marginalization. Because the costs of data collection are generally very high, many countries are precluded from consistently updating their demographic information on people with disabilities. Indeed, country or regional disability data presented in this chapter may be outdated or incomplete, due to the challenges routinely faced with disability data.

Estimates of disability by gender and by urban and rural areas are readily available for the United States and represent a major opportunity for future work. The forthcoming WHO/World Bank *World Report on Disability* will contain new data on the prevalence and nature of disability, together with the environmental factors that often make life harder for women and men experiencing health conditions associated with disability. The report is scheduled for release some time in 2011. Its release will provide essential information to those involved in urban planning. WHO and other federal statistical organizations in each country of the world should commit to keeping data on people with disabilities—and in particular women with disabilities—consistently updated and readily available to support urban planning that accommodates the specific needs of this population.

Table 7.2 provides estimates of the proportion of people with disabilities in selected countries of Asia and the Pacific region. Australia, Turkey, Vietnam, Bangladesh, and China have the highest percentage of disability (20 percent, 12.3 percent, 6.4 percent, 5.6 percent, and 5 percent, respectively). However, sources and dates for data availability vary considerably.

Table 7.2. Disability in Asia and the Pacific Region as a Percentage of Total Population*

Country and Percentage (with data source)	Definition of Persons with Disabilities
	East and Northeast Asia
China 5%: 1987 National Sampling Survey on Disability	*Law of the People's Republic of China on the Protection of Disabled Persons (1990)* A person with disabilities is one who suffers from abnormalities of or loss of a certain organ or function, psychologically or physiologically or in anatomical structure and has lost wholly or in part the ability to perform an activity in the way considered to be normal.
Hong Kong, China 4%, excluding intellectual disability: 2005 Census, Statistics Department	*Census and Statistics Statistics Department (2000)* Under the framework of the survey, "persons with disabilities" were defined as those who (1) had been diagnosed by qualified health personnel (such as practitioners of Western and Chinese Medicine, including herbalists, bone-setters and acupuncturists) as having one or more of the following seven conditions, or (2) had perceived themselves as having one or more of the first four of the following seven conditions which had lasted, or were likely to last, for a period of six months or more at the time of enumeration: (a) restriction in body movement; (b) seeing difficulty; (c) hearing difficulty; (d) speech difficulty; (e) mental illness; (f) autism; (g) mental handicap.
Japan 5%	*Article 2 of Basic Law for Persons with Disabilities; Article 4 of Law for the Welfare of Physically Disabled Persons; Operational Definition Used for Persons with Intellectual Disabilities; Article 5 of Mental Health and Welfare Law of Mentally Disabled* Persons with disabilities are those whose daily or social life is substantially and continuously limited due to physical, intellectual or mental disability. Persons with physical disability are persons over 18 years of age who have physical disability which comes under one of those physical disabilities enumerated in the law, and who have received a certificate for persons with disabilities from the governor of local governments. Persons with intellectual disabilities are persons who have intellectual disability manifested during the developmental period (birth to 18 years of age) and have functional deficits in

Table 7.2. Continued

Country and Percentage (with data source)	Definition of Persons with Disabilities
Japan (continued)	skills for daily life which require supportive services. Persons with mental disabilities shall be persons who have schizophrenia, psychotic disorders due to psychoactive substance use, mental retardation, personality disorders, and/or other mental disorders. Persons with developmental disabilities are persons who have developmental disability and whose daily and social life are substantially limited by the disability.
Mongolia 3.5%: 2005 National Statistical Office of Mongolia	*Provisions No. 3 of Law on Social Security of the of the People with Disability defines people with disabilities as:* Citizens of Mongolia, foreign residents who live officially in Mongolia, and the stateless persons whose physiological and mental impairment is transmitted through genetically and non-genetically, congenital defect, post-injection complication, lost control of voluntary movement functions reasoned from accidents and impossible to labor in ordinary circumstances, have visual, auditory and speech disability, as well as mentally retarded and psychologically impaired are investigated and registered by Medical and Labor Certification. This definition is used in Mongolia for official statistics.
Republic of Korea 4.6%: Ministry of Health and Welfare	An individual whose daily life and social life in the community are limited by physical or mental disabilities for a long time.
	Southeast Asia
Indonesia 1%: Ministry of Social Affairs, Central Board of Statistics	Person having physical and/or mental deficiencies which can hinder or restrict that person's ability to function properly.
Cambodia 2.4%: National Institute of Statistics, Ministry of Planning 3.9%: World Bank	Any citizen who lacks any physical organ or capacity or suffers any mental impairment which causes decent restrictions on his/her daily life or activities such as loss of limbs, quadriplegia, visual or hearing or mental impairment.

(continued on next page)

Table 7.2. Continued

Country and Percentage (with data source)	Definition of Persons with Disabilities
Lao People's Democratic Republic 8%	[no definition available]
Malaysia 1%: 1958 government data	*Based on 1980 WHO definition* Any peson unable to ensure by himself, wholly or partly, the necessities of a normal individual and/or social life as a result of a deficiency, either congenital or not, in his physical or mental capabilities. For the purpose of the registration, the following six categories are applied: physically disabled; deaf; blind; cerebral palsy; learning disabled; and others.
Philippines 1.2%: 2000 National Census of Housing and Population	*Magna Carta for Disabled Persons, Republic Act 7277 (1995)* Those with restriction of different abilities, as a result of a mental, physical or sensory impairment, in performing an activity in the manner or within the range considered normal for a human being.
Singapore 3%, excluding intellectual disability: 2003 Ministry of Community Development, Youth and Sports	Those whose prospects of securing, retaining places and advancing in education and training institutions, employment and recreation as equal members of the community are substantially reduced as a result of physical, mental, intellectual, developmental or sensory impairments.
Thailand 1.7%: 2002 Disability Survey	A person with physical, intellectual or psychological abnormality or impairment as categorized and prescribed in the Ministerial Regulations, impairments in terms of sight, hearing or communication, physical and locomotion, mentality or behavior, and intellectual or learning disability.
Vietnam 6.4%: 2004–2005 Ministry of Labour—Invalids and Social Affairs	By definition of this Ordinance, irrespective of the causes of the disability, persons with disabilities are defined as defective in one or many parts of the body or functions which are shown in different forms of disability, and which reduce the capability of activity and cause many difficulties in work, life and studies.

Table 7.2. Continued

Country and Percentage (with data source)	Definition of Persons with Disabilities
	South and Southwest Asia
Bangladesh 5.6%: 2005 National Forum of Organizations Working with the Disabled; Handicap International	*The Disability Welfare Act (2001) defines disability as:* Disability means any person who (a) is physically crippled either congenitally or as result of disease or being a victim of accident, or due to improper or maltreatment or for any other reasons became physically incapacitated or mentally imbalanced, and (b) as a result of such crippling or mental impairment—(1) has become incapacitated, either partially or fully; and (2) is unable to lead a normal life. Any person having disability described hereunder shall be included in the meaning and scope of the definition under subsection (1) of this section. (a) Visual impaired means any person who has: (1) no vision in any single eye, or (2) in both the eyes, or (3) visual acuity not exceeding 6/60 or 20/200 (Snellen) in the better eye even with correcting lenses; or (4) limitation of a field of vision subtending an angle of 20 degrees or worse. (b) Physically handicapped refers to a person who has— (1) lost either one or both the hands, or (2) lost sensation, partly or wholly, of either hand, or it is so weaker in normal condition that the situations stated under subsection 1 (a) and (b) are applicable to this case or (3) lost either one or both the feet, or (4) lost sensation, partly or wholly, of either or both feet, or it is so weaker in normal condition that the situations stated under subsection 1 (a) and (b) are applicable to this case; or (5) has physical deformity and abnormality, or (6) has permanently lost physical equilibrium owing to neuro-disequilibria. (c) Hearing impairment means one has loss of hearing capacity in better ear in the conversation range of frequencies at 40 decibels (hearing unit) or more, or damaged or ineffective otherwise. (d) Speech impairment means loss of one's capacity to utter/pronounce meaningful vocabulary sounds or it is damaged, partly or wholly, or dysfunctional. (e) Mental disability means (1) one whose mental development is not at par with his chronological

(continued on next page)

Table 7.2. Continued

Country and Percentage (with data source)	Definition of Persons with Disabilities
Bangladesh (continued)	age or whose Intelligent Quotient is far below the normal range, or (2) has lost mental balance or is damaged, partly or wholly. (f) Multiple disabilities refer to one who suffers from more than one type of above stated impairments. (g) Any other type of impairment to be defined and declared by the National Coordination Committee.
Bhutan 3.4%: 2005 Population and Housing Census of Bhutan	[no definition available]
India 2.1%: 2002 Census quoted in National Policy for Persons with Disabilities 1.8%: 2002 National Sample Survey Organization	*National Policy for Persons with Disabilities (2006)* A person with restrictions or lack of abilities to perform an activity in the manner or within the range considered normal for a human being was treated as having disability. The policy excluded illness/injury of recent origin (mobility) resulting in temporary loss of ability to see, hear, speak, or move.
Maldives 3.4%: 2003 Ministry of Gender, Family Development and Social Security	[no definition available]
Nepal 1.6%: 2001 CBS, NPC, and UNICEF Survey	A person unable to perform livelihood due to physical deficiency, weakness or dystrophy whether inborn or due to accident or disease is defined as disabled.
Pakistan 2.5%: 1998 Nation Census Report 7%: 1980 WHO Survey	*The Gazette of Pakistan (Statutory Notification SRO 627(1)/88)* For the quota system "disable person" means a person on account of injury, disease or congenital deformity is handicapped in education or for undertaking any gainful profession or employment in order to earn his livelihood, and includes a person who is blind, deaf, physically handicapped or mentally retarded.
Turkey 12.3%: 2002 Disability Survey	*Turkish Disability Law (put in force May 7, 2005)* A group of people who lost their physical, mental, psychological, emotional, and social

Table 7.2. Continued

Country and Percentage (with data source)	Definition of Persons with Disabilities
Turkey (continued)	abilities to an extent that prevents them meeting the demands of daily life because of diseases or accidents that either exist in birth or happen later in life and who need special care, protection, rehabilitation, guidance and support services.

	North and Central Asia
Kazakhstan 3%: 2006 State Statistical Agency	*Law on Social Protection of Disabled Persons* Person unable, partly or totally, to implement certain actions as a result of losing work ability due to illness, trauma or inborn defect.

	Pacific
Australia 20%: 2003 SDAC Survey by Australian Bureau of Statistics Survey of Disability	*2003 Survey of Disability, Ageing and Carers (SDAC)* A person has a disability if he/she has a limitation, restriction or impairment which has lasted, or is likely to last, for at least six months and restricts everyday activities. This includes: loss of sight (not corrected by glasses and contact lenses); loss of hearing where communication is restricted; or an aid to assist with, or substitute for, hearing is used; chronic or recurrent pain or discomfort causing restriction; difficulty in learning or understanding; mental illness; head injury; stroke or other brain damage; incomplete use of feet or legs.
	Disability Discrimination (1992) For the anti-discrimination law, disability in relation to a person, means: (a) total or partial loss of the person's bodily or mental functions; or (b) total or partial loss of a part of the body; or (c) the presence in the body of organisms causing disease or illness; or (d) the presence in the body of organisms capable of causing disease or illness; or (e) the malfunction, malformation, or disfigurement of a part of the person's body; or (f) a disorder or malfunction that results in the person learning differently from a person without the disorder or malfunction; or (g) a disorder, illness or disease that affects a person's thought processes, perception of reality,

(continued on next page)

Table 7.2. Continued

Country and Percentage (with data source)	Definition of Persons with Disabilities
Australia (continued)	emotions or judgment or that results in disturbed behavior; and includes a disability that: (h) recently exists; or (i) previously existed but no longer exists; or (j) may exist in the future; or (k) is imputed to a person.
Cook Islands 0.7%: National Disability Database	One who has a form of impairment/disability whether physical, mental, or intellectual and whose behavior is abnormal at times.
Fiji	*1994 Fiji National Council for Disabled Persons Act (FNCDP), Both Policy and Data Collection Purpose* Persons who as a result of physical, mental or sensory impairment are restricted or lacking in ability to perform an activity in the manner considered normal for human beings.
Kiribati	*Kiribati National Disability Survey, 2004* Persons with hearing or visual impairment, mental health problems, physical and/or intellectual disability.
Solomon Islands 3.5%	[no definition available]

*Certain terms used in this table (e.g., crippled; handicapped) are considered to be discriminatory terms. However, they are used here because the language was extracted directly from legislation or policies from each country.

Source: United Nations. 2006. *Disability at a Glance: A Profile of 28 Countries and Areas in Asia and the Pacific.* Bangkok, Thailand: United Nations, ESCAP.

Table 7.3 displays 1996 disability data by gender available from fourteen countries of the European Union. Figure 7.1 shows that among the European population aged 16 to 64 years, almost 15 percent of women and 14 percent of men reported either a moderate or a severe disability. Differences between men and women are larger for those with moderate levels of disability.

For the Eastern Mediterranean Region, 2002 data are available for twelve countries indicating low and high estimates of the total population of people with disabilities. These data are presented in Table 7.4.

For Africa, as with other regions or countries in the developing world, data on disability are very fragmented or outdated; only a few countries, mainly in eastern and southern Africa, have compiled recent informa-

Table 7.3. 1996 Percentage of Population Reporting Severe, Moderate, or No Disability in European Union Countries by Sex and Age Group, 16–64

Country	Women with Disability (%)				Men with Disability (%)			
	Severe	Moderate	None	Total	Severe	Moderate	None	Total
Belgium	4.2	8.7	87.1	100	5.0	7.9	87.1	100
Denmark	4.8	15.4	79.8	100	4.6	10.1	85.3	100
Germany	4.0	12.9	83.1	100	5.2	12.4	82.6	100
Greece	3.2	5.5	91.3	100	3.5	4.2	92.4	100
Spain	3.0	7.0	90.0	100	3.6	6.2	90.3	100
France	6.0	9.8	84.3	100	6.0	8.8	85.2	100
Ireland	2.2	8.8	89.0	100	2.7	8.1	89.3	100
Italy	2.4	5.7	91.9	100	2.1	5.4	92.5	100
Luxemburg	4.1	11.4	84.6	100	4.6	12.9	82.5	100
Netherlands	6.8	14.0	79.2	100	4.7	11.4	83.9	100
Austria	3.4	8.5	88.2	100	3.1	10.1	86.8	100
Portugal	8.2	11.9	80.0	100	6.7	9.9	83.4	100
Finland	5.8	18.4	75.9	100	6.7	15.0	78.3	100
United Kingdom	5.1	14.5	80.5	100	6.4	11.6	82.0	100
Average	4.3	10.6	85.1	100	4.7	9.3	86.0	100

Source: EUROSTAT 2001. *Disability and Social Participation in Europe.* European Commission. Luxembourg.

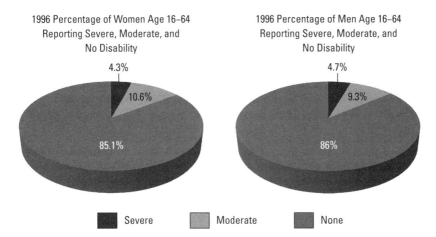

1996 Percentage of Women Age 16–64 Reporting Severe, Moderate, and No Disability

1996 Percentage of Men Age 16–64 Reporting Severe, Moderate, and No Disability

Severe   Moderate   None

Figure 7.1. Disability estimates by gender in fourteen countries of the European Union.
Source: EUROSTAT. 2001. *Disability and Social Participation in Europe.* European Commission. Luxembourg.

Table 7.4. 2002 Disability Population Estimates in Countries of the Eastern Mediterranean Region

Country	Low Estimate	High Estimate
Djibouti	7,000	69,300
Egypt	2, 608,500	6,979,500
Iran	725,200	1,940,400
Jordan	196,100	524,700
Lebanon	133,200	356,400
Morocco	1,113,700	2,979,900
Syria	10,600	1,366,200
Tunisia	358,900	960,300
West Bank and Gaza	125,800	336,600
Yemen	193,000	1,910,700
Total	8,491,700	24,165,900

Source: Metts, R. 2004 . Disability and Development. Background Paper Prepared for the Disability and Development Meeting, World Bank, November 16, 2004.

tion. Much still needs to be done to obtain disability data from central and western African countries, but funding for this remains a problem. The 2007 Kenya National Survey for Persons with Disabilities (KNSPD), however, should serve as a prototype of a successful partnership with numerous other organizations, including the World Bank. Table 7.5 provides KNSPD information collected from nearly 15,000 households across all of Kenya's sixty-nine districts. Respondents were evenly divided by sex: 49.6 percent were male and 50.4 percent female. Slightly more females than males resided in rural areas.

Table 7.5. Number and Percentage Distribution of People with Disabilities in Kenya by Age, Sex, and Residence: Survey of 15,000 Households

	Male		Female		
	%	Number	%	Number	Total
Age Group					
0–14	50.0	15,153	50.0	15,178	30,329
15–24	50.5	7,276	49.5	7,244	14,620
25–34	48.1	4,523	51.9	4,880	9,402
35–54	49.2	5,301	50.8	5,473	10,774
55+	49.5	3,359	50.5	2,406	4,765
Do not know	45.7	365	54.3	435	800
Residence					
Urban	50.1	7,240	49.9	7,201	14,441
Rural	49.5	27,837	50.5	28,413	56,250

Source: *Kenya National Survey for Persons with Disabilities: Preliminary Report*. 2008. Nairobi: National Coordinating Agency for Population and Development.

The International Disability Rights Monitor (IDRM) *Americas Regional Report* released in 2004 provides a compilation of disability as a percentage of total population in numerous countries in the Western Hemisphere. Table 7.6 summarizes this information. Essentially, the majority of the countries in the Western Hemisphere reported disability rates of under 10 percent. Survey methodologies varied, however, making data

Table 7.6. Disability in the Western Hemisphere

Country	Definition of Persons with with Disabilities	Proportion of People with Disabilities	Data Source
North America			
Canada	—	12.4%	2000 PALS
Mexico	—	1.84%	2000 Basic Census
		2.31%	2000 Extended Census
United States	Activity limitations	19.3%	2000 Census
South America			
Argentina	—	7.1%	2005 Encuesta Nacional de Personas con Discapacidad—ENDI
Bolivia	Impairment-based	0.9–1.2%	2001 Census
		10%	Ministry of Health and Sports
Brazil	Activity limitations	14.5%	2000 Census
Chile	Impairment-based	5.3%	2000 Social Economic Survey
	Activity limitations	21.7%	2000 Quality of Life and Health
	Impairment-based	2.2%	2002 Census
		12.9%	2004 Encuesta Nacional de Discapacidad (ENDISC-CIF)
Colombia	Impairment-based	1.85%	1993 Census
		6.4%	2005 Census
Ecuador	—	12.14%	Ecuador: La Discapacidad con Cifras. INEC-CONADIS, 2005
Paraguay	—	—	2002 Census
		1.0%	2005 DGEEC

(continued on next page)

Table 7.6. Continued

Country	Definition of Persons with with Disabilities	Proportion of People with Disabilities	Data Source
Peru	—	1.3%	1993 Census
		13%	1993 Specialized Rehabilitation Institute
Suriname	—	2.7%	1980 Census
	—	—	2003 Census
Uruguay	—	7.6	2003/2004 National Disability Survey
Venezuela	Impairment-based	4.2%	2001 Census
Central America and the Caribbean			
Bahamas	—	6.0%	2001 BLCS
Belize	Impairment-based	5.7%	2000 Census
Bermuda	—	4.5%	2000 ?
Costa Rica	Impairment-based	5.4%	2000 Census
Dominica	—	1.1%	2002–2005 Census
Dominican Republic	—	—	2002 Census
		4.2%	La Discapacidad en la Republica Dominicana, ONE-CONADIS, 2006
El Salvador	—	1.6%	1992 Census
		6.6%	2000–2002, Encuesta
		4.1%	2005 Registro Nacional de Personas Naturales
Guatemala	—	6.2%	2002 Census
Guyana	—	9%	1994 Census
	—	2.2%	2002 Census
Honduras	—	2.6%	2002 Multipurpose Household Survey
Jamaica	—	6.2%	2001 Census
Nicaragua	—	12.5%	? Census
		10.25%	2003 ENDIS
Panama	Impairment-based	1.8%	2000 Census

Source: Modified from International Disabilities Rights Monitor (IDRM). 2004. *Regional Report of the Americas.* Chicago: International Disability Network/Center for Internaitonal Rehabilitation.

reliability a matter of concern. Additional information on those with disabilities in the United States is provided separately, as follows.

The American Community Survey (ACS) is a continuous data collection effort conducted by the U.S. Census Bureau. It is used to produce annual estimates at the national, state, and local level on the characteristics of the U.S. population. The survey provides federal, state, and local governments with information for the administration and evaluation of government programs. It also provides data users with timely information each year on demographic, housing, social, and economic statistics that can be compared across states, communities, and population groups. The survey contains disability questions relevant to major forms of disability (e.g., auditory, visual, cognitive, ambulatory) and addresses self-care and independent living. Since 2005, yearly estimates have been available for geographic areas with populations of at least 65,000. Geographic areas with populations of 20,000 or more are available using three years of ACS data. Geographic areas with populations of less than 20,000 using five years of data were made available on December 14, 2010.

Table 7.7 and Figure 7.2 display information on disability prevalence in the United States by gender, age, and distribution by urban, metropolitan (principal cities), and rural areas. Similar proportions of women and men with disabilities are found among the populations aged 18 to 64. Slightly higher numbers of males with disabilities are seen under age 18 and seem to be found above age 64, although the total population of females in this table is higher for the above age 64 group. Both females and males with disability are similarly distributed between urban and rural areas in the United States, with slightly more women with disability living in urban areas.

Urban Planning and Disability Status

Understanding the concerns and multiple needs of women with disabilities requires knowledge of the diverse nature of their disabilities and the intersection with their various identity markers (Beijing Platform for Action 1995: paragraph 46). Women with disabilities may be blind or have low vision; be deaf or hard of hearing; or have a learning, developmental/intellectual, physical, mental/psychiatric, and/or other form of hidden disability. These will intersect with identity markers such as gender, age, race, ethnicity, culture, language, faith, religion, and spirituality. Further, women with disabilities generally face challenges navigating systems and structures designed without their input. For women with disabilities, it can be difficult to have a healthy lifestyle while living

Table 7.7. United States Civilian Noninstitutionalized Disability Population

	Total Population	Urban	Metropolitan Statistical Area Principal City	Rural
Total	301,472,074	230,570,633	99,766,479	70,901,441
Male	147,545,278	112,247,170	48,580,247	35,298,108
≤18 years	38,041,645	28,941,999	12,269,684	9,099,646
Disability	1,826,100	1,363,274	579,548	462,826
No disability	36,215,545	27,578,725	11,690,136	8,636,820
18 to 64 years	93,184,758	71,487,274	31,740,352	21,697,484
Disability	9,471,954	6,816,908	3,020,815	2,655,046
No disability	83,712,804	64,670,366	28,719,537	19,042,438
≥65 years	16,318,875	11,817,897	4,570,211	4,500,978
Disability	5,843,874	4,136,397	1,653,680	1,707,477
No disability	10,475,001	7,681,500	2,916,531	2,793,501
Female	153,926,796	118,323,463	51,186,232	35,603,333
≤18 years	36,316,708	27,673,631	11,802,428	8,643,077
Disability	1,081,017	811,497	350,948	269,520
No disability	35,235,691	26,862,134	11,451,480	8,373,557
18 to 64 years	95,996,466	74,207,368	32,828,701	21,789,098
Disability	9,582,633	7,187,868	3,258,493	2,394,765
No disability	86,413,833	67,019,500	29,570,208	19,394,333
≥65 years	21,613,622	16,442,464	6,555,103	5,171,158
Disability	8,345,132	6,416,340	2,700,921	1,928,792
No disability	13,268,490	10,026,124	3,854,182	3,242,366

Source: *2009 American Community Survey*. Washington, D.C.: U.S. Census Bureau.

in an urban setting. Women with disabilities face significant barriers in accessing adequate housing and services (*Women's Right to Adequate Housing and Land* 2004), yet much of the research on this population living in urban environments concentrates on barriers to employment, which is only one component of a much broader agenda (Haniff-Cleofas and Khedr 2005a, 2005b).

One of the first things that should come to mind during urban planning is accessibility, a very important issue for people with disabilities and for older adults. Accessibility is often understood within the context of medical approaches. For example, women of all ages with disabilities often have difficulty physically accessing health services due to limitations with facility design and space and a lack of adjustable medical equipment (Mitra 2006: 236). Accessibility in this sense is important

Noninstitutionalized Females
with Disabilities

Noninstitutionalized Males
with Disabilities

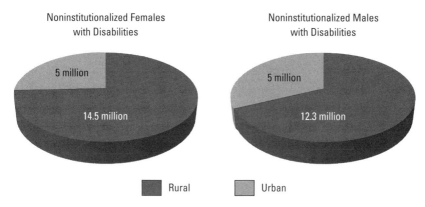

Figure 7.2. U.S. rural and urban distribution of population with disabilities in 2009.
Source: *2009 American Community Survey*. Washington, D.C.: U.S. Census Bureau.

for people with disabilities. However, applying the medical approach to accessibility for people with disabilities, and in particular women with disabilities, does not always ensure their full and equitable access to housing, transportation, social/recreational activities, health services, education, employment, and other forms of social participation.

Unlike the medical model, the social model of disability acknowledges that a person with a disability may be disadvantaged because of social, environmental, physical, and political factors (Mitra 2006). The following sections describe briefly three well-known models of disability care, all of which are relevant to urban planning.

The Medical Model

This medical model of disability generally reflects the belief that disability is a defect that must be cured, treated, or fixed so that persons with disability will be able to function more "normally" in society. In this approach, barriers relevant to women with disabilities are not addressed in a holistic way, and the relationship between gender and disabilities is usually not taken into account. Women's medical conditions are used to describe barriers, generally physical in type, that prevent women from performing their activities of daily living; medical conditions are also used to define the services and supports they need. The medical model of disability is currently known as the "old paradigm" and stands in contrast to the social model of disability (Mitra 2006: 237; Pfeiffer 2001; Parsons 1975). It is important, however, to emphasize that the medical model of care continues to evolve toward a center-based approach, which allows for the integration of complementary and alternative approaches to care.

The Social Model

The social model of disability directly links to community living, care coordination, and integration of services and supports for this population. In the United States, the social model of disability care highlights the discriminations faced by people with disabilities and the segregation they suffer through sensory, attitudinal, cognitive, physical, and economic barriers. In this model, the experiences faced by people with disabilities are perceived as similar to those suffered by racial and ethnic minority groups and include extraordinarily high rates of unemployment, poverty, welfare dependency, school segregation, inadequate housing and transportation, and exclusion from many public facilities (Mitra 2006: 237; Pfeiffer 2001).

The Capability Approach

The capability approach is seen as one of the most comprehensive approaches toward an inclusive life in society. In this approach, the capabilities open to people with disabilities—for example, services and supports such as accessible transportation, and accessible and affordable housing—are understood to be affected by the environment in which people with disabilities live as well as their personal characteristics. The cost of achieving a given capability varies depending on how the environment was planned and built. The costs associated with making cities accessible to those with mobility limitations, for example, vary considerably from country to country depending on the availability and need for assistive technology, and on the design and maintenance of the local physical environment (Mitra 2006: 242–43).

Table 7.8 provides scenarios illustrating approaches and perspectives under the medical, social, and capability models of disability care. The scope, process, direction, and outcomes of health will likely differ depending on which model guides policy and which determinants of health, disease, and functional status are chosen. Choices will eventually drive health-care costs, quality of life, and full integration in community life.

Achieving Successful Planning and Sustainable Environments

Evidence shows that taking gender into account during urban planning and policy development results in the building of a more sustainable,

Table 7.8. Scenarios Illustrating Approaches and Perceptions Under Disability Models of Care

Scenario	Medical Model*	Social Model	Capability Approach
Woman with intellectual disability	"This patient should see a psychiatrist to get some medicine or treatment to improve her condition."	"It is good that this person lives in the community with support from her family members."	"It is important that this person lives in the community with support from her family members. There are multiple opportunities and approaches to enhance her skills and abilities to help her live a meaningful and productive life in the community."
Woman using a wheelchair	"There might be a treatment that this patient can seek with a doctor that will make her walk like everybody else does."	"It is important that this person lives in the community with access to supports and services she needs. Ramps should be built and accessibility ensured to facilitate her participation in community life."	"It is good that this person lives in the community with access to supports and services she needs. Her community is prepared to provide her with affordable and accessible transportation, ramps to facilitate her entrance into buildings, an accessible office for her job, and plenty of opportunities for social inclusion and participation in community governance."
Woman with hearing impairment	"With all the research going on, science will soon present this patient with a cure."	"Sign language should be learned by all of us to facilitate communication with this person."	"Sign language should be learned by all of us to facilitate communication with this person. There are numerous opportunities for this person to enjoy and actively participate in her community life. There are also opportunities for us to learn and benefit from affordable sign language training."

*The medical model continues to evolve toward a person-centered care that allows for the integration of complementary and alternative approaches to care.

equal, and accessible environment for all members of society (Burgess 2008; Greed 2005). The same rationale can be applied to the specific needs of women with disabilities.

Governance and Development

Substantial progress has been made in increasing women's access to power and decision-making. Between 1998 and 2008, the proportion of women in national assemblies increased by 8 percent to the current global average of 18.4 percent, compared to an increase of just 1 percent in the two prior decades (UNIFEM 2008). Despite this current rate of increase, developing countries are not expected to reach gender equality until 2045. For urban environments to be sustainable, there must be equal participation of women and men in urban planning, management, and governance. Political accountability to women begins with augmenting the number of women in decision-making positions. Governance reforms may be needed to supply public organizations with the incentives, skills, information, and procedures to address women's specific needs (UNIFEM 2008–2009).

A growing number of urban governance programs and tools have been created to improve women's participation and empowerment. These programs and tools target women of diverse backgrounds and levels of education (UN-HABITAT 2009b). These targeted groups must include women with disabilities. Even when women with disabilities are actively involved in their communities, they often suffer from low visibility during urban planning processes. Policymakers and planners often fail to recognize women with disabilities and their specific needs (Hannif-Cleofas and Khedr 2005a, 2005b). Projects implemented without adequate consultation with this population group can result in programs that are not accessible or are discriminatory.

Women with disabilities also face challenges when accommodations for their specific needs are lacking; these may relate to accessible transportation, attendant care, sign language interpretations, alternative information formats (e.g., large prints, Braille, or disks), and others. Because women with disabilities are frequently not heard, they may feel discouraged from participating in community work. In addition, these women often cannot afford to volunteer much of their time to community work. Local authorities and public officials should strategize on how to support the participation of women with disabilities in committees, boards, commissions, and working groups. Providing them with transportation, childcare, and perhaps some type of financial support may be a reasonable solution that may allow environments to benefit from their contributions.

Economic Growth

Inclusion of women in the workforce in urban areas results in economic benefits that extend to rural and global economies. The promotion of entrepreneurship empowers all women, but it is particularly important for those with disabilities. Entrepreneurship considerably helps improve their living conditions and status within their households. Empowerment of women provides them with access to capital, resources, credit, land, technology, information, and health and support services. Unfortunately, the United Nations estimates that, worldwide, only 25 percent of women with disabilities are in the workforce (UN-HABITAT 2009a).

Improving reproductive health, childcare, and young women's access to training, education, and technology can increase economic opportunities and growth worldwide. Commitment to programs responsive to gendered disability is important for local or public officials to help meet these goals.

Safety

Numerous countries are taking a gender-based approach to working with community groups and are including networks of women in planning for safe cities and urban developments. In areas throughout the world, women still experience a high degree of insecurity and vulnerability due to violence in both public and private environments. South Africa has one of the highest rates of violence against women in the world, with reports in 2007 of 124 rapes out of every 100,000 people (UN-HABITAT 2009b). Data from the *Women and Community Safety Guide* of the Women Against Violence Society of Cowichan Valley, British Columbia, indicate that about 60 percent of Canadian women feel concerned about walking alone in their neighborhoods after dark; 76 percent are worried about waiting for or using public transit after dark; 83 percent fear walking alone to their car in a parking garage; and 39 percent do not feel comfortable being home alone at night (Drusine 2002).

In disaster situations, violence against women increases considerably, with widespread reports of sexual exploitation in settings for displaced people and an increase in domestic violence in post-crisis situations. Integrating a gendered approach into local and national crime prevention policies can protect women against violence. Making women the center of urban safety planning and articulating strategies for their safety increase the likelihood that women will fare better in their communities (Khosla 2005).

Literature documents the seriousness of violence and abuse against women with disabilities and the lack of accessible domestic violence services (Nosek et al. 2001). Numerous forms of violence against women with disabilities have been reported, including physical, sexual, and emotional abuse as well as disability-specific violence such as destruction of medical equipment and communication devices; withholding, stealing, or overdosing medications; physical neglect; and financial abuse (Powers, Hughes, and Lund 2009). Recent evidence supports earlier findings that maltreatment by personal assistants and caregivers remains a unique problem faced by women with disabilities (Nannini 2006). Caregivers have being found to withhold medicine and assistive devices, such as wheelchairs or braces. They have also been reported refusing to help with daily needs such as bathing, dressing, or eating.

Violence and abuse against women with disabilities negatively affect women's ability to work, live independently, and maintain their health (Haasouneh-Phillips 2005). Younger age, more education, less mobility, and higher levels of social isolation and depression were key characteristics found in 84 percent of women with disabilities who suffered from violence in a study published in 2006 by Nosek and colleagues (Nosek et al. 2006).

Critical components of a well-planned community include services that address violence against women, as well as other safety-promoting features. Local or public officials and urban planners are responsible for ensuring that environments are safe for women, including those with disabilities; women with disabilities have the right to urban services, resources, and facilities that are safe and structured for their needs.

Housing

Access to affordable and durable housing is an important means of empowering all women. Although women with disabilities are more likely to be institutionalized than men with disabilities (*Women's Right to Adequate Housing and Land* 2004), for those who qualify for community living, having access to affordable, accessible, and durable housing is of prime importance.

Worldwide, women with disabilities are more likely to have lower incomes than those without disabilities and than men with disabilities and, therefore, are more likely to rely on government support programs. To qualify for these programs, including in-home support, a series of medical and socioeconomic criteria may apply. For example, those who suffer from mental disorders may need first to spend a period of time in a psychiatric facility. Others may not qualify for personal care assistance. To complicate things, cultural and religious beliefs make it more challenging for some women with disabilities to select personal caregivers. If a woman with disabilities remains single, lives with her extended family, and also chooses not to participate in a personal assistance program because she does not find it to be person-centered (i.e., culturally competent and respective of her preferences), then she may not qualify for housing support.

Sanitation, Health, and Support Services

Compared to people living in rural areas, those living in urban areas tend to have greater access to social and health services, higher literacy rates, and longer life expectancy. Nevertheless, urban living is also associated with numerous challenges that may affect people's health and health care (Sclar and Northridge 2001), with some people suffering disproportionately from poor health. Nearly every large city has pockets of both wealth and extreme poverty; some people over-consume health care and pay high costs for it while others lack the most basic care for financial and other reasons.

Although disability in an industrialized country is characterized differently from that in a developing country, the percentage of persons affected by disabilities (some 10 percent of the population) is generally similar. As many as one in four households in developing countries has a family member with a physical or mental impairment; half of those are generally females. The causes of impairment often reflect the extent of poverty in a country. In developing countries, impairment may be caused by lack of primary health care; disease or chronic illness; lack of safe drinking water; poor sanitation; pollution; home, transportation, and work accidents; or natural and artificial disasters, including armed conflicts. Many are impairments that, in industrialized countries, can be corrected medically or for which technical aids, devices, or assistance is available to facilitate the normal activities of daily living and participation in working life.

Designing, planning, and implementing water and sanitation programs brings multiple benefits to communities and positively affects women with disabilities. According to the United Nations, less than half the population in urban communities of Africa, Asia, and Latin America have water piped into their homes and less than one-third have adequate sanitation (UN-HABITAT 2009a). Because women generally take responsibility for fetching water and spend more hours than men at home or in their neighborhoods, women are more likely to be directly exposed to environmental hazards from poor sanitation and, consequently, are more likely to acquire and spread diseases resulting from poor drainage, contact with human or animal feces, or contact with decomposing materials. When family members become sick, women also bear the greatest burden as caregivers (UN-HABITAT 2009a). For women both with and without disabilities, living in urban areas means facing numerous health risks such as infectious diseases (e.g., HIV/AIDS), which are highly prevalent in developing countries; chronic, noncommunicable diseases; conditions fueled by tobacco use, unhealthy diets, and physical inactivity; alcohol abuse; road accidents; violence; and crime. These risks result from a complex interaction of various social and health determinants associated with insufficient infrastructure and services that affect the health of the poor and slum dwellers (WHO 2010e, 2010f).

Women generally live longer than men and experience more of the disabilities associated with advanced aging. Rates of mental illness, including depression, are higher among women. The presence of debilitating conditions such as chronic noncommunicable diseases (e.g., asthma, cardiovascular diseases, diabetes, and obesity) is also higher among women, with stroke associated with higher rates of severe disability among women than among men. Sex- and gender-based violence as well as disaster-related situations may leave survivors with permanent and disabling injuries.

Rapid urban growth has been associated with increased inequality of access to skilled care during childbirth and to emergency care for both rich and poor women with or without disabilities. Poor women who live in slums frequently lack access to basic health services such as these, rarely receiving appropriate care during pregnancy and childbirth. In developing countries, they are, for example, less likely than rich women to undergo cesarean sections and to have access to a skilled nurse or midwife during childbirth. In India, women with physical disabilities are not even eligible to receive reproductive health services because they are considered to have no marriage prospects (USAID 2010).

Neglect, lack of or limitations with medical care, and less access to food and related resources lead to higher mortality rates for girls with disabilities. A study conducted in Nepal found that the survival rates for boys several years after they had polio was twice that for girls, despite the fact that there are no gender differences in prevalence of the disease (USAID 2010).

Since 1975, there has been a fourfold increase in the number of natural disasters, mostly climate-related, such as tsunamis, tropical cyclones, earthquakes, and flooding. About 14 percent of the urban population in developing countries live in low-elevation zones, which are more prone to these natural disasters (UN-HABITAT 2009b). Women often bear the burden of preparing for and responding to these increasingly common environmental threats. They also bear the brunt of their effects, being more likely to die or suffer serious consequences from natural disasters. During crisis situations, women face enormous challenges in meeting their families' basic needs—acquiring food and water, fuel for cooking and lighting, and wood or other building materials to rebuild their homes. As key players in building resilience in areas affected by disasters, women can mobilize communities and help public officials reduce the costs associated with reconstruction.

Typically, more women than men live with disabilities that shape the way they prepare for, cope with, and respond to natural hazards, disasters, and other emergency situations. Disaster situations compound the social effects of disability, particularly for women and girls who already face a number of other barriers. For example, rates of sexual assault and partner violence may increase in post-conflict and post-disaster situations. Cultural norms that limit women's personal mobility may also deter women with disabilities from successfully accessing support services or post-disaster resources. Women disability activists are increasingly challenging disaster risk managers to consider the gendered dynamics of disasters in emergency preparedness, relief, and reconstruction.

Federal, state, and local authorities and communities should be prepared to respond to the needs of all people including women, children, older adults, and people with disabilities during emergency situations. In 2004, the U.S. federal government adopted a policy ensuring that supports needed by individuals with disabilities are integrated into emergency preparedness planning and implementation by federal, state, local, and tribal governments and private organizations. To this end, the Office on Disability of the U.S. Department of Health and Human Services developed a toolkit to provide guidance to state managers on the steps to be taken to meet the needs of people with disabilities during emergency preparedness and response strategies (US DHHS 2004). In the United States this toolkit has served as a valuable resource to guide states and communities in preparing for such events. Currently, forty-eight states have emergency and preparedness plans that include guidelines on meeting the needs of people with disabilities.

Although this toolkit is designed for U.S. systems and strategic approaches, it has numerous components that can be adapted to other countries' needs. The toolkit provides information on the basic infrastructure needed to prepare and respond to emergencies, and this basic infrastructure reflects common practices or standards to be shared and used across countries. The toolkit has been translated into Spanish and is being used by the Regional Health-Care Training Center of Panama City to support the development of a similar tool for that country and potentially for Central America. The Regional Health-Care Training

Center was established in 2007 as part of a health diplomacy initiative and partnership between the U.S. Department of Health and Human Services and the Ministries of Health of Central America. The author of this chapter was one of the key leading officials working on the establishment of this training center.

Education

Women living in poor and heavily populated environments tend to have children at an earlier age (UN-HABITAT 2009b: 127). This often precludes them from gaining an education, and from seeking, holding, and benefiting from quality jobs. Young women living in such areas also are more likely to stay home to look after their children or sick relatives and to do household chores. These findings also apply to women with disabilities. According to a 1998 study, the global literacy rate for adults with disabilities is as low as 3 percent, with a 1 percent rate for women with disabilities (VSO 2010). In addition, less than 5 percent of children and young persons with disabilities have access to education and training. Girls and young women with disabilities face significant barriers to participating in social life and development (United Nations 2010b).

In the United States, the federal Individuals with Disabilities Education Act (IDEA) governs how states and public agencies provide early intervention, special education, and related services to children with disabilities; the act, which identifies thirteen categories of disability, addresses educational needs from birth to age 21 (U.S. Department of Education n.d.). Schools are required to provide all services that children with disabilities need, not just educational services. For example, if a child needs catheterization or help eating, those services must be provided. Moreover, each child has an Individualized Educational Program that is approved by the parents and the school. With the passage of the No Child Left Behind Act in 2001 (U.S. Department of Education 2010) and the development of the New Freedom Initiative that same year (US DHHS n.d.), a commitment was made to provide individuals with disabilities with a high-quality education and to ensure that they have equal opportunities to benefit from services. Despite these protective laws, improvements in access to education for this population are still needed. Students with disabilities continue to be held to lower expectations academically; young people with disabilities are employed at a much lower rate than their counterparts; a shortage of special education teachers and the inability of regular education teachers to address the needs of students with disabilities remain concerns; and many students with disabilities have limited or no access to needed assistive technology or to the Internet and other forms of communication.

Workforce and Employment

In 2003, 40 percent of the world's 2.8 billion workers were women, an increase of nearly 200 million from the prior decade, according to *Global Employment Trends for Women,* an analysis of female employment by the UN ILO (United Nations International Labour Office 2004b). In an earlier report, women's share of professional jobs was shown to have increased by just 0.7 percent between 1996 and 1999 and between 2000 and 2002, and women were significantly underrepresented in management compared to their overall share of employment (United Nations International Labour Office 2004a). More recently, women's share of managerial positions in almost sixty countries has been found to range from 20 percent to 40 percent (Robinson 2004), which is in contrast to prior reports that consistently showed the share of women in managerial positions to rarely exceed 20 percent. Such an increase has not occurred, however, for women with disabilities. For example, in academic positions the presence of women with disabilities is small; even when women with disabilities are part of academic environments, they tend to be less visible than others who do not have disabilities. One study focusing on the career development of women with physical and sensory disabilities found these women to be passionate about their work, perseverant in the face of internal and external barriers, self-confident and self-reliant, conscious of their coping strategies, internally motivated, and highly committed to helping people grow in their careers (Noonan et al. 2004). These women also showed considerable skill in turning challenges into opportunities for personal and professional development. These findings imply that women with disabilities are likely to be very successful in leadership or managerial positions if offered or exposed to them.

Women remain more likely than men to have low-productivity, low-paid, and vulnerable jobs with limited or no social protections, basic rights, or voice at work. Unequal pay for equal work remains a problem worldwide, with occupational segregation common and women's involvement in economic decision-making rare (O'Reilly 2003). Low participation of women in the workforce is associated with billions of dollars in losses per year. Reports by the United Nations show that, in 2007, Asia and the Pacific regions lost $42 billion due to restrictions in women's access to employment and another $16 to $30 billion due to gender gaps in education (United Nations Economic and Social Commission for Asia and the Pacific 2007: 105). When women are allowed greater access to and control over resources, they allocate more of these resources to food and other benefits associated with children's health and education. This is true for both developing and developed countries (World Bank 2007: 107), suggesting that increased participation of women in the workforce not only leads to economic growth but significantly contributes to the health and well-being of their families.

Generally, people with disabilities are much more likely to face difficulties in entering the labor market, with women with disabilities being half as likely to have jobs compared to men with disabilities. These women often experience unequal hiring and promotion opportunities, as well as unequal access to training, credit, and other resources.

Transportation

Public transportation must be responsive to the needs of people with disabilities to allow this population to participate in urban communities. To meet daily household needs, women worldwide generally depend on public transportation (WHO 2008a: 145). Studies in urban environments in numerous countries have shown that whereas 11.6 percent of households headed by men had cars, only 1.62 percent of woman-headed households had them (WHO 2008a).

Better transportation in urban environments is an issue of gender equality because it helps to address women's limited access to social and economic opportunities and to health services, resources, and information (Riverson et al. 2005: 5). When women are excluded from public transportation due to overcrowded buses or inadequate sidewalks, access to workplaces may be delayed or blocked and crimes such as theft, sexual attacks, and harassment may increase (Riverson et al. 2005: 5).

Although urban environments are designed and built to facilitate transportation by cars and/or public transit, neither option completely meets the specific needs of women with disabilities. Offering specialized services and having conventional services and facilities accessible should be part of urban planning for healthy communities. Because public transportation is relatively affordable, this is generally how women with disabilities get to work, school, volunteer positions, medical appointments, shopping, and socializing. A major challenge women with disabilities face with public transportation is the need to plan and coordinate services far in advance: In some places, these services must be booked as long as two weeks ahead. Although women with disabilities may usually be able to use the metro and buses, they might not be able to do so when it is raining or snowing. Accessible cabs are an option that the vast majority of women with disabilities cannot afford.

For women with disabilities living in large urban areas and subjected to violence, limited or no accessible transportation may prevent them from leaving abusive relationships. Availability of accessible information is a critical means of communication for people with all types of disabilities but in particular those who are blind or deaf or who have vision or hearing deficits. Accessible telecommunication also is critical for this population, allowing them to obtain essential transportation and other day-to-day services.

In the United States, the Americans with Disabilities Act of 1990 (ADA) prohibits discrimination and ensures equal opportunity and access to transportation for persons with disabilities. In addition, the U.S. Federal Transit Administration (FTA) works to ensure nondiscriminatory transportation in support of its mission to enhance the social and economic quality of life for all Americans (US FTA 2010).

Conclusions

Successful urban planning and development must be built upon both gender equality and disability equality, both of which are associated with sustainable urbanization. When urban design addresses gender and the needs of specific populations, such as women with disabilities, and promotes equal and diverse opportunities for all, greater social and economic benefits can be achieved worldwide. Consulting community members when making urban planning and development decisions is becoming standard procedure for all levels of government. The active participation in such consultations of women and of people with disabilities, and in particular of women with disabilities, will help identify and implement good practices that address disability issues in urban planning, development, and governance.

The views expressed in this chapter are those of the author and do not necessarily represent the views of the U.S. Department of Health and Human Services or the U.S. federal government.

Chapter 8

The Health and Well-Being of Immigrant Women in Urban Areas

DeAnne K. Hilfinger Messias

Human migration and the growth of cities are interconnected local and global phenomena affected by social, economic, and political forces in the sending, transit, and receiving countries that play out in the lives of individuals, families, and communities. For some women, migration provides opportunities to lead productive and fulfilling lives in welcoming, safe, and healthy urban environments and therefore is worth the sacrifices and the difficulties of separation from family, language, culture, and country of origin. For other women, the migration experience is fraught with risk, fear, abuse, exploitation, and significant damage to their physical, mental, and social health and well-being. For most immigrant women, migration and settlement—and in some cases, return migration—occur within fluid, in-between spaces of transition and ongoing social, cultural, economic, and identity adaptations and adjustments (Donnelly 2006; Messias 2010). Immigrant women's health is intimately connected to the context of these in-between, intercultural spaces as well as to the physical and social environments in which they live. To be effective, health promotion efforts, health and social services, and related policies in urban areas must take into account the diversity and complexity of immigrant women's lives and migration experiences.

This chapter provides a broad overview of the intersections of migration, gender, and health in urban contexts, drawing on evidence and examples from the international literature. The chapter begins with a brief presentation of commonly used migration terms and classifications followed by an examination of migration flows and the growth of urban areas. The discussion then turns to the interactions of gender, migration, health, and urban environments, with emphasis on salient immigrant women's health issues, and concludes with recommendations for health-care providers, systems, and researchers, as well as poli-cymakers, urban planners, and administrators.

Classifications of Migration and Migrants

Human migration is the process of leaving one place, moving to an-other, and settling there. Migration occurs both within and across national borders. Transnational migrants, defined as persons living out-side their country of birth, constituted 3 percent of the world popu-lation in 2005 (UNFPA 2006). Migrants are commonly classified into several basic types (e.g., voluntary migrants, refugees and asylum seek-ers, and irregular migrants). Although these terms and classifications are important and useful, they are not universally adopted or accepted and may not adequately reflect the diversity of contexts and conditions involved in women's migration decisions and experiences. (See the Global Migration Group [2008] for detailed definitions and descrip-tions of the migrant classifications.)

The distinction between *voluntary* and *forced* migration implies the presence or lack of free choice in the migration process. In theory, vol-untary migrants move of their own free will, often seeking better em-ployment, educational opportunities, and improved access to resources and health and social services for themselves and their families. Eco-nomic and labor migrants are generally considered voluntary migrants, a very broad category that ranges from rural peasants fleeing deteriorat-ing economic, environmental, and social conditions to highly educated professionals seeking better-paying jobs outside their country of origin.

Forced migration includes the cross-border movement of *refugees* and *asylum seekers*, who leave their homes fleeing war and persecution due to race, religion, national or tribal membership, or political positions. In the past thirty-five years, 2.6 million refugees from Central and South America, Europe, Africa, and the Middle East have been resettled in the United States (US DHHS 2009b). Forced migration also includes human trafficking for forced labor and the sex trade, often involving women and girls. *Internally displaced persons* are forced migrants who migrate within a region or country but do not cross national borders.

Irregular migrants, often referred to as undocumented, clandestine, or illegal immigrants, are individuals who lack legal status in a transit or host country as a result of either undocumented entry or visa expiration (Global Migration Group 2008). Irregular migrants may have left their country of origin as either voluntary or forced migrants. Their irregu-lar status contributes to heightened vulnerability and exposure to abu-sive conditions. Irregular migrants often live in substandard housing and work without any type of labor or health protections and undocumented female immigrants are particularly at risk for sexual and physical abuse (UNFPA 2006). Overall, women face more barriers to regular migration than men, increasing women's likelihood of resorting to clandestine migration and contributing to their risks of falling prey to trafficking or smuggling schemes. Women constitute most of the trafficked population, estimated at between 700,000 and 4 million people per year (UNECA 2006).

Gender, Migration, and the Growth of Urban Areas

Both rural-to-urban and transnational migrants are major contributors to the burgeoning urban population worldwide. Rural poverty and the lack of educational and economic opportunities in rural areas contribute to the migratory flow to cities. As is discussed in the introduction to this book, approximately 3.5 billion persons—more than half of the world's population—currently reside in urban areas (United Nations 2010b). During the latter half of the twentieth century, rapid urbanization transformed demographic distribution and settlement patterns across the globe, including the massive rural-to-urban migration flow in China, in which 210 million persons have left the rural farms and villages to work in urban factory, construction, and transportation jobs (Ford 2010). By the end of the twentieth century, the rate of urbanization in Latin America was considerably higher than that in either Asia or Africa. As a result, 75 percent of the Latin American population now live in burgeoning urban areas characterized by huge social disparities between rich and poor and a lack of adequate housing and infrastructure to support the rapid influx of rural migrants (Dufour and Piperata 2004). By 2030, 81 percent of the world's urban dwellers will reside in urban areas of the developing world. In Africa and Asia, urban growth is expected to double between 2000 and 2030 (UNFPA 2007).

Internal movement and international migration—for employment, education, family reunification, or environmental or political reasons—contribute to population growth in urban and peri-urban areas around the globe. A majority (60 percent) of the world's international migrants live in more economically developed regions. One of every ten persons living in developed regions is a migrant, compared to one out of every seventy in less-developed regions (Global Migration Group 2008). A related demographic trend is the voluntary or forced migration of indigenous peoples, including women and youth, to urban areas. In many countries the majority of indigenous peoples now live in urban areas (UN-HABITAT 2010a).

Child fostering or circulation, the practice of parents sending their children to live with relatives and friends, is part of a common social and economic survival and improvement strategy and a contributing factor to rural-to-urban migration (Leinaweaver 2007). Child fostering is a long-standing cultural practice in many regions of Latin America and Africa (Gozdziak 2008). Parents send their children to live with others for a variety of reasons, including to strengthen family social ties; as a result of illness, death, or separation of parents; and to further the economic or educational aims for the child. Young girls from rural areas are often sent to cities to serve as domestic workers in the homes of relatives or acquaintances.

Although women make up half of all transnational migrants, they outnumber male migrants in more developed countries (Global Migration Group 2008). Gender patterns vary among and across migrant streams: Families may migrate as units; men may migrate first, followed by women and children; or women may migrate independently (Li 2003). The increasing feminization of migration is attributed to factors ranging from changing gender norms and expectations to the transformations in global agricultural practices, variable labor market dynamics, and increasing competition for goods and services (Fry 2006). Furthermore, the rise of female-specific forms of migration including the commercialized migration of domestic workers, the migration and trafficking of women in the sex industry, and the organized migration of women for marriage also contribute to increasing feminization of migration (Carling 2005).

Immigrant women often encounter divergent gender roles, expectations, and values in their interactions with host society social structures in public and private spaces (Remennick 2004; Rodriguez 2007). The effect of migration on women's status and gender roles varies and may be influenced by both macro- and micro-level factors. At the individual level, national origin/ethnicity, social class, educational level, occupation, language skills, religion, marital status, sexual orientation, presence or absence of extended family in the host country, and immigration status all factor into an immigrant woman's gender roles, expectations, and status. Macro-level factors include labor market conditions; the social, political, cultural, and religious context; and the status of women in both sending and receiving societies (Ahmad, Modood, and Lissenburgh 2003).

Due to the double-negative effect of gender and immigration status, educated immigrant women have lower returns from their education than do native women. Immigrant women educated in their home countries frequently encounter significant barriers to employment when their degrees are not valued or recognized in host nations. Even in relatively immigrant-friendly contexts, such as Canada, immigrant women tend to earn less than nonimmigrant women. This earning gap is larger than that between immigrant and nonimmigrant men and persists over time (Stewart et al. 2006). In reviewing Canadian income data, Li (2003) found little indication that immigrants were less productive than native-born Canadians, yet there was strong evidence that immigrants encounter unequal opportunities based on gender, race, and other factors such as education and language. Specifically, immigrant women of visible minority origin suffered the largest negative economic impact.

Push and Pull Factors in Urban Migration

Migration is most often considered a development issue related to disparities in income levels and economic opportunities in transnational and rural/urban contexts. The confluence of *push and pull* factors is a traditional framework for explaining human migration. Individual women's migration decisions and experiences reflect complex interactions at multiple levels, from the individual, family, and local community to national and international economics, policies, and politics. Global climate change is another force contributing to internal, regional, and transnational migration (Podesta and Ogden 2007).

Women's migration motives, patterns, and behaviors relate to personal, work, and family contexts as well as to the broader economic, social, political, and environmental contexts of both sending and receiving nations. Limited employment opportunities for decent and well-remunerated work, rampant unemployment, and poverty are major factors pushing immigrants out of sending countries. Human rights abuses, including violence, social exclusion and discrimination, inequities and disparities, and the lack of or unequal access to basic resources and services also contribute to out-migration. Labor demands and cross-border wage differentials are major pull factors in receiving countries (Global Migration Group 2008).

Enhanced access to opportunities and resources is a magnet that attracts immigrants to urban areas. Cities offer migrants a wider range of employment opportunities and more easily accessible resources and services (e.g., basic sanitation, transportation, education, health care, arts, and recreation). Urban areas with long-standing ethnic/immigrant populations attract new waves of immigrants with their established social, communication, and labor networks and ethnic subeconomies that offer access to employment and a more familiar context for the cultivation of social capital and integration into the broader national economy (Li 2003; Menjívar 1997, 2000).

Migration push and pull factors are often complementary. For women in developing countries, poverty is frequently the push factor, and the pull factor is the "care deficit" of middle-income women abroad (Ehrenreich and Hochschild 2002). In China, the skewed birth rate resulting from the official one-child policy and cultural preferences for the male baby, in combination with the massive rural-to-urban migration flow, has resulted in a shortage of women in the Chinese countryside, attracting North Korean defectors willing to risk their lives to cross the border into China seeking opportunities for marriage, domestic employment, or work in the urban sex industry (Demick 2010). The recent wave of migration from rural states in southern Mexico to new immigrant settlement areas in the southeastern United States also resulted from the convergence of push and pull factors in the two countries (Lacy 2009; Mohl 2003). Beginning in the mid-1990s, increasing numbers of rural Mexicans moved northward, pushed out by rising unemployment and a rapidly deteriorating rural economy exacerbated by neo-liberal international trade policies and drawn by labor needs in tourism, food processing, construction, and other low-paying, unskilled positions of the booming economies in southeastern U.S. cities. Despite the lack of established Latino settlements in the cities of these nontraditional, non-gateway states, the lower cost of living compared to that in more traditional receiving areas (e.g., California, Texas, and New York) was an attraction for Mexican and Central Americans from "new" sending areas with no prior family or community connections in the United States (Lacy 2009).

There is no doubt that out-migrants, from manual and domestic workers to professionals, scientists, and health-care workers, constitute a labor and intellectual drain on developing economies. However, many immigrants do contribute directly to the development and economic stimulus of their home countries through the monetary remittances they send home (UNFPA 2006). For many less-developed nations, labor export is, in fact, an important development strategy aimed at reducing local unemployment, enhancing the balance of payments, and procuring investment capital (Castles 2004).

Governments intentionally implement policies and incentives to encourage or deter migration. The Philippines actively encourages out-migration through formal and informal incentives (Parreñas 2001). For example, the out-migration of poor women to work as domestic workers overseas is fostered through training programs on how to operate household appliances (Ehrenreich and Hochschild 2002) and for-profit, diploma-mill nursing schools cater to Filipino students lured by the opportunity of migration (Baumann and Blythe 2008).

The formal and informal reception of immigrants in receiving societies ranges from welcoming to hostile. In Canada, Newfoundland and

Labrador has the lowest immigrant retention rate (36 percent) among the Canadian provinces. Faced with a declining and aging native population and recognizing the global trend of urbanization, with more and more people, immigrants included, moving to large cities, the provincial government began to pursue strategies to actively recruit and retain more transnational immigrants and stimulate economic, social, and cultural development (Gilroy 2005). In contrast, the case of Japan, an island nation with a high degree of racial/ethnic homogeneity, exemplifies global migration in the context of an outsider-resistant, unwelcoming society. Several waves of global migrants began arriving in Japan during the economic boom in the mid-1980s. The immigrants included Vietnamese refugees and unskilled foreign labor, primarily Japanese descendants from Brazil and Peru, fleeing the high inflation, lack of employment, and generalized economic turmoil in Latin America. The reception of foreign workers and refugees was highly contested within Japanese society, particularly by individuals and groups intent on preserving racial/ethnic homogeneity. But in the face of labor needs, official policy responses included an amendment in 1989 to the Immigration Control and Refugee Recognition Act that allowed descendants of Japanese emigrants (*Nikkeijin*) to enter and work in Japan as unskilled foreign laborers (Asakura and Murata 2006; Yamanaka 1993).

National policies and collective responses to immigrants and their needs do not always reflect the human rights approach to migration and migrant rights promulgated through international agreements and conventions, such as the 1951 United Nations Convention on the Status of Refugees and recent reports by the Global Migration Group (2008). Nativism and xeno-racism are on the rise across the globe, from the United States and Europe to South Africa, Asia, and Latin America.

Manifestations of nativism and xeno-racism in Europe include pan-European racism directed against asylum seekers and migrant workers, an increased monolingual focus and diminishing public tolerance of nonnative languages, rising Islamophobia, and stricter requirements for residency and citizenship (Fekete 2009). In the United States, the increasingly polarized immigration debate has been fueled by the high level of irregular immigrants coupled with the recent economic recession. The divergent immigration policy initiatives under consideration by individual states and the U.S. Congress include proposals for immigration management through higher levels of border control, the deportation of millions of undocumented immigrants, and options for status regularization and paths to citizenship. Economic and cultural nativism is increasing across the country. Economic nativism targets immigrants, particularly irregular immigrants, based on the perception that they are taking jobs, housing, and resources away from native-born citizens.

Cultural nativism is apparent in the anti-immigrant discourses and representations in the popular media, as well as English-only propositions (Lacy 2009). In an increasingly globalized world, it is not yet clear what the social, economic, and political impact of rising nativism in traditional receiving countries will be on future transnational migration patterns and practices.

Immigrant Women's Health in Urban Areas

A wide range of social and environmental determinants (e.g., housing conditions, air and water quality, exposure to pollutants) affect the health of city dwellers. Among immigrant women, these social and environmental conditions interact with a host of other individual, cultural, behavioral, and lifestyle factors (e.g., nutrition and diet, physical activity, smoking, alcohol and drug use), all of which may operate in different ways in the context of migration and urban life. A prime motivator behind migration is the desire for better living conditions, economic status, lifestyle, and personal development for immigrants and their children. When these expectations for a better life are at least partially realized, positive effects on women's individual and collective health status may ensue (Evans 1987). However, for immigrant women living in urban environments characterized by poverty, squalid living conditions, violence, lack of sanitation, and exposure to infectious diseases, the risks for poor physical, mental, and environmental health are exponentially higher. Declining immigrant health status over time is commonly attributed to processes of acculturation, which involve adaptive changes in behaviors, beliefs, and values of individuals or groups resulting from cross-cultural contacts (Marin and Gamba 1996). Women's migration to urban areas is often accompanied by decreased levels of moderate or vigorous physical activity, an increase in sedentary behaviors, and unhealthy dietary changes, leading to increased cardiovascular disease risks (Torun et al. 2002; Stafford 2010). Other factors contributing to poor or deteriorating immigrant health include barriers in accessing health services due to language or cultural differences, lack of information and understanding of the health-care systems in the host country, and lack of skills in navigating health-care financing and service systems. For example, among immigrants with limited prior exposure to formal health-care services in their host nations, improved access and utilization of health services in the receiving society may lead to the identification of previously undiagnosed conditions, which would be reflected in the data as an apparent worsening of immigrant health (Messias and Rubio 2004).

The lack of fair and just reception and treatment of immigrants is a human rights issue in many receiving societies (Global Migration Group 2008). Living in a xenophobic and anti-immigrant environment—one that forces undocumented immigrants through dangerous border crossings, increases the risk of exploitative working conditions and mistreatment by employers and landlords, and contributes to fear of dominant society institutions and representatives from the police to health-care providers—can have a negative impact on immigrants' mental and physical health (McGuire and Canales 2010).

The heterogeneity among immigrants, the complexity of migration patterns, and the multiple environmental and social factors operating in urban settings make it difficult, if not impossible, to formulate generalizations about the health status of immigrant women in urban areas. However, the international research on immigrant women's health points to several important concerns, which often are manifest across immigrant groups and settings. These concerns include the health impact of immigrant women's work; social transitions and the degree of isolation or integration within host societies; immigration-related stress, violence, and abuse; and health-care access barriers, specifically the lack of accessible, linguistic, and culturally competent health care. The following sections present brief overviews of these health issues, illustrated with examples from the international literature.

Gender, Migration, Work, and Health

Women's participation in transnational migration has increased steadily in recent decades, and women now make up half of all international migrants, outnumbering male immigrants to more-developed countries (Global Migration Group 2008). The evidence clearly indicates that "migration is not a 'gender-neutral' phenomenon: men and women display differences in their migratory behaviours and face different opportunities, risks and challenges, including factors leading to irregular migration; vulnerability to human rights abuses, exploitation, and discrimination; and health issues. The experience of female migrants differs from that of men from the moment women decide to migrate" (Global Migration Group 2008: 45).

Historically, the migration of women was associated primarily with family reunification. Beginning in the late twentieth century, women's migration was associated with increasing labor opportunities in both formal and informal markets (Agustín 2003). Female migrants are major participants in the broader urban service sector, including hotels and tourism, food service, and sex work, and in manufacturing, particularly in free trade zones and *maquiladoras* (foreign-owned and operated export assembly plants). However, many women migrate primarily for traditional "women's work." In cities around the globe, immigrant women have become a major domestic labor source for cleaning, cooking, housekeeping, and caring for children, the elderly, the sick, and the disabled. In Western Europe and North America, the higher demand for paid domestic labor is largely a function of the increasing participation of middle-class women in outside employment. The irony of immigrant domestic work is that many women leave their homes and their children to engage in work that enables other women to seek employment outside the home to maintain or raise the living standards of their families (Parreñas 2001). In turn, many immigrant women pass on the direct care responsibilities for their own children or parents to other female relatives—or, with their remittances, hire a lower-income domestic worker at home. The result is an interconnected "global care chain" that stratifies gendered caregiving by class, ethnicity, and immigration status (Hochschild 2002).

With migration, women's own domestic work burden may increase quantitatively and qualitatively. The case of Jewish immigrants from the former Soviet Union (FSU) provides an example of the triple burden of immigrant women's work (Remennick 2004). In the 1990s approximately 500,000 Jewish women from the FSU migrated to Israel. The majority were highly educated professionals who had actively participated in the FSU labor force. One result of this massive migration and resettlement was occupational downgrading and de-skilling as these immigrant professional women found their employment opportunities rarely matched their educational and skill levels or the gender preferences and expectations of the Israeli workforce. With this substantial occupational, economic, and social downgrading in Israel, these highly educated women faced "double-shift service work (for a wage and at home) . . . a common destiny for immigrant women of any origin, be it Third World or east European, in western countries" (Remennick 2004: 97). In addition, they frequently took on the role of caregiver for elderly immigrant parents or in-laws, who faced significant language and cultural barriers in navigating Israeli society and the health-care system. Similarly, Latin American immigrant women with higher socioeconomic and educational levels who are accustomed to having domestic servants in their home countries may struggle with the unexpected burden and stress of their personal domestic workload in the United States (Messias 2001).

Among some immigrant groups, home and family work remains women's priority and is integrally associated with their personal health perspectives. Findings from research with diverse South Asian immigrants in Canada indicated that these women equated health with the ability to perform their multiple expected caregiving roles for their children, husbands, and elderly in-laws (Bottorff, Johnson, and Venables 2001). Caring for others regularly took priority over caring for self, and the value of personal health was the ability to do their family work and not be a burden to others. Fulfilling this traditional role as the primary caregiver for the extended family did create challenges for some immigrant women. Being productive and completing their family work responsibilities were associated with health and happiness, as "not being able to complete one's duties could potentially cause family disharmony as well as feelings of uselessness, laziness, and tension, reinforcing feelings of ill health" (Bottorff, Johnson, and Venables 2001: 396).

Work and employment often dominate immigrant women's lives, and, at the same time, their work and migration status expose them to increased risks. Immigrant domestic workers, trafficked women, and those in irregular status are the most vulnerable to abuse of human and labor rights (Global Migration Group 2008). Employment in gender-segregated sectors (e.g., the textile industry) and the informal economy (e.g., working in the homes of private employers) increases immigrant women's vulnerability to health risks, exploitation, and lack of legal protections. The garment industry is a major employer of migrant women worldwide. Health risks among garment workers include ergonomic and environmental factors (e.g., inadequate workstation design and seating, poor lighting, inappropriate match of size of machinery for workers). In the United States, California is the current center of apparel manufacturing, and the vast majority of sewing operators in California are immigrant Hispanic and Asian women. Findings from a descriptive study of female monolingual Cantonese-speaking garment workers ($n = 100$) seeking health care at an occupational health clinic in California documented a high prevalence of work-related musculoskeletal disorders, including musculoskeletal pain, headaches and vision problems, allergies, and lower extremity pain and swelling (Burgel et al. 2004). Not surprisingly, a majority (66 percent) of these women self-reported health status as either "fair" or "poor."

Social Transitions and Immigrant Women's Health

Migration transitions and the accompanying changes in immigrant women's daily lives, work, social and leisure practices, and identities have implications for individual, family, and community health (Messias 2010). For example, among immigrant women from traditional rural agricultural societies with more communal and noncompetitive social structures (e.g., Pacific Islanders), the concomitant migration and urbanization transitions to independent, individual-oriented, competitive, and industrialized urban societies may involve significant educational, economic, social, and health disparities (Stafford 2010). Social support deficits, experiences of discrimination, and the degree of integration with or isolation from the dominant society all affect immigrant women's health.

The stress of being an "outsider" may be compounded by the separation from family and friends and the absence of readily available female support systems and role models. Women accustomed to well-established female social networks and participation in regular family gatherings in their home societies may find immigrant life lonely, boring, and lacking meaningful social interactions (Rodriguez 2007). Social isolation can contribute to immigrant women's feelings of inadequacy, conflict, guilt, and loneliness, and to clinical depression (Shattell et al. 2010) and entry into the labor market does not necessarily increase immigrant women's social networks. In a study of highly educated immigrant Pakistani women who had lived in the United Kingdom for over twenty years, Rodriguez (2007) noted wide variability in the degree of social integration. Some women reported a loss of informal social capital in the private sphere, but others found they were able to increase their social capital in the public space through contacts with host-country institutions (e.g., schools, the health-care system). The differing abilities of individual Pakistani immigrant women to negotiate the structural constraints of the home and host countries provided evidence that exposure to different cultural values per se does not necessarily result in migrant women's social emancipation.

Social, cultural, linguistic, and environmental barriers often separate immigrants and impede or hinder their active engagement in host communities. Community-based research conducted in a new receiving community in the southeastern United States indicated that lack of communication and trust was a major barrier to the effective integration of recent Latina immigrants into the local community (Barrington, Messias, and Weber in review). For example, immigrant women reported difficulties communicating with their children's teachers and concern about the lack of access to spaces where their children could play safely or participate in sports or cultural activities. Members of the host community reported little direct contact with the immigrants yet considered them a source of competition for local economic, social, educational, and health resources. Social isolation within the emergent immigrant community was also evident. Interviewees indicated that communal living arrangements (e.g., large groups of single men or multiple families living together in a single dwelling) and the high concentration of Latinos in apartment complexes and trailer parks did not automatically generate meaningful social relationships or mean that women knew each other well or considered local acquaintances as friends.

Pregnancy and motherhood are important developmental and health transitions in women's lives that may have additional layers of complexity in the context of migration, when immigrant women may be separated from their families of origin and traditional pregnancy, birthing, and child-rearing practices. In their study of the motherhood experiences of Thai women in Australia, Liamputtong and Naksook (2003) reported immigrant women's isolation and loneliness and concerns about separation from and lack of support from extended family. Thai immigrants married to Anglo-Australian men reported spousal conflicts regarding traditional Thai child-rearing practices. Being an immigrant mother involved challenges to the women's cultural-based mothering practices, their social relationships, and their identities.

The lack of broader community engagement has serious implications for immigrant women's health and well-being. The physical, linguistic, and social isolation of many immigrant women in urban areas results in limited opportunities to foster meaningful social connections, develop broader networks, and take full advantage of community resources. At the same time, immigrant women who challenge or break with their traditional cultural values and practices may incur psychological or social risks, and increasing acculturation may create tension or social distance within families or immigrant communities. Women's transnational migration experiences may involve multiple ongoing social and personal transitions, fluid identities, and constant comparisons between competing perspectives on class, culture, and women's work and health (Meleis et al. 2000).

Stress, Discrimination, and Violence: Immigrant Women's Mental Health

Everyday life of immigrant women in urban areas involves myriad stressors of varying dimensions. These stressors range from the hassles of daily family life in the context of settling into and navigating unfamiliar terrain, systems, language, and cultural norms, the emotional toll of loneliness and social isolation, and work- and economic-related stresses to experiences of overt discrimination, social stigma, and violence. Gender- and immigration-related stress, discrimination, stigma, violence, and abuse are among the most troubling issues related to immigrant women's mental and physical health and well-being. The cumulative ongoing stress of adaptation, daily hassles of immigrant women's employment and family responsibilities, social isolation, and exposure to difficult and stressful living conditions, employment conditions, and violence contribute to poor health and diminished well-being.

Depression and other forms of psychological distress may be associated with immigrant women's experiences of migration stress and discrimination. For women who migrate without their children, the separation, whether temporary or long term, may result in psychological consequences, including major depression. In a study of depression among Latina immigrant mothers in the United States, the odds of depression among those who were separated from their children were 1.52 times those of immigrant women who currently resided with their children (Miranda et al. 2005). Another study, which looked at depression and stigma-related concerns about mental health care and utilization of mental health services among low-income immigrant and U.S.-born black and Latina women ($n = 15,383$), demonstrated significant differences among immigrant and ethnic-minority women as compared to U.S.-born white women (Nadeem et al. 2007). Among women who screened positive for depression, black immigrant groups from Africa and the Caribbean were more likely than U.S.-born whites to endorse stigma concerns related to mental health care (i.e., being embarrassed to talk about personal matters with others; being afraid of what others might think; facing potential disapproval among family members).

Immigrants from more visible ethnic-minority groups encounter higher risks of discrimination and stigma. In the host society, the level of openness and acceptance of cultural diversity is an important factor in the social integration of immigrants. South Asian women in the United Kingdom, both Muslims and non-Muslims, reported being subjected to scrutiny or discrimination regarding their dress (e.g., wearing *Hijab*, saris, or Punjabi suits). The Muslim women also reported religious discrimination, both direct and indirect, in the context of employment, education, and housing. They encountered employer discrimination, including issues with employers related to their ability to observe religious rituals such as prayers, breaking the fast in Ramadan, and taking religious holidays (Ahmad, Modood, and Lissenburgh 2003).

Exposure to racism, discrimination, and human rights abuses associated with immigrant women's nationality, immigration or social status, and gender may occur throughout the migration and settlement experiences. For many immigrant women, particularly those risking illegal border crossing and travel through hostile environments or those subjected to various forms of violence and extortion by smugglers, the migration journey itself is the most dangerous and stressful part of the migration experience (McGuire 2001). The stress of urban settlement can also exact a high emotional toll. Urban areas may expose women to increased vulnerability for domestic, workplace, and community-

level violence and abuse rooted in gender inequalities, labor exploitation, and human rights violations. Immigrant women are likely targets
of exploitation and mistreatment by employers, but due to fear of retal-
iation and financial necessity they may suffer in silence rather than report workplace abuses (Bottorff, Johnson, and Venables 2001). Latinas
in the U.S. South reported discrimination and sexual harassment as
their major workplace concerns (SPLC 2009). Community health promoters reported several violence-related health concerns among Cape
Verdean immigrant women in the United States (De Jesus 2009). Community and domestic violence, loss and isolation, economic injustice,
immigration-related issues and abuse, unequal gender-based power relations, and cultural taboos were among these immigrant women's most
salient health concerns.

With regard to intimate partner violence, immigrant women face
systemic and structural barriers as well as legal and policy obstacles in
disclosing their situation and accessing information and services. Consequently, abused immigrant women may suffer serious mental and
physical health effects resulting from staying in relationships, often
with their children, for prolonged periods of time (Alaggia, Regehr,
and Rishchynski 2009). Despite their multiple risks of exposure to family and workplace stress and violence, immigrant women may be hesi-
tant, embarrassed, or ashamed to discuss personal concerns related to
work or occupational safety, cancer, sexuality, mental health, and family
tensions or violence with health-care providers.

Health-Care Access Issues

Common barriers immigrant women face in accessing host-country
health services include language, culture, cost or insurance status,
lack of information and understanding of the health-care systems in
the host country, transportation, and a lack of skills necessary to effectively navigate health-care service and financing systems. Immigrants to
newer receiving cities are likely to encounter more social, cultural, and
linguistic barriers than those in cities with long-established immigrant
communities. Smaller cities and those without a history of immigrant
reception are less likely to have access to bilingual staff or experienced
and trained interpretation services at health and social service facilities
(Lacy 2007; Parra-Medina et al. 2009; Springer et al. 2010).

Some immigrant health-care access issues are similar to issues encountered by native-born women as they engage with health-care providers and systems. As findings from a recent study indicated, even in
Canada, a nation with nearly universal health coverage, the barriers im-

migrant women faced in accessing health and social services were similar to those faced by Canadian-born family caregivers with low incomes and limited flexibility in juggling the multiple responsibilities of home, employment, and family care-giving demands (Stewart et al. 2006). However, the immigrant women faced additional barriers and burdens due to lack of cultural sensitivity, language barriers, and the absence of support from family due to geographical separation.

Immigrant women who do not speak the dominant language of their health-care providers face significant language and communication barriers when health services lack appropriate language assistance (e.g., interpretation services and translated written materials). The lack of cultural and linguistic competency among individual providers and within the health-care system is a major access barrier and quality-of-care concern. Unequal treatment related to language barriers has been associated with disparate health-care access and health outcomes among immigrants and non-native language speakers (US DHHS 2001; Divi et al. 2007).

All health-care encounters involve some degree of transcultural exchange, but in the case of immigrants, the overt cultural barriers and degree of difference and dissonance in cultural expectations between providers and patients are amplified significantly. Findings from research on the health and care needs of immigrant Muslim women in Newfoundland, Canada, indicated the lack of cultural and religious specificity of the limited health information available to meet the immigrants' needs during pregnancy, labor, delivery, and the postpartum period (Reitmanova and Gustafson 2008). The researchers noted that maternity health services did not adequately meet the immigrant Muslim women's needs for culturally and linguistically appropriate information and emotional support. Further, the local health-care system was not prepared to anticipate and respond to certain expectations and preferences of Muslim women, including their preference for a female attendant for labor and delivery. The lack of accommodations for family involvement and support in health and illness practices and in decision-making processes can be a major barrier for members of immigrant and refugee groups accustomed to family decision-making (Grewal, Bottorff, and Hilton 2005; Springer et al. 2010).

Experiences of discrimination, insensitivity, and lack of awareness and knowledge of immigrant women's cultural and religious practices within health-care systems further contribute to social isolation for these women. Johnson and colleagues (2004) conducted a large ethnographic study of health-seeking behaviors among South Asian women in Canada. The sample included health-care providers with extensive prior experience serving South Asians and immigrant women of diverse religious affiliations (Sikh, Hindu, Muslim, Christian) from India, Pakistan, Bangladesh, Fiji, and eastern Africa. The researchers noted patterns of disjuncture and difference between the immigrants' perspectives and those of the health-care providers. In contrast to the immigrant women's stories of race, racism, and discrimination in their health-care experiences, the providers tended to couch their discourse in notions of equal treatment and cultural appropriateness. Providers' *othering* perspectives and practices reflected culturalizing, racializing, and essentializing the views and explanations of the South Asian women. Examples of essentializing included stereotypical over-generalizing about culture, race, social background, and immigrant women's health-care practices and the tendency to create; oppositional binaries of "us and them" and "good and bad." Providers presented culturalist explanations of South Asian women's lack of responsibility and lack of motivation in participation in health practices such as cancer screenings. As noted by the researchers, "Rather than looking at barriers inherent in the system such as the lack of female health care providers and limited clinic hours, the health care providers used women's personal characteristics (e.g., shyness, passivity) that they labeled as cultural to explain lack of participation in health programs" (Johnson et al.: 262).

Given these diverse access barriers, it is not surprising that utilization rates of preventive care, such as cancer screenings, tend to be lower among immigrant women. In the United States, some of the differences in immigrant women's cancer screening rates are clearly associated with availability or type of health insurance coverage and access to a usual source of care (Echeverria and Carrasquillo 2006; Parra-Medina et al. 2009). A study of immigrant women's health status and access to health care in Texas found undocumented Latinas had lower educational and income levels than documented immigrants and were less likely to have health insurance and a regular health-care provider (Marshall et al. 2005). Remennick (2004) reported lower rates of breast cancer screening among Ashkenazi Jewish immigrants in Israel, despite risks due to prior environmental exposure and behavioral hazards in the USSR. The women attributed their lack of participation in regular breast cancer screening activities to lack of time due to multiple employment and family responsibilities and to the attitude that cancer is a risk but nevertheless a remote one.

Recommendations for Practice, Policy, and Research

If immigrant women living in urban areas are to achieve their potential for health, much work must be done in the areas of outreach and education among immigrant communities, health-care service delivery, policymaking and implementation, and research. Health-care providers, researchers, and policymakers should consider women's migration transitions and experiences from holistic, lifecycle, and human rights frameworks. This approach includes ongoing assessment and support for the health of women and girls before they migrate, throughout the migration process, in the context of their situations in host countries, and, when applicable, upon return to country of origin (Messias 2010). The following four broad recommendations provide a platform for building integrated efforts in practice, policy, and research: (1) Engage communities to foster the social integration of immigrant women and their families through outreach and partnerships; (2) address access and communication barriers through capacity building at all levels of health and social service provision; (3) develop, implement, and monitor policies to assure the basic human rights of immigrants locally and globally; and (4) expand interdisciplinary and transnational research endeavors to include more innovative, community-engaged, participatory approaches to immigrant women's health.

Engaging Communities

Efforts to promote and enhance immigrant women's health must extend beyond individual-level interventions and engage broader communities of immigrants and nonimmigrants alike to create healthy urban environments and address social and structural determinants of health. Effective social integration is necessary if immigrants are to be productive members of their communities of destination. Community-based outreach to immigrant women is an effective approach to raise awareness, educate, and increase participation in health and social service programs. The use of community health workers, lay health educators, or health promoters (*promotoras de salud* in Spanish) is a culturally and linguistically appropriate approach to reach disadvantaged or hard-to-reach groups, including immigrant women. A key characteristic of such outreach workers, whether volunteer or paid, is that they share ethnic, linguistic, social, cultural, and life experiences with the community they serve (US DHHS 2007).

Immigrant women often have difficulty navigating host-country health, social, and educational services because they lack the appropriate language and literacy skills. Partnership initiatives involving immigrant-serving organizations, health and social service providers, educators, and librarians can contribute to enhancing immigrant women's interactions and integration with educational and health-care services. To better meet immigrant women's health needs and the health needs of their family members, programs must be designed in ways that address language, informational, transportation, attitudinal, and network barriers and concurrently advance intersectoral and interagency communication and collaboration (Stewart et al. 2006). Mobile clinics are an alternative model of care delivery that may ameliorate some of the access barriers immigrant women face in urban areas (Guruge et al. 2010). It is also imperative that sending communities be engaged in the migration process and that women and the families they leave behind receive the education, preparation, and support they need prior to and throughout their migration experiences. Immigrant women's transnational health resources and practices need to be acknowledged by health-care providers, who also should explore the personal and cultural meanings and utility of these resources for individual women's health (Clark 2002; Messias 2002).

Community-based and collectively administered programs and services may be an appropriate and cost-effective approach for immigrant women. Such programs may be more acceptable than individually focused interventions, particularly in relation to issues that may be considered sensitive in some immigrant communities (e.g., mental health, depression, family violence, sexuality). Urban coalitions can facilitate communication and coordination among providers of health and social support services for vulnerable immigrant women, including trafficked women and girls and victims of sexual and domestic violence. Policymakers and urban planners must consider immigrant civic integration as a priority in planning and designing public spaces and resources for education, health, and leisure activities.

Improving Institutional Capacity and Addressing Language and Communication Barriers

There is increasing recognition of the importance of recognizing patient diversity in the provision of health care and the need to address inequities in the provision of health care related to race/ethnicity, gender, language, and culture. Providing health-care services for diverse groups of immigrant women requires effective partnerships with immigrant communities as well as institutional and individual commitments to change the ways in which services are provided. Institutional capacity for care that is sensitive and responsive to gender, social, cultural, religious, and linguistic needs must involve all levels of service providers. Cultural awareness and sensitivity are necessary but clearly not sufficient in understanding the ways in which migration, gender, culture, and other factors shape immigrant women's responses to health, illness, and health care. As others have argued, culture is embedded in fluid networks of meanings situated within social, economic, political, and historical processes that play out in power differentials and inequities in health-care settings (Anderson and Reimer Kirkham 1998). Cultural competency in health-care settings must be viewed as a multidirectional phenomenon involving interactions between patients, providers, staff, and the environment.

Substantial evidence from research and practice supports the need for improved language access through the provision of formal, qualified interpreting services within a supportive health-care environment (Flores 2005; Smedley, Stith, and Nelson 2003). Language access is part of organizational cultural competency and must include the availability of bilingual providers and staff members or trained, qualified health-care interpreters, as well as the provision of translated written materials at appropriate levels of literacy and cultural and linguistic competency training for all staff. In the United States, it is imperative that providers at all levels of service understand and participate in the implementation of the National Standards for Culturally and Linguistically Appropriate Services in Health Care (US DHHS 2001).

Because effective interpreter-mediated communication requires awareness and skillful attention on the part of providers and interpreters, institutions must regularly train and update staff on language and cultural communication awareness, skills, and competencies. Immigrant women and their families need appropriate orientation and explanations to become fully aware of their personal rights to language interpreter services; to understand the roles of all parties in an interpreted encounter; and to have the opportunity to provide feedback regarding the quality and appropriateness of language interpretation services. At the policy level, current national and local standards and guidelines need to be reviewed, debated, and possibly revised to better reflect the actual language assistance needs of patients, providers, and interpreters, and to ensure the most effective practices.

Effective cross-cultural communication skills involve more than language assistance. In communicating with immigrant women, providers accustomed to the standard format of Western medical health history need to be encouraged to adapt their communication style to more narrative formats. To better serve the health-care needs of immigrant women and their families, providers should be encouraged and enabled to modify their communication styles (e.g., by asking fewer interrogative questions and adopting a more open-ended questioning approach), become better listeners, and involve immigrant women's family members more. Other communication barriers in caring for immigrant women include the reluctance of many immigrant women to disclose "family matters" with outsiders and their embarrassment, shame, or guilt in discussing personal health concerns (e.g., sexuality, mental health). In contrast to the strong individual orientation of Western societies, immigrant women from more collective societies whose roles are focused on caring for others may be reluctant to talk about themselves or may not conceptualize their personal health issues in an individualistic framework. It is imperative to ensure privacy and take measures to reduce the potential stigma of mental health care among immigrant populations (Nadeem et al. 2007).

Promoting and Assuring Immigrant Women's Rights

The assurance of basic rights, including education, housing, employment, and health care, is necessary for the effective integration of immigrant women and their families into the social and cultural lives of the cities in which they settle. At the local and global level, policymakers must develop, implement, and monitor policies to ensure the human rights of immigrants. Immigrant women's needs must be addressed in developing and implementing national and international immigration law. Although most migration policies are not designed to discriminate against women, in practice women often face significant barriers to legal migration, particularly due to restrictions imposed on visas for female-dominant occupations (Global Migration Group 2008). The inclusion of domestic employment under national labor law and codes is a first step in protecting the rights of immigrant domestic workers around the world.

National and local health policies rarely focus attention on the specific health concerns of immigrants. The rise of anti-immigrant public discourses, racist groups, and overt violence against immigrants in the United States prompted McGuire and Canales (2010) to exhort health-care professionals to disrupt these anti-immigrant discourses and address the invisibility of immigrants and their health and human rights in their professional policy statements and practices. Health and social service providers working with immigrant women must be encouraged to take seriously their roles as patient advocates, cultural brokers, and social justice workers (Messias, McDowell, and Estrada 2009).

It is imperative that health and social service providers, policymakers, and researchers recognize that in immigrant communities around the globe, violence against women, whether it be sexual, domestic, or workplace violence, is not an inherent attribute of culture but rather "must be understood in the context of White supremacy, patriarchy, colonialism, and economic exploitation of marginalized communities, not as if such violence is inherent in the culture" (Sokoloff and Dupont 2005: 47). The exploitation of immigrant women, whether in the context of employment or human trafficking, "requires strong government responses in the areas of prevention, protection, and prosecution" (Global Migration Group 2008: 46).

Advancing Immigrant Women's Health Through Research

Research in the area of immigrant women's health requires innovative, interdisciplinary, and transnational approaches to examine the impact of migration on health among specific immigrant populations. Analyses of immigrant women's health must go beyond descriptions of current health status to examine relationships between health status and social, behavioral, cultural, and environmental factors such as immigrants' legal and citizenship status, length of residence in the host country, country of birth, and access to and utilization of local and transnational health and social services. In conducting research with immigrant women, investigators must critically examine the cultural appropriateness, reliability, and validity of health and illness measures that were originally developed and designed for use with nonimmigrant populations.

Large national data sets provide evidence of population trends but often do not distinguish between subsets of immigrants; therefore, the heterogeneity and diversity of immigrant women are often not evident in analyses of these data sets. More research is needed to better understand the health impact of migration policies, migration practices, and health outcomes of migrant and receiving populations. Participatory, community-based research with women in sending, transit, and receiving countries is needed to further understand the perspectives and experiences of diverse groups of immigrant women.

In conclusion, the complex interactions of migration processes, urban environments, health-care systems, and national and international policies may either contribute to or ameliorate health disparities among immigrant women. Migration and settlement in urban areas can afford women greater economic autonomy and independence and social and educational advancement, thus contributing to the advancement of gender equality and women's empowerment in both sending and receiving countries. Increasing collaboration and partnerships between immigrant women, community organizations, urban planners, policymakers, health-care providers, and health and social service agencies at all levels of service will contribute momentum to local and global efforts to attain health for all.

PART III

Models of Excellence

Chapter 9

Women's Health in the Urban Community: National Institutes of Health Perspective

Vivian W. Pinn and Nida H. Corry

Every week, 3 million people in the developing world migrate to cities, including large numbers of women (UN-HABITAT 2009b). As has been described in previous chapters, the pace of urbanization in many low-income settings exceeds local government capacity to provide basic amenities; as a result, urbanization in many places has resulted in the creation of vast urban slums, where a third of all households are headed by women (UN-HABITAT 2009b). This chapter discusses U.S. National Institutes of Health (NIH) initiatives and priorities in response to this phenomenon. After setting the stage with a review of the effects of urbanization on women's health, the chapter discusses the Office of Research on Women's Health (ORWH) research agenda and priorities; Fogarty International Center (FIC) programs; other NIH initiatives; and the larger federal framework within which the NIH works to address the needs of poor urban women in developing countries.

Women and Urbanization

Gender Inequality in the Urban Setting

Households headed by women frequently suffer disproportionately in cities in the developing world. In fact, global urban poverty has become highly feminized because poor, urban women tend to have low-paying jobs, high illiteracy rates, and fewer years of formal education. In addition, they are more vulnerable to intimate partner violence and are often forced to juggle family caretaking with work responsibilities. Social and political factors often make it difficult for women to own a home or land or to obtain credit to start small enterprises. For women, unstable housing has the combined potential to decrease food security and sustainable development and further compound ill health related to slum dwelling (Kothari 2003; Benschop 2004). Data suggest that health on average is better in urban than rural settings, due to more stable employment and better access to health services, clean water, and sanitation. However, these average findings mask wide socioeconomic differentials. When the data are *disaggregated*, urban poor often face health risks nearly as severe as those of rural villagers and sometimes worse, including high rates of infectious diseases and mental disorders, such as depression and anxiety, for which prevalence rates among women are double those for men (Harpham 2009: 112). In addition, urban areas have a higher incidence of breast cancer, perhaps due to increased risk factors, such as dietary factors, increasing age at first live birth, and lifestyle (e.g., alcohol use, activity levels) (Byrne 1996).

One specific aspect of urban health services that needs priority attention is reproductive health, which includes pregnancy, HIV/AIDS, birth, maternal health, and fertility (Harpham 2009: 111). Impoverished urban women are significantly less likely than their more affluent counterparts to have access to reproductive health or contraception and, not surprisingly, have higher fertility rates. In addition, the data suggest that urban poor women have very little access to information needed to make informed decisions about reproductive health, including protection against sexually transmitted infections (STIs), such as HIV/AIDS (Sai 1993; USAID 2004). HIV/AIDS is commonly thought to be prevalent among urban poor due to specific risk factors, such as sexual initiation at a younger age and more reported forced or traded sex. An array of urban conditions influence the spread of HIV or the severity of the illness, including overcrowding and high population density; inequitable spatial access and city form; competition over land and access to urban development resources; pressure on environment resources; and urban development capacity (Dyson 2003). In addition, data suggest higher rates of violence by an intimate partner in urban settings, especially slums. Gender inequality and alcohol use, which are pronounced in many urban settings, are recognized as key determinants of violence against women (Goebel, Dodson, and Hill 2010).

The *urban setting* itself is a social determinant of health. In this setting, living and working conditions especially among urban poor women may result in unsafe water, unsanitary conditions, poor housing, overcrowding, hazardous locations, and exposure to extremes of temperature creating health vulnerability. *Gender inequality* is another powerful social determinant of health, as it is a fundamental structure of social hierarchy that shapes access to health care. Consequently, women in urban settings face the double burden of gender and an urban environment, which poses compounded social and structural challenges to achieving and maintaining good health (Goebel, Dodson, and Hill 2010).

Aging and Urban Women

Between 1998 and 2050, the proportion of older people in urban communities of developing countries will have multiplied sixteen times, from about 56 million in 1998 to over 908 million in 2050 (UNFPA 2002). By 2050, older people will constitute one fourth of the total urban population in less-developed countries. In almost all societies, women form the greatest percentage of older people, and women are most often the caregivers for the elderly. However, with increased urbanization and greater numbers of women entering the workforce, women are less likely to be at home during the day to spend time with older relatives. This issue requires additional gender-responsive programs and services to assure the support and well-being of aging women living in urban centers. To effectively target resources and develop gender-responsive programs and services, there is a need to provide evidence-based tools for assessment and intervention. Therefore, the effects of urbanization on women's health should be a focus of any global health research agenda.

Office of Research on Women's Health Mission

The mission of the NIH is to discover knowledge that will lead to better health for everyone. As the primary federal agency in the United States for conducting and supporting medical research, the NIH accomplishes this mission by supporting and conducting both basic and applied biomedical and behavioral science research. Located centrally within the Office of the Director, the Office of Research on Women's Health (ORWH) has the mission of improving women's health through scientific investigation focusing on women and by raising the awareness of the scientific community about the importance of sex and gender factors in both basic and clinical research, along with their implications for women's health care. Recognizing the growing importance of the effects of urbanization and lifespan issues on global women's health, the ORWH included specific discussions about relevant topics in its preparation of a strategic plan for the next decade of the twenty-first century (US DHHS 2010).

The ORWH was established in 1990 to respond to scientific, advocacy, and congressional concerns about the lack of inclusion of women in biomedical research studies funded by the NIH. In order to systematically address these concerns, ORWH initially developed a research agenda that focused on gaps and emerging areas in women's health and sex/gender factors. Programs to promote biomedical career development for women, including research policy and health and science careers, were created. ORWH led the NIH efforts to implement its clinical research inclusion policy requirements. In recent years, ORWH has developed and implemented innovative interdisciplinary research and career development programs and has encouraged researchers to address race/ethnicity, effects of poverty, urban and rural living, understudied populations, and other factors that contribute to the health status and outcomes among different populations of women. The women's health research community embraces a comprehensive perspective that includes access to medical services and the effects of poverty and the environment on the health of women and their families.

ORWH Strategies for Women in Urban Areas

The ORWH celebrated its twentieth year at the NIH with the launch of the new strategic plan that identifies research priorities for the next decade. This plan incorporates suggested research initiatives that could improve the health of urban-dwelling women in developing countries, especially when poverty is a critical factor, through research and capacity building (US DHHS 2010).

ORWH has focused on improving women's and girls' health across the lifespan, encouraging NIH-funded research to incorporate sex/gender determinants, health disparities/differences, and diversity—themes applicable to women's health in any country. Innovative interdisciplinary research at ORWH has shifted the emphasis from the biological, disease-specific model to look at other factors that affect the health of women, including behavioral, social, community, racial/cultural, and environmental influences. Geographic location, occupational responsibilities, level of poverty, and access to health-care services are important factors in shaping an effective medical research approach. ORWH recognizes that public health or medical interventions are insufficient to address a range of diseases, including HIV/AIDS. Research that engages the community can enable a more complete understanding of the constellation of factors that contribute to the overall health and quality of life of urban women. Empowering women—who often serve as the portal to the health of their families and communities—to contribute to research and benefit from the results can change the fundamental ways women relate to their bodies and understand gender identity, and can ultimately improve health outcomes for the community as a whole.

Overarching themes in ORWH's research agenda include the prevention and treatment of diseases and conditions that affect women, the biological and behavioral bases of sex and gender differences, basic and clinical research methodology, and quality-of-life issues. In addition, ORWH develops research collaborations and partnerships with other NIH institutes and centers (ICs) to maximize resources, increase impact, and raise the visibility of emerging research issues in women's health. Initiatives have focused on the inclusion of women and minorities in clinical research to acquire sex/gender-specific data. Other initiatives have focused on promoting educational and career development with the purpose of both attracting and advancing girls and women throughout their scientific careers and encouraging both men and women to sustain careers in women's health research.

Within the broader context, ORWH is considering new paradigms that can advance research on women's health and sex differences in future years. The agenda-setting process addressed several basic questions: What progress has been made? Which scientific issues, emerging technologies, and areas of research are poised to advance over the next ten years? What partnerships and interdisciplinary approaches can improve the health of women and girls around the world? How can research results best be translated to benefit women's health and prevent, diagnose, or treat chronic and infectious diseases? How can the scientific workforce capacity be increased in developing countries to ensure that women are included at all levels and trained to be leaders in the research and health-care delivery communities?

A paradigm shift will inherently include a shift in emphasis from vulnerability to resilience, focusing on the ability of women to cope with serious threats to health and adapt to changing circumstances. For example, strengthening social support networks, self-esteem, autonomy, and connections with competent leaders and individuals in the wider community may build resilience among women and improve the health of the urban poor in the next decade (Harpham 2009: 115). Such a paradigm would need to identify specific opportunities and define methods to address them. ORWH will encourage these considerations in the design of research to explore new scientific approaches and applications that can improve the health of future generations of women, their families, and their communities—including those who continue to migrate to cities, both within the United States and in other countries around the world.

ORWH facilitated a series of regional meetings with leading experts in women's health issues to identify scientific challenges and gaps in knowledge and then to develop recommendations for future research. Working groups were utilized to focus discussions on specific content areas. Among these, and relevant to discussions of women's health in urban communities of the world, were a working group on women's global health and another on understudied populations including urban women and women who suffer from the effects of poverty. These working groups are discussed in more detail later in this chapter.

ORWH Updated Research Agenda

The 2010 strategic plan, *Moving into the Future with New Dimensions and Strategies: A Vision for 2020 for Women's Health Research,* incorporates several overarching strategies that reflect a commitment to global health for women, particularly in developing countries and urban poor communities (US DHHS 2010). Among these strategies are the following:

- *Create strategic alliances and partnerships to maximize the domestic and global impact of women's health research.* It would be beneficial to expand global strategic alliances and partnerships aimed at improving the health of women and girls throughout the world.
- *Employ strategic communications of research findings and health messages to enhance understanding, credibility, and application of scientific information derived from women's health research to improve public health and health care.* Since cultural and racial/ethnic diversity is a reality of our national and international societies and communities, information about women's health research and related issues should be disseminated in culturally appropriate ways in order to educate, explain, and promote healthy behaviors and public health. Multiple media strategies, along with employing the latest communication technologies, should be considered in communications research to determine how to best reach diverse audiences on a global and national level.
- *Employ innovative strategies to build a well-trained, diverse, and vigorous women's health research workforce.* This strategy involves a two-pronged approach. One is to devise programs to increase and enhance the roles of women in science, research, public health policy, and health leadership to support the scientific research enterprise. The second is to ensure that both men and women researchers understand and will pursue global research that addresses health issues of women.

Global Women's Health Research for the Coming Decade

As referenced earlier, ORWH facilitated a working group on women's global health to inform the development of the 2010 NIH strategic plan for women's health and sex differences research. This working group discussion took place at a scientific workshop hosted by the University of California, San Francisco (UCSF) in May 2009. This working group discussion was co-chaired by experts from UCSF and the University of California, Los Angeles (UCLA) and NIH representatives from the National Institute of Allergy and Infectious Diseases (NIAID) and the Eunice Kennedy Shriver National Institute of Child Health and Human Development (NICHD).[1]

The discussion reviewed sex- and gender-based disparities in disease and injury throughout a woman's lifespan, particularly in the areas of health risks and health needs. The participants recognized that women have less opportunity to enjoy good health and have greater needs due to childbearing and longevity, as well as more responsibilities in providing health services, and are also less likely to possess the power to bring about changes in these circumstances. Specific areas where global disparities are particularly acute were highlighted, such as in maternal mortality, unsafe abortion, and maternal disability. Participants also looked at health conditions that almost exclusively affect women in developing countries, including female genital mutilation, obstetric fistula, chronic conditions (and deaths) associated with indoor cooking fires, and the interaction of infectious diseases such as malaria and HIV/AIDS with pregnancy (Buvinić et al. 2006).

Discussions centered around three subtopics of women's health: (1) maternal, sexual, and reproductive health, (2) chronic diseases, and (3) infectious diseases, considering questions such as: What should be the priorities for research in this area? How should the priorities be set? And, how could research be structured to achieve maximum impact on women's health in developing countries?

Based on discussions about the status of women's global health, the working group formulated a series of recommendations for funding agencies in the following areas (Table 9.1).

1. *Implementation science.* Funding agencies are encouraged to support innovative, translational research to facilitate the implementation of evidence-based and sustainable interventions in developing countries to improve women's health. Improvements in health are characterized by decreased maternal morbidity and mortality and increased access to health care. Research should focus on preventive strategies to reduce risk for reproductive, chronic, and infectious disease and on development of standards of practice for conducting culturally sensitive research that ensures effective interventions.

2. *Sexual/reproductive health.* Research is needed on the determinants, long-term consequences, and effective strategies to eliminate or reduce

Table 9.1. Examples of Recommended Strategies on Global Women's Health and Understudied Urban Populations

Area of Focus	Overall Recommendation
	Global Women's Health
Implementation science	Support innovative, translational research to facilitate the implementation of evidence-based and sustainable interventions in developing countries to improve women's health.
Sexual/reproductive health	Research is needed on the determinants, long-term consequences, and effective strategies to eliminate or reduce critical understudied conditions that affect female children and adolescents in developing countries. Longitudinal studies could determine cumulative effects on women across the lifespan.
Mechanisms of disease risk across the lifespan	Research is needed on the biological, environmental, behavioral, and physical factors that contribute to or protect against chronic diseases, including mental illness, in women, as well as research that explores their mechanisms of action.
Infectious diseases	Research is needed to understand the increased susceptibility of women in the developing world to various infections, including malaria, human immunodeficiency virus, human papillomavirus, and sexually transmitted infections.
Capacity building in developing countries	Research capacity in developing countries could be enhanced through mentorship programs, research training programs, career and leadership development for women, and building supportive institutional environments to encourage health professionals to continue working in their own countries.

critical understudied issues that affect female children and adolescents in developing countries, including early sexual trauma, female genital mutilation, exploitation and trafficking, coerced sex, unwanted pregnancy, gender-based violence, and early marriage. Longitudinal studies could determine cumulative effects on women across the lifespan. One important area of focus would be the development and evaluation of new and improved contraceptives that are appropriate and sustainable for developing countries to address unwanted pregnancy among the

Table 9.1. *Continued*

Area of Focus	Overall Recommendation
	Understudied Urban Populations
Participation and inclusion of understudied groups of women in various research designs	Develop new technologies and methodologies for remote data collection; new measures, statistical approaches, and sampling methods in small samples; and strategies to overcome time/distance/literacy/differently abled/social role barriers to research participation.
Incorporate considerations of place, space, and context	Increase measurement of specificity and detail to identify culturally contextual factors that distinguish the influential factors and risk details within groups. Disaggregation of data is needed.
Role of trauma in health outcomes	A biopsychosocial research agenda for understudied women needs to encompass the role of trauma on health outcomes.
Health communication and literacy	Identify how women access health care and health information as a function of their different statuses. Examine and identify effective ways to use women's existing social networks to disseminate health information and translational findings from research.

Source: U.S. Department of Health and Human Services. 2010. *Moving into the Future with New Dimensions and Strategies: A Vision for 2020 for Women's Health Research.* NIH Publication No. 10-7606. Bethesda, Md.: Public Health Service, Naitonal Institutes of Health, Office of Research on Women's Health.

young, marginalized, and poor. In addition, behavioral research was identified as vital to understanding factors underlying the expanded use of contraceptives in developing countries.

3. *Mechanisms of chronic disease risk across the lifespan.* Research is needed on the biological, environmental, behavioral, and physical factors that contribute to or protect against chronic diseases (including mental illness) in women and should explore their mechanisms of action. Many other factors, such as poverty, the environment, and unequal social status, negatively affect women's health. To address these disparities, research should focus on early life events and exposures (including in utero), family and intergenerational causes, and lifestyle factors that uniquely affect women. Because chronic depression among women in developing countries has been particularly neglected, research is needed that identifies both protective and risk factors for de-

pression, as well as best practices for prevention and treatment within a range of cultural, political, and economic contexts.

4. *Infectious diseases.* Research is needed to understand the increased susceptibility of women in the developing world to various infections, including malaria, HIV, human papillomavirus (HPV), and STIs. Research on the biological factors that may contribute to this increased susceptibility can help explain sex differences in infectious diseases. For example, it would be useful to study the pathways of behavioral and hormonal changes across the menstrual cycle and lifespan that can influence infectious disease susceptibility. This research would lead to a greater understanding of how women are affected differently and can lead to sex- and gender-appropriate prevention, diagnostic, or treatment models. Also needed is research on the physiologic mechanisms of transmission of HIV and other infectious diseases through breast milk, since breastfeeding is so important for children's health in resource-constrained environments. The group also noted that pregnancy and compromised nutritional status may place millions of females at increased risk for disease.

5. *Capacity building in developing countries.* A major problem affecting developing countries is human capital flight, or "brain drain," of health researchers, medical practitioners, and health program managers. To help slow or reverse this trend, research capacity in developing countries could be enhanced through mentorship programs, research training programs, leadership development for women, and building supportive institutional environments to encourage health professionals to continue working in their own countries. Recommendations in this area also included the implementation of a resource center of information technology, standardized definitions, methodologies, and data on women's health, which could be easily accessed and shared to enhance research among many disparate populations around the world.

Understudied Populations Research for the Coming Decade

The working group that focused on women and girls who are underrepresented in research studies due to their vulnerable societal statuses or other reasons met at Northwestern University in Chicago in October 2009. The session was co-chaired by experts from UCLA, West Virginia University, George Mason University, Howard University Hospital, the University of Wisconsin–Madison, and representatives from NICHD, the National Institute of Diabetes and Digestive and Kidney Diseases (NIDDK), and the National Center on Minority Health and Health Disparities (NCMHD).[2]

This discussion group addressed the diversity of understudied or underrepresented groups in research and the unique configuration of risk and protective factors found in particular populations of women. The participants considered such subgroups as racial/ethnic minority women, immigrant women, women in urban and rural areas, women with disabilities, and women living in poverty. The discussion focused primarily on the identification of crosscutting research issues and overarching themes that would be applicable to most groups of understudied women. The working group developed the following recommendations for funding agencies to consider (see Table 9.1).

1. *Increase participation and inclusion of understudied groups of women in biopsychosocial, biomedical, and other research designs.* Approaches to improve representation of understudied groups include (1) developing new technologies and methodologies for remote data collection; (2) developing new measures, statistical approaches, and sampling methods in small samples to include understudied subpopulation groups of women; and (3) developing strategies to overcome time, distance, literacy, differently abled, and social role barriers in order to enhance and increase participation of understudied groups of women in various research designs.

2. *Incorporate considerations of place, space, and context in studies of women's health.* Measurement of specificity and detail needs to be increased to identify culturally contextual factors that distinguish the influential factors and risk details within groups; thus, disaggregation of data is a key factor.

3. *Integrate a focus on the role of trauma in health outcomes of understudied groups of women.* A biopsychosocial research agenda for understudied women needs to encompass the role of trauma on health outcomes. For example, research should focus on the "gendered" nature of trauma and the ways that women's experiences of trauma influence lifespan and intergenerational outcomes.

4. *Improve health communication and literacy.* Relatively little evidence is available to inform "best practices" for improving the health literacy levels of women from understudied subpopulation groups. Therefore it is important to identify how women access health care and health information as a function of their different statuses (e.g., socioeconomic status, geography, age, sexual orientation, and differently abled). In addition, research should examine and identify effective ways to use women's existing social networks to disseminate health information and translational findings from research. One specific suggestion included investigating methods for the improvement of women's and girls' health literacy through the use of public campaigns and activities, similar to

those that teach women about appropriate ages for health screening and vaccination activities.

Fogarty International Center Programs

ORWH collaborates with the Fogarty International Center (FIC) at NIH, which supports and facilitates global health research conducted by U.S. and international investigators, builds partnerships between health research institutions in the United States and abroad, and trains the next generation of scientists to address global health needs. The FIC supports research and research training programs that focus on the needs of low- and mid-income countries dealing with both communicable (e.g., HIV/AIDS, malaria) and noncommunicable (e.g., tobacco addiction, brain disorders) diseases and disorders, and the FIC research portfolio also includes population health, environmental health, and research ethics.

Global Research Initiative Program for New Foreign Investigators

The research training and capacity-building programs at FIC include the Global Research Initiative Program for New Foreign Investigators in Basic/Biomedical Sciences and Social Sciences (GRIP), for which ORWH is a partner. This program promotes re-entry of NIH-trained developing country investigators into their home countries as part of a broader program to enhance the scientific research infrastructure in developing countries. Consequently, "second-generation" training occurs when these foreign scientists return home and contribute to the training of the next cohort. In addition, this program aims to stimulate research on a wide variety of high-priority health-related issues in these countries. Examples of GRIP-supported research topics relevant to women's health include the association between widow inheritance and HIV infections; iron supplementation in HIV-infected women in Mexico; the use of antenatal corticosteroids; and Balkan endemic nephropathy in women.

FIC Clinical Research Scholars and Fellows Program

The FIC Clinical Research Scholars and Fellows program (FICRS-F) responds to the acute need for future U.S. clinical investigators to contribute to research that will address issues in global health. The FICRS-F provides highly motivated U.S. medical and graduate students in the health sciences the opportunity to experience one year of mentored clinical research training at distinguished low- and middle-income country research institutions at which NIH has active programs. Each U.S. student is paired with a low- or middle-income-country student, who also receives training as an equal partner. The program includes a postdoctoral program for medical residents and fellows, as well as for scientists with doctoral degrees engaged in health-related postdoctoral programs. The majority of scholars and fellows in this program are women (65 percent).

Medical Education Partnership Initiative

One of the newest FIC programs, the Medical Education Partnership Initiative (MEPI), with support from the ORWH, the NIH Office of the Director, the NIH Office of AIDS Research, the Office of the U.S. Global Aids Coordinator and other U.S. government agencies, was designed to build research and clinical capacity in sub-Saharan African countries. Additional collaborators include seventeen NIH ICs, the Centers for Disease Control and Prevention (CDC), the U.S. Department of Defense, and the U.S. Agency for International Development (USAID) at the Department of State. Institutions in countries that receive the President's Emergency Plan for AIDS Relief (PEPFAR) support three major goals: to increase the number of health-care workers who work in HIV/AIDS prevention, treatment, and care by 140,000; to strengthen the medical education system in these countries; and to retain faculty of medical schools and clinical professors.

Other Fogarty International Center Initiatives

The AIDS International Training and Research Program (AITRP) supports research on women's health that examines sex and gender differences related to antiretroviral treatment access, AIDS-related mortality and long-term survival rates, and risk for HPV infection. In addition, the research addresses cultural notions of sexual reputation and factors that may have a differential impact on HIV-infected women. A recent maternal health study in the medical journal *The Lancet* found that 61,400 maternal deaths worldwide were attributable to HIV in 2008 (Hogan et al. 2010). Further, one of the key priorities for the Office of AIDS Research's FY2011 Trans-NIH Plan for HIV-Related Research is to translate HIV-related research from bench to bedside to the community, focusing on both epidemiological studies and information dissemination. The special populations targeted by this plan for the reduction of HIV-related disparities include women and girls of various racial and ethnic populations in a global setting (Office of AIDS Research, NIH 2010).

Researchers at the University of KwaZulu-Natal, Durban recently released promising findings from the CAPRISA 004 trial, which assessed the safety and effectiveness of a candidate antiretroviral microbicide gel containing 1 percent tenofovir, a nucleotide reverse transcriptase inhibitor widely used in the treatment of HIV, for the prevention of HIV acquisition in women (Karim et al. 2010). This study, supported by multiple NIH ICs, was conducted from May 2007 to March 2010 at an urban and a rural clinic in KwaZulu-Natal, South Africa, and employed a two-arm, double-blind, randomized, placebo-controlled trial design. Findings indicated that tenofovir gel reduced HIV acquisition by an estimated 39 percent overall and by 54 percent in women with high gel adherence. The protective effect of coitally-related tenofovir gel use was apparent soon after initiation and peaked at 50 percent following 12 months of gel use. Notably, this protective effect was evident irrespective of sexual behavior, condom use, herpes simplex type 2 virus infection, or urban/rural differences. The study found no increase in the overall adverse event rates, no changes in viral load, and no tenofovir resistance in HIV seroconvertors. The researchers called for additional studies to corroborate these findings and to compare the safety, effectiveness, adherence, and/or cost of coitally-related tenofovir gel with daily tenofovir in either the oral or gel formulation for HIV prevention. The authors posit that "this antiretroviral microbicide could potentially fill an important HIV prevention gap, especially for women unable to successfully negotiate mutual monogamy or condom use" (Karim et al. 2010).

The FIC also supports studies focused on mental health, a critical issue for women in developing countries. A program entitled "Brain Disorders in the Developing World" funds research grants to study brain disorders across the lifespan in low- and middle-income nations. The purpose of the grants is to build sustainable research capacity in these countries to address nervous system development (sensory, motor, cognitive, and behavioral), function, and impairment throughout life and to lead to diagnostic, prevention, and treatment strategies that are applicable worldwide. Research areas related to women's health include postpartum depression, the interface of psychiatric disorders and HIV in women, and the effects of neurotoxins/neurotoxicants in the home. Several other NIH ICs and ORWH partner in this program.

NIH Initiatives in Climate Change/Environmental Health

In May 2009, *The Lancet* termed climate change "the biggest global health threat of the 21st century" (Costello et al. 2009). Urban environments, because of concentrated populations, are most vulnerable to extreme weather events caused by climate change. In addition, as greenhouse gases accumulate in the atmosphere, extreme weather conditions threaten to take an exceeding toll on women, who make up a large share of the world's poor.

In recent years, reports by international organizations such as the United Nations have highlighted the disproportionate impact of climate change on the world's women. Greater poverty, less power over their own lives, less recognition of their economic productivity, and an unequal burden in reproduction and child raising cause women to face additional challenges as the climate changes. Women and girls in many developing countries constitute the larger share of the agricultural workforce and have access to fewer income-earning opportunities, thus limiting their mobility and increasing their vulnerability to weather-related natural disasters. One of the recommendations of the United Nations Population Fund report on climate change was to bring a better understanding of population dynamics, gender, and reproductive health to climate change and environmental discussions at all levels (UNFPA 2009: 4–6).

In 2008, the FIC coordinated a planning group to assess the research questions in health and medicine that climate change presents. This Trans-NIH Working Group on Climate Change and Health actively involves sixteen NIH ICs who are working to identify research needs and priorities for an NIH research agenda on this topic. In January 2009, an interagency working group, led by the National Institute of Environmental Health Sciences (NIEHS), was formed to identify areas for strategic research on the linkage between climate change, the environment, and human health to develop a general conceptual model for research coordination. The recommendations of these two groups will guide the NIH in the development of a research portfolio that is science driven and relevant to the need for prevention and intervention to protect human health from climate change on the national and global level.

Recently, the interagency working group, led by NIEHS, completed a report entitled *A Human Health Perspective on Climate Change*, which identified gaps in knowledge of the consequences for human health of climate change, as well as mitigation and adaptation, and suggested research to address these gaps (Portier et al. 2010). The report noted that children, pregnant women, and the elderly are, in general, more susceptible to diseases linked to climate change and that poverty typically makes people more vulnerable to many of the health effects of climate change. Poverty is a factor largely due to inadequate access to health care, as well as to displacement, often to urban communities. The authors emphasized that a "broad-based, trans-disciplinary research portfolio" is needed to undertake this type of research, which will help us "develop the proper tools and make informed choices that will ultimately result in better health and better lives for the citizens of the United States and of the world" (Portier et al. 2010).

Another component of the ORWH strategic planning process carried out at UCSF in May 2009 was a working group on women's health and the environment. This session was co-chaired by experts from UCSF, Kaiser Permanente, Asian Communities Reproductive Justice, and NIH representatives from NICHD, NIEHS, and the National Cancer Institute (NCI).[3] This group developed recommendations that included identifying a broad range of underexplored environmental factors that affect women's health across the lifespan, including those related to climate change. A second focus was on funding research to evaluate how public policy can address environmental influences on women's health. Another, applicable to women living in large cities of developing countries, was to support community-based research that would increase the quality and usability of research. In addition, this type of research should build capacity among researchers and members of the community to prevent and mitigate negative environmental effects on women's health.

Clinical Trials for Women in Developing Countries

The NIH Revitalization Act of 1993 (Public Law 103-43) included language to ensure that women and racial/ethnic minorities and their subpopulations are included in all human-subject research funded by the NIH. This law was based on the concerns of advocates, scientists, and members of Congress about the lack of inclusion of women in NIH-funded biomedical research studies on health conditions that affect both men and women. The act requires Phase III clinical trials to include women and minorities and their subpopulations in such numbers that a valid analysis of differences in intervention effect can be completed. Outreach efforts and programs to recruit these groups into clinical studies were called for by the law, with cost not permitted as an acceptable reason for exclusion of these groups. Consequently, NIH now has a policy based upon the implementation of this law.

Current trans-NIH tracking mechanisms in the scientific review of individual grants do not capture the economic status of participants, nor geographic location, such as urban or rural environment. To meet the NIH policy regarding inclusion of "minorities," utilization of the classification policies of the U.S. government Office of Management and Budget (OMB) is required (U.S. OMB 1997). Non-U.S. participants in clinical research should be categorized according to the OMB classification scheme as if they were domestic participants. The law is clear that there are no exceptions to policy implementation, so that NIH-supported studies conducted outside of the United States must meet the requirement of identification of sex/gender and of race/ethnicity of their participants.

Enrollment statistics for recent clinical research reflect the commitment of NIH to women's health on a global level. The years 2002 through 2008 witnessed an increase of participants in non-U.S. protocols of Phase III clinical trials from 30,111 to 201,473, with 53.5 percent enrolled female participants in 2008. The total enrollment in *all* non-U.S. clinical research studies conducted in 2008 was 1,277,728 (8.3 percent of total enrollment), and females made up 57.1 percent of all non-U.S. subjects (ORWH 2009: 116, 123).

Numerous clinical research studies at the international level are currently being conducted on diseases of documented high prevalence in urban settings, including breast cancer, cardiovascular disease, obesity, trauma and violence, depression, and HIV/AIDS. A comprehensive list of these studies is available online at www.clinicaltrials.gov, a site sponsored by the NIH that provides consumers, as well as health professionals, with up-to-date information about the availability, status, and location of clinical trials for a wide range of health issues.

Many of the current NIH programs are highly relevant to women in developing countries; for example, the NICHD efforts to reach women worldwide include addressing the impact of pregnancy on maternal obesity, preventing maternal mortality in developing countries, and preventing HIV transmission during pregnancy. Many clinical research studies rely both on NIH investigators from the United States and NIH-funded researchers in other countries.

National Institutes of Health Top-Down Support

NIH director Francis Collins has identified global health as one of five areas of focus during his tenure. Collins noted in his inaugural address that global health research "should be a conversation with other countries, but not one in which the great United States tells the world what the answers are without listening to their experiences" (Collins 2009). Collins follows the lead of previous NIH directors who supported global health, including Harold Varmus, who served as a co-chair on the recent Institute of Medicine (IOM) report that issued recommendations for the U.S. commitment to global health to the new administration (IOM 2009). In addition, former NIH director Elias Zerhouni was announced as a special science envoy to the Muslim world for the administration of the president of the United States (National Science Foundation 2009).

Federal Global Health Perspective

The U.S. government's Global Health Initiative (GHI), a six-year $63 billion initiative to improve and expand access to health services globally, has a strong focus on improving maternal, newborn, and child health and, via a series of trans-GHI principles, supports implementing GHI programs through woman- and girl-centered approaches. In support of this objective, the GHI will encourage long-term systemic changes to remove barriers and increase access to quality health services for women across their lifespan, for example, supporting integrated health services, improving training of health providers on gender issues, and engaging civil society to address gender equity in health care. Through the GHI, the U.S. government is pursuing a comprehensive "whole-of-government" approach to global health, led by a committee composed of the heads of the USAID, NIH, CDC, and the U.S. Global AIDS Coordinator, thus engaging the full federal science community in this effort.

Within the U.S. Department of Health and Human Services, the Office of Global Health Affairs serves as liaison to the World Health Organization and promotes the health of the world's population by advancing the global strategies and partnerships set forth by the Secretary of the U.S. Department of Health and Human Services. Federal government efforts are linked to the Millennium Development Goals of the United Nations, the world's time-bound and quantified targets for addressing extreme poverty in its many dimensions—income poverty, hunger, disease, lack of adequate shelter, and exclusion—while promoting gender equality, education, and environmental sustainability (United Nations Development Programme n.d.). NIH and ORWH are operating within this dynamic, multidimensional federal framework that reinforces initiatives and priorities that can assist in addressing the needs of poor urban women in developing countries.

Future Directions

Scientists, advocates, and health-care providers have participated in creating a dynamic, interdisciplinary, science-based approach for future endeavors that address prevention, detection, and treatment of illnesses and health conditions among women of all races, cultures, and ages in diverse environments and different geographic settings. The newly revised NIH research agenda on women's health for the first time includes specific discussions related to urbanization and globalization that can encourage both investigators and funding agencies to address deficiencies in our understanding of these issues.

In the next decade, ORWH and its NIH partners will continue to address gaps in knowledge, build a flexible framework for evolving research priorities, and integrate new knowledge into scientific, health professional, and public health education that can be globally applicable. A long-term focus will be *sustaining* public and personal health interventions by building competencies needed to overcome the specific health challenges of urban environments for girls and women in developing countries around the world. NIH enters the next decade prepared for the broader challenges inherent in creating synergy in the global community through research and scientific capacity building that will ultimately result in improved health of girls and women, their families, and their communities.

The authors appreciate the contributions to this chapter of members of the NIH Fogarty International Center, including Deputy Director Michael Johnson, M.D., Susannah Cleary, Ph.D. (NIH/NINDS), Rachel Sturke, Ph.D., M.P.H., M.I.A., and Nalini Anand, J.D., M.P.H.; members of the ORWH staff, including Deputy Director Janine Clayton, M.D., and Indira Jevaji, M.D., M.S.L. The authors also appreciate the editorial assistance of Jennifer M. Bishop and Mary Lou Rife of Educational Services, Inc.

Chapter 10

Transforming Urban Environments

Diane Cornman-Levy, Grace R. Dyrness, Jane Golden,
David Gouverneur, and Jeane Ann Grisso

Our personal experiences as advocates, activists, and academicians have illuminated women as the center of community change and the architects of strong social networks that can spark community transformation. In this chapter, we describe exciting models of change in poor urban communities. We begin by telling our stories—stories that represent real life experiences of urban transformation. As we reflect on these models of success, common themes emerge, both positive and negative. These themes lead us to discussions of possible barriers to sustainability as well as practical principles that we believe will improve the likelihood of success. But, first, our stories.

The following pages describe some exciting examples of urban transformation, both in cities in the United States and in developing countries. The pivotal role of women in community change emerges in every setting.

More Than Just a Vegetable Garden

The City of Philadelphia has more than 40,000 vacant lots, many of which are magnets for trash and crime as well as symbols of hopelessness. A majority of these lots are located in poor neighborhoods throughout Philadelphia—neighborhoods where children, youth, and families struggle with hunger, violence, decent housing, lack of sustainable jobs, and poor health.

The statistics are at best bleak. At 24 percent, the poverty rate in Philadelphia is the third highest rate among large U.S. cities. In 2009, community organizations in Philadelphia reported a 50 percent increase in the number of families seeking food assistance and a major gap between the demand for food and the availability of food through food cupboards (Federation of Neighborhood Centers 2009). More families are going hungry. Mothers deal with the daily struggle of keeping their children safe and finding programs that will promote the healthy development of their children. Families feel isolated from "mainstream" society. All of these factors create an environment of high stress and hopelessness.

In spite of those daunting realities, women throughout Philadelphia are organizing to create better lives for themselves and for their children. The driving force behind the work of many women is their children. Like all mothers, they want the best for their children and they will do what it takes to build a better life for them.

In the winter of 2005, community leaders—all of whom were women—from a low-resource neighborhood in Central North Philadelphia organized a meeting to discuss the challenges they faced, including violence, lack of healthy food, and lack of positive programs to engage their children, especially their teenagers. They discussed the vacant lots in their community, lots that attracted violence and trash. They voiced their frustrations about the lack of investment in their communities. They talked about how wonderful it would be to have a large grocery store in their community that would provide healthy food and jobs for community members. As the discussion evolved, new ideas developed. The women started asking questions about the vacant lots: Why can't we transform them into gardens? How about creating urban farms? As the ideas flowed, the energy and creativity in the room intensified, and soon a vision emerged of an urban farm that would not only produce affordable, healthy food for their families, but also provide learning opportunities for the children.

The brainstorming session led to a written strategic plan for securing land for the urban farm. The women organized themselves and reached out to potential partners with expertise in urban farming, land acquisition, and health and nutrition. Within six months, the women had secured a parcel of land. Community members and their partners volunteered to clean up the land and prepare for the first plantings. By the spring of 2005, a dozen vegetable beds were formed. This once vacant piece of land transformed into a working urban farm producing fresh produce for the community.

The community leaders continued to meet and discuss next steps. During the discussions, the women expressed their continued concern for engaging their older children in positive activities and keeping them off the streets. Soon the idea of a youth-led urban agricultural business emerged. Youth would learn how to transform vacant lots into urban farms. They would learn how to manage the farms and run socially responsible businesses. As they grew healthy food for their communities, they would also learn how to plant, nurture, harvest, package, and distribute vegetables, herbs, fruit, and flowers; sell produce and garden-related products (e.g., cookbooks, calendars) to local communities, restaurants, and stores; design and conduct nutrition programs; design marketing materials (i.e., Web site, newsletters, brochures); manage finances; communicate effectively; apply character strengths to solve problems; and build healthy relationships through teamwork, networking, sales presentations, and customer service. Figures 10.1 and 10.2 show teen community members harvesting and selling produce grown in their urban gardens.

In 2006, these community youth came together and created a new business, Teens 4 Good. The brainstorming of community leaders had planted the seed that turned one vacant lot into a garden and then into a youth-led urban agricultural business. Today there are eight urban farms in sixteen low-income neighborhoods that employ 150 youth per year and harvest more than 5,000 pounds of produce—enough to supply five families of four with vegetables for one year. Teens 4 Good continues to grow because it is owned by the youth and the community, who build the capacity of youth to become engaged, productive leaders of the future. Now those teens and their mothers have a new and exciting vision for the future. They want to create a national model of youth-led urban agricultural businesses. They will use twenty-first century skills to build the leadership capacity of at-risk youth while developing models of local food systems that bring fresh, affordable produce to their neighborhoods.

Ties That Bind

Manila, the capital of the Republic of the Philippines, is a city of more than 20 million people. Not only is it is the largest city in the Philippines, but it is also the most densely populated city in that country and, by some accounts, in the world. About 40 percent of all Filipinos live in abject poverty, and in Manila the poverty is palpable. Sections of the city are home to informal settlements consisting of small houses made of a variety of materials, from plywood to, in the most dire of cases, cardboard. Roof after roof extends across the horizon of the largest slum areas, zinc sheets held down with old tires, stones, and anything else that will help keep the roof from blowing off during the strong typhoon winds that pass through every monsoon season. People courageously try to make a living, working mostly in marginalized occupations such as house helpers, construction workers, laundry washers, ironers, and scavengers. Others set up small businesses selling vegetables or fish in the market stalls,

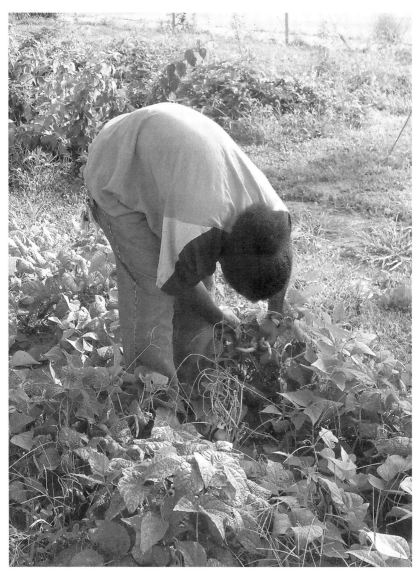

Figure 10.1. One of Teens 4 Good founders harvesting cucumbers in the group's urban farm. (Photo courtesy of Diane Cornman-Levy.)

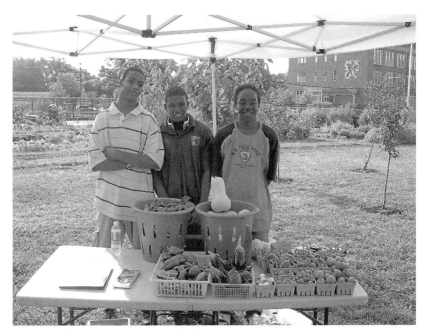

Figure 10.2. Teens 4 Good youth selling their produce at a neighborhood farmers' market. (Photo courtesy of Diane Cornman-Levy.)

brewing local beer, running small gambling houses, or cooking meals for workers who cannot go home to eat. This is how Aling Lita lives.

Aling Lita has four children. She lives with her family in a house in one of the resettlement areas, sites set up just outside the city by the government as a means of moving people out of the squatter settlements within Manila. Yet Aling Lita relies on the opportunities for work that are available in the city and commutes back and forth to the resettlement area. She washes clothes for wealthier people in Manila. Her husband is a shoe shine person, an extremely precarious occupation that brings in very little money on a daily basis. Their house is a one-room structure made out of plywood with one bed, a small table, a chair, and a kerosene stove for cooking. There is no bathroom in the house, although there are facilities available outside.

Women like Aling Lita form strong social networks that support them in their daily lives and help them while they negotiate the complex issues of survival and caring for and educating their children. The networks become a source of solidarity for these women and become a springboard for community transformation. They are a key strategy for coping for many women. Most of the networks develop from activities

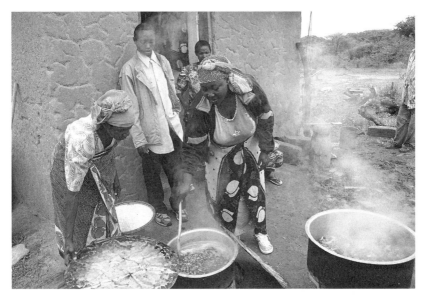

Figure 10.3. Women working together in Tanzania. (Photo courtesy of Donald E. Miller.)

around the home. Groups of women who cook meals to sell within the slums support one another even amid competition for customers. Thus, if one woman becomes ill and cannot cook, the others cook for her and deliver the food to her customers so she will not lose them. This is true for women in much of the developing world, such as the two women pictured in Figure 10.3 working together in Tanzania.

For Aling Lita in Manila, relying on her friends and neighbors to help her when she gets sick, or to care for a sick child while she goes into the city to wash clothes, is vital for her survival. Supporting one another becomes a means of creating a safety net, of providing help just when it is needed. Only in this way can women like Aling Lita keep their jobs and customers. And they will do the same for their friends.

These networks at times become the source of women's entertainment and leisure. It is here they can share the latest gossip and news, provide tips for getting jobs or customers, and simply laugh and tell jokes. Often this occurs around the local water spigot or in the market. The hard work of living in a slum or squatter settlement does not allow much time for leisure. Women become resourceful and take advantage of times when they are together to enjoy themselves. One of Aling Lita's neighbors was vehemently opposed to the suggestion that her daughters should go to the water spigot and do the hard job of washing laundry: Why in the world would she want that? It would deny her the one chance she has of being with her friends! While washing clothes or sitting in the market stall, women build ties that bind.

To an outsider it may seem that Aling Lita is living in dire poverty, with few material possessions, struggling to keep food on the table for herself and her family. But she feels that she is doing well. To her, the city is the place where she pins her hope for the future of her children. That is the reason she came to the city, to provide opportunities for her children. Now, in spite of the struggle and hard work, she says a dream of hers is being achieved: "Here it is, it has been realized. It was difficult, but I am very thankful that we now have our own house. This was my dream. Now I have my own place" (Dyrness 1978: 63).

Aling Lita's story echoes in many cities around the world where women rely on one another to survive. These are courageous, industrious, entrepreneurial women. Even homeless women seek ways to connect and build solidarity among themselves, by watching one another's children, providing sounding boards for airing common concerns, and communicating vital information about job possibilities or services that can be utilized. Women depend on their network of friends to survive the harsh realities of their lives.

In addition to creating a tapestry that holds the community together, these networks can also be a springboard for transforming even the most desperate living situations by providing the solidarity needed when advocating for change. Indeed, they often become the basis of community organizing. Aling Lita and her friends in a Manila slum talked together about the lack of services they were getting from the government (such as no trash collection) and decided to stage a demonstration in front of the police department to bring notice to their predicament. They took their babies and sat in the police station and refused to budge until they were guaranteed a truck for garbage collection, using their role as mothers and providers to join together for the good of the community and in their own self-interest. Because they had already learned to rely on one another for the small things, they were ready to join efforts for the larger, community-wide changes that they believe need to happen. Working together is a strategy they have learned for survival; but much more than that, it is a way to thrive and improve the lives of their families and their communities.

Medellín: From War Zone to a Place of Peace and Hope

The story of Medellín is about optimism and the belief that cities can change in a very short period, improving the quality of life in poorer communities. Medellín is the second largest city in Colombia, with a population of 3.5 million. Nestled in a narrow Andean valley at an elevation of 3,000 feet, Medellín gained world attention in the 1980s as the epicenter of the production and trade of cocaine, giving leverage to drug cartels and making it one of the most violent cities on the planet. Most of the crime occurred as a result of vendettas between the drug lords, particularly within poorer, informal neighborhoods located on the steep slopes of the Medellín valley. In these poor neighborhoods, a high percentage of the population engaged in drug-related activities. They were not often pursued by the police due to the difficult accessibility, which made them off-limits for nonresidents and authorities alike. The violence became so severe that many residents died and others were forced to flee.

In less than a decade, Medellín has experienced one of the greatest environmental and civic transformations in history. It has become a unique example of how urban change may occur despite the most adverse conditions. This success story stems from an unusual synergy among talented politicians, public officials, community leaders, and creative professionals.

For decades, Colombia had been plagued with violence. Millions of its citizens left the country in search of better living conditions. The violence and disruption severely affected Colombia's reputation and its economy. The guerrilla movement, which began in the late 1940s, initially sought structural social reform. To fund their work, the guerrilla movement gradually embraced drug trafficking, gaining immense wealth and political leverage. The drug cartels took control of vast rural areas of the country where the drug labs and transportation bases were located, making driving between the major urban centers a high-risk activity. In addition to the original guerrilla organizations, rival groups entered the drug business, increasing the level of conflict and corruption.

In the late 1990s major changes occurred in the political arena including, in particular, the emergence of a highly qualified political leadership committed to restoring governance. Presidents Cesar Gaviria and Alvaro Uribe were crucial figures in this era. Restoring functioning government also included the implementation of Plan Colombia, which included financial, military, and strategic support from the United States in the war on drugs as well as extradition treaties for drug-related crimes. A turning point was certainly the incarceration, escape, and death in 1993 of the Medellín drug lord Pablo Escobar, who was thought to be one of the richest men in the world at the time.

The new constitution of 1991 also introduced important political and administrative reforms, including strengthening the decentralization process and providing municipal governments with greater autonomy, financial muscle, and a legal framework. These reforms led to new laws that facilitated urban planning and offered the technical and managerial tools to implement urban changes, and they set the framework for the emergence of new political figures at municipal and regional levels. This was certainly the case of Sergio Fajardo, a highly qualified, outspoken, and high-energy math professor who was elected mayor of Medellín in 2003 after campaigning on a political platform totally independent from the traditional parties.

Fajardo, along with architect Alejandro Echeverri, who was appointed by Fajardo as director of city planning, orchestrated an effort from 2005 to 2009 to create a model of urban transformation. The main objectives were to significantly reduce the crime rate in Medellín, offer the best facilities to address social inequalities, improve education and access to information, and use local resources to foster commercial enterprises to generate alternative sources of income. The mayor's team proclaimed that if the social division were to be closed, the poor areas of the city required the best of everything that could be offered. This, they stated, could be attained through coordinated planning and interventions in design carried out by the best-qualified professionals they could attract, while engaging a community normally mistrustful of public officials and political groups.

Their first goal was to reduce isolation and ensure accessibility and connectivity. They envisioned the use of sky lifts, or gondolas, that would provide quick access to the community without disrupting the dense urban fabric. They designed a gondola system—pictured in Figures 10.4 and 10.5—called Metro-cables, since they were linked to the city's Metro mass transit system. They placed the Metro-cable stations in the heart of the distressed neighborhoods. These stations and the public spaces around them quickly catalyzed urban change. The new plazas became meeting places and hubs of activity. The people living closest to these new transportation modes quickly upgraded their homes by adding such commercial activities as small shops, restaurants, and Internet centers.

The city plan also included development of a wide array of recreational and cultural facilities, including schools, amphitheaters, and community centers. Most amazing were the quality and quantity of new schools, which often housed technical training programs that helped boost small, competitive enterprises. The mayor's team also constructed iconic buildings known as "park-libraries," as pictured in Figure 10.6. Most of these were designed by young Colombian architects who had won these commissions through design competitions.

Neighboring barrios, although located at similar elevations, were separated by ravines and gorges. These barrios were populated by groups who had migrated from different regions of the country, many of which became warring communities controlled by different drug lords.

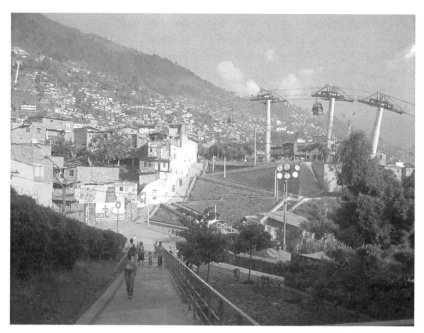

Figure 10.4. Zigzagging terraces and Metro-cable pillars, Barrio Santo Domingo, Medellín, Colombia. (Photo courtesy of David Gouverneur.)

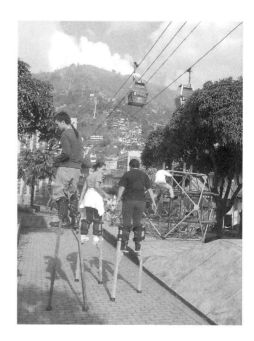

Figure 10.5. Promenade under Metro-cable alignment, Barrio Santo Domingo, Medellín, Colombia. (Photo courtesy of David Gouverneur.)

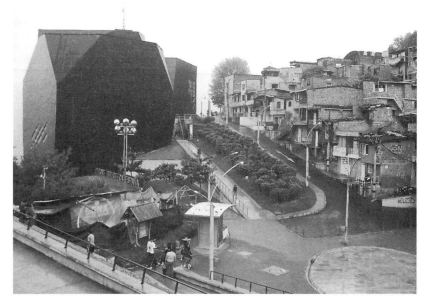

Figure 10.6. Public Library/Community Center and open spaces, Barrio Santo Domingo, Medellín, Colombia. (Photo courtesy of David Gouverneur.)

Corpses, resulting from violent confrontations, were commonly found in the gorges. To open these communities, urban designers connected the neighborhoods with pedestrian bridges over the ravines, allowing adjacent communities to gain access to their neighbors, Metro-cable, and community facilities. The bridges were anchored by small-scale parks, designed primarily for youth and children, which included such facilities as skateboard parks and climbing walls. In addition, the designers removed housing located in the flood plains of the ravines and built replacement housing on safe locations in the same barrios. As a result of these changes, areas around the once-dreaded gorges became linear parks of fun and peace.

The results were astonishing: The power of the vision and the quality of the designs transformed the neighborhoods into lively interconnected communities. An important feature of this program was its managerial framework that incorporated public and community participation and continuous maintenance of the new facilities and public spaces. In the process, the elected officials had to overcome major administrative problems, mainly corruption, which eroded municipal funds, as well as red tape and resistance to changing the old ways of doing things, which made it almost impossible to induce significant urban changes in short periods. To overcome these problems, the mayor introduced major re-forms to assure transparency in public administration and recruited new, well-trained personnel. In addition, the mayor directly coordinated multiple municipal agencies that had not previously worked together.

Community outreach and engagement were critical. No one had seen a gondola before in Medellín. Residents from the barrios could not have envisioned the use of gondolas as a means of transportation, nor the scope of the buildings and spaces that were to be redesigned. However, once the physical changes were completed, the community responded with vigor and creativity to the new challenges, helping to think beyond and actively participating in the new programs and projects. Notable was the adaptability of the buildings and open spaces to the local conditions, including the topography, the density of homes, and the climate and culture.

To increase attendance at cultural and recreational events and provide work for young people, youth were offered jobs distributing flyers in their neighborhoods to promote concerts and other events. One boy knocked on the door of a single mother who had raised three children. She received the flyers and thanked the boy. As he departed, she broke down in tears. Some months earlier, that very boy had killed her oldest son. She contacted Mayor Fajardo and told him: "Sergio, nothing will bring my child back to life, but had this initiative been carried out years before, many mothers would still have their kids around, I will go to the concert" (Echeverri 2008).

The impact of this urban transformation has been celebrated worldwide, and the current municipal government continues the vision and programs created by the Medellín community. It is important to note, however, that despite the significant changes at the national level, such changes as have occurred in Medellín have not occurred in many other cities. In nearby Cali, for example, a strong and visionary municipal leadership has not yet emerged. And, in Cali, there has not been a significant reduction in the levels of violence nor have residents been able to improve living conditions or boost sustainable economic activities. As demonstrated by the story of Medellín, powerful and enlightened leadership and urban visions that stem from community aspirations, accompanied by creative managerial frameworks to implement and support changes, can make a real difference.

The Power of Demonstrating Success

Mantua had long been referred to as "The Bottom" in the Philadelphia area. Unfortunately, sometimes names say it all, and "The Bottom" summed up how many people saw this part of the city. Once thriving, Mantua had suffered a significant population loss in tandem with years of neglect and blight.

Jonny Durham, a bus driver for the Southeastern Pennsylvania Transportation Authority, responded to the problem by organizing a grassroots group committed to turning the community around one block and one child at a time. The group was thirty people strong—all of them men, some of whom had been in prison. They remained steadfast in their collective effort to give back to Mantua in spite of significant obstacles and a dearth of resources. They were aware that as men they had been absent from the fabric of the community for many years. Crime, violence, drugs, personal struggles, and life's complexities had kept many of them away from the day-to-day struggle of running the community. That task had been driven for years by the women of the neighborhood. By their own admission, the men felt they had abdicated responsibility—now they were on a mission to give back. In the minds of these men, a connection to the community was clearly long overdue; the men hoped their work would create a tangible legacy.

The group requested several murals from the Philadelphia Mural Arts Program, and they identified a large parcel of land with two walls facing each other on which the murals could be painted. The walls had peeling paint, graffiti, and a large lot in between—almost half a block long—filled with trash and debris. Nearby was a recreation center, with its field covered in broken glass. Jonny wanted the tallest wall to be a mural of Ms. Jones—the matriarch of the neighborhood. A community leader and a block captain, she had lived in Mantua for fifty years and saw the community as extended family. She and others in the neighborhood invited Mural Arts leaders into their homes and not only taught them about the history of the community but also demonstrated the roles of women leaders in a community and the impact they made using little available resources. In Jonny's mind, Ms. Jones symbolized a person who was not just the glue of the community, but the spirit.

Community residents met about the project. They wanted to connect the wisdom of the seniors with the energy and potential of young people. They also loved African-American quilts and felt strongly about connecting the murals to the theme of quilting. A quilt brings parts together, piece by piece, and, like a successful community-led project, reflects the input of dozens if not hundreds of participants. Community residents and Mural Arts staff created a design that would feature a mural of Ms. Jones with a beautiful quilt on one wall and, on the other wall, a mural composed of pictures of neighborhood children selected because of their academic achievements. Figure 10.7 depicts these murals.

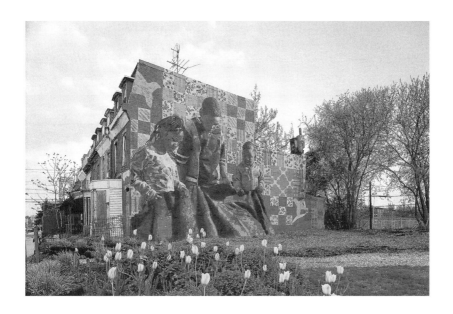

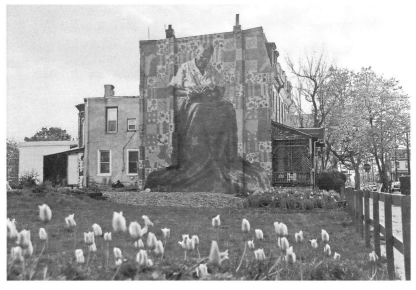

Figure 10.7. *Holding Grandmother's Quilt*: Murals designed by community residents and the Philadelphia Mural Arts Program in the Mantua section of Philadelphia. One wall features Ms. Jones, a community leader and matriarch. The other wall features neighborhood children selected because of their academic achievements. (© 2004 City of Philadelphia Mural Arts Program/ Donald Gensler and Jane Golden, Photos by Jack Ramsdale.)

The community also wanted to clean up the large lot between the walls, but it was a difficult project and the city would not take it on. So, volunteers started cleaning up the area, and that galvanized other neighbors. As the painting of the murals began, neighbors volunteered to help every day. Excitement began to spread throughout the Mantua community. Fueled by the momentum, the group went to a city councilwoman to plead for new equipment for the nearby recreation center. She agreed to provide funding for the equipment, and the group went on to ask for help from local nonprofits, including the Philadelphia Green Program and the Urban Tree Connection, which worked on city lots. Both organizations agreed to lend a hand. A resident with a bulldozer came over after work to remove the heavy debris, like tires.

Halfway into the project the group decided to have a volunteer day to help build community spirit. Over 300 people came—people of all ages and all races. Residents brought food, and the men barbequed.

Eight months after it was begun, the project was completed. In the Mural Arts Program, it is always an exhilarating moment when the scaffolding comes down and the entire community is brought together to celebrate all that has gone into the project. The dedication of the murals was a huge celebration—with dancing, drill teams, poetry, and speeches from multiple neighborhood leaders, including Ms. Jones and Jonny.

After dedications like these, murals often take on a life of their own as neighborhood landmarks, icons, and continual sources of pride and renewal. Some murals become locations for ongoing teaching and learning or the foci of increased city services, social services, and community development. In Mantua, the men who started this project were so inspired that they asked the city to turn one of their mural-decorated buildings into a community center. The city ultimately sold them the house for one dollar. This group proceeded to renovate the house, and today the building houses a community center that offers a range of services—everything from coaching to tutoring and to providing the community with information about housing and jobs. The group now has its own nonprofit organization and is raising money to keep its programs active within the community.

The creation of a mural and its dedication become major, life-affirming events. They draw widespread positive attention, but much more importantly, these moments give people a chance to see themselves represented with honor and dignity. The experience promotes both individual and communal self-esteem. The making of a mural enters the collective memory as an extraordinary, transformative moment in a neighborhood's history.

The changes in Mantua were just one example of changes that have occurred in Philadelphia, and they underscore the importance of an integrated, grassroots approach to community development. Changing the physical landscape and partnering with different agencies and departments can have a truly profound impact on communities. Murals are not a panacea for all the problems of a city, but they can play a central, catalytic role in healing the wounds of an urban environment. The creative, unifying act of mural-making, in the midst of chaos, can unleash the energy for a full-scale community renaissance.

Potential Barriers to Sustainability

Many exciting and effective programs are created through strong coalitions, charismatic leaders, and broad community support. However, just as often, many are not sustained or do not evolve to address different issues as funding or interest declines. Although these diverse stories focus on positive change, we recognize potential threats to sustaining such change. Having shared rich stories from different cultural and professional perspectives, we both recognize the positive change that can blossom and potential threats to sustaining change—threats that should be anticipated and mitigated from the beginning.

Gentrification is one threat to sustaining change, which may have different effects in developing countries as compared to industrialized nations. In developing countries, even in slums and barrios, most residents own their dwellings. Although they may have started off by squatting on the land, as the barrios get organized they are often able to negotiate ownership rights. Thus, the added value derived from urban transformation benefits the original residents as their property translates into increased land value, new amenities, and new commercial enterprises within the existing buildings. In contrast, in urban ghettos in developed nations, residents usually live in public housing or rent their homes. In these circumstances, urban improvements tend to translate into higher taxes and rents and displacement of the original tenants. For this reason, it is important to foresee the possible negative effects of urban revitalization and plan for ways to avoid them. Such plans may include establishing a percentage of affordable housing in areas of urban improvements, developing programs to help renters purchase homes, or acquiring vacant land and derelict buildings before property increases in value. Another potential negative effect of gentrification is the displacement of the previous community leaders by new urban residents. Weakening the traditional leadership in this way might work against the sustainability of urban transformation programs once the initial changes have been achieved. Thus, it is important to support the original leaders as visible communicators and managers of new projects, making sure they have real and important roles in future planning.

Corruption is another important threat that community leaders have to face. The leaders, as the stories of Manila's slums and Philadelphia's urban farms illustrate, are often poor women who are struggling to improve their lives and those of their families. According to Transparency International, corruption is rarely an isolated phenomenon but more often is systemic and widespread. Corruption often permeates every level of society and threatens sustainable development, fair business practices, and good governance. When poor women are asked to pay a bribe to the police in order to keep their microbusinesses going, it is difficult for them to engage in any savings plan, much less move into a sustainable future. Bribes are a common practice in many parts of the world, including inner cities of the United States, where, for example, gang members extort a payment for "protection" from other gangs. Unless strategies are implemented to mitigate against corruption, it becomes doubly difficult for poor women to become self-sufficient and enjoy a higher quality of life.

In the story of Medellín, the new mayor did a lot to address corruption in city government. He successfully implemented major reforms to assure transparency in public administration. He recruited new, well-trained personnel who were committed to the plan and the shared vision of transformation. In addition, the mayor directly coordinated multiple municipal agencies that had not previously worked together, ensuring not just collaboration, but also his direct oversight.

A third threat to sustaining new community initiatives is the effect of frequent changes in political leadership, which can be inevitable and very disruptive. Transitions frequently occur not just among senior leadership positions, but at all levels, particularly in low-resource communities. For example, immigrant women working as street vendors in Los Angeles reported that one of the challenges they face is changes in city office personnel. Just when the women would build a relationship with the head of the Community Development Department, for example, that person would have another job opportunity or would be transferred to another position. The new director may not understand the project, and a lot of time is lost in trying to rebuild those relationships—time that is costly for the women.

Transitions can be devastating for grassroots, nonprofit organizations and the communities they serve. The difficult struggle to maintain funding usually means that only a few people, and typically a single charismatic leader, can be employed. The capacity to adequately train and nurture new leaders and develop an orderly plan of succession does not exist. Thus, when a leader dies or moves on, the organization often fails, which can represent a tremendous loss for the community.

Not all transitions in leadership and partners are negative. Some transitions are planned for and contribute to sustainability. In the story of Philadelphia's urban farms, the women turned their project over to well-trained young persons, who continued and expanded the work. In Medellín, mayors can serve only one term. There, the widespread support for the city's transformation meant that any elected leader had to commit to carrying it forward, and the community residents and new leaders made sure that it happened.

Practical Principles for Successful Urban Transformation

This first principle for successful urban transformation is that of sustainable change. The likelihood of sustained change is greater if members of the community are engaged from the beginning and involved in all aspects of planning, implementation, and evaluation. In the story of the urban farms, the ideas and priorities came from women in the community. Sustainability is enhanced if the interventions build economic and social capital and the capacity for further change. That is exactly what the women did. They engaged young people and helped them develop a business, with the proceeds going back to their business so they could expand and train additional youth. This approach stems from community-organizing principles that promote community ownership, capacity, and power.

Outside organizations and individuals can partner with community members to leverage resources for the community, but the ideas and strategies for implementing the ideas should come from the community. If the interventions generate funds, distributing resources back to the community can help to further develop economic and social capital in the community and continue the change process. In Philadelphia, the urban farm initiative Teens 4 Good continues to grow because it is owned by the youth and the women leaders who make sure to continue to build the capacity of youth to become engaged, productive leaders of the future. A large percentage of the profits are reinvested to support the development of new farms and food systems to ensure that urban farms are viable economically. The group's vision of the future—to create a national model of youth-led urban agricultural businesses—may or may not be realized, but working toward it will continue to inspire and energize them as other creative ideas emerge. Promoting sustainable change is challenging but essential to improving the lives and opportunities for women and their families in urban communities.

Women are the center of change—a second key principle. The leadership of women is pivotal for the welfare of poorer communities. In the story of urban farms in Philadelphia, it was the women who developed capacity-building, transformative initiatives. Their drive was indispensable for the success and continuity of social programs. The women came together because they were fed up with what they saw in their neighborhood—the graffiti, the vacant lots, and empty, decaying buildings. Instead of being overwhelmed by a sense of defeat from seeing a community beset by seemingly insurmountable problems, they chose to see the potential that remained alive within it.

As the story of Aling Lita demonstrates, it is often the women who sustain family and cultural values—values that counter violence and corruption. They develop community networks of friends to support one another through difficult times. While washing clothes or sitting in the market stall, women develop friendships, building ties that bind. Their networks create a tapestry that holds the community together, creating a springboard for transforming even the most dire living conditions by providing the solidarity needed when advocating for change.

Although men carried out the projects in Mantua that led to the murals, they were clear from the beginning that women were the pioneers in the effort to improve the community and provide new opportunities for children. Many of the men had been in prison, in the military, or incapacitated by drugs, alcohol, or homelessness. It was once said that there were entire blocks in Mantua without male residents. The men organized to give back to the community and recognized the long-standing leadership roles held by women in Mantua. That is why they chose Ms. Jones to be portrayed in the mural, wishing to honor her fifty years of commitment and leadership in Mantua.

A third important principle for successful urban transformation is to develop an integrated strategy that addresses multiple problems. Most tough social and environmental problems result from many interrelated factors. Developing issue-specific programs like HIV care does not take advantage of the energy and creativity that multidisciplinary efforts can generate. For example, the epidemic of childhood obesity in low-resource urban communities results from multiple environmental and social factors, such as decreased access to healthy food in schools, corner stores, and fast food restaurants. Access to healthy food is also diminished through pricing disparities and the lack of local grocery stores. Finally, targeted advertising plays an important role. The other side of the energy equation involves increasing physical activity. That is difficult, particularly in lower-resource urban communities where many schools have eliminated or greatly reduced recess, there are no safe parks or playgrounds, urban design is often not exercise-friendly, and transportation systems do not link to safe recreational areas. Further, in communities where many people are without jobs or the hope of jobs, the underground economy flourishes and contributes to unsafe streets. Ideally, policy and environmental changes to address childhood obesity should involve multiple sectors and be designed to affect more than just obesity. The changes could also result in reduced crime rates, healthier environments, a greater sense of belonging, reduced disparities, and enhanced economic development. In the Philadelphia urban farms initiative, the women leaders understood that urban farms could increase access to fresh fruits and vegetables in communities without supermarkets. They also recognized that transforming trash-filled, vacant lots could reduce crime, injuries, and the availability of drugs. And finally, they realized that training young people to take over the urban farms as businesses could provide green jobs, a sense of pride, and economic development.

Key to integrating interventions across sectors is interdisciplinary partnerships. Success stories often encompass interdisciplinary efforts and are the result of synergy among different urban stakeholders, including community leaders, politicians, professionals, developers, and the like. In the story of the murals and the men in Mantua, the men knew that they needed to partner with a number of different groups, including the Philadelphia Mural Arts Program, the Philadelphia Green Program, various government agencies, and elected politicians. In Medellín, the mayor brought together the best architects, urban planners, engineers, government officials, transportation experts, as well as community leaders and residents. The synergy among these groups produced dramatic physical and social transformation of the poorest areas of the city. Building partnerships also extends to one's immediate neighborhood. In Manila, women worked in a wide range of informal jobs that could collapse if they became ill. Some of the jobs were in direct competition with each other, such as vendors in a market or sidewalk food stalls. Yet the women took care of one another.

Successful urban interventions usually require the participation of a coalition or network that includes diverse talent and skills. Academia, community organizations, and institutions can help tap financial, technical, and managerial resources that poorer communities may not attain on their own. Building partnerships and sustaining them requires trust, mutual respect, a common vision, and most of all, time.

Finally, it is important to demonstrate success and develop a coherent vision with leaders from the neighborhood. A first step is to work with community partners to elect an area or setting in the neighborhood where change is possible, an area that is accessible and visible, anchored on good public space. Then community change efforts should be focused on that place, with work to bring in, for example, highly visible public art, high-quality community services, and economic development through programs to tap local small business and entrepreneurial skills. Demonstrating success will build hope. A small success can generate widespread attention and excitement, and a cascade of positive changes often ensues. This was true for all of the stories. The murals inspired community residents in Mantua to rebuild their recreation center and rehabilitate an empty and decaying building to house a nonprofit organization. When residents of the barrios of Medellín saw the gondola and the new public space around the Metro stations, they were galvanized to create new enterprises and improve their homes. In Philadelphia the vision of urban farms producing healthy vegetables and fruits inspired the women to expand their work and train youth to create new businesses based on the farms.

A Theme for Change

In these challenging circumstances, women often become the leaders for community change. They organize, demand services, and support one another. They have strong social ties. Aling Lita and her friends in Manila had already learned to rely on one another to help with daily problems. And they had developed important social networks that led to discussions of the problems they faced. As a result, they decided to demonstrate together about the lack of basic services (i.e., trash collection). By taking their babies and refusing to move, they used their roles as mothers and providers to join together for the good of the community and in their own self-interest.

The tenacity and commitment of women leaders, in partnership with diverse stakeholders, can lead to profound urban transformation. We have provided just a few examples, from creating urban farms that provide fresh vegetables and jobs to honoring senior matriarchs through murals that catalyze further community development. In spite of daunting realities, women in poor urban communities continue to organize to create better lives for themselves and their children.

Chapter 11

Bearing Witness: Women in Cities as Agents of Transformation for God

Grace R. Dyrness

The women of Dolores Mission Church in Boyle Heights, Los Angeles, gathered together in the early 1990s to share the personal stories of tragedy and sorrow that prevailed in their community as a result of gang violence. Fear and pain permeated the neighborhood, and the women were tired, sad, and desperate, anxious to put a stop to the violence. As they met weekly in their parish Christian-based communities to study the scriptures, they discussed what relevance these sacred words had for them in their own situation. They came to understand that they needed to reach out to these "homeboys" (the local word for gang members) and let them know that violence would not be tolerated anymore and that they would work hard to provide alternatives for these youth. As the women began to put the meaning of the Gospels into practice, they held peace vigils on the corners of the community every Friday, praying for protection and the end to violence, and signaling to the homeboys that their actions would not be tolerated. At the same time, a group of these women worked with the parish priest to find jobs for the kids. To their dismay, few businesses would employ gang members—kids with tattoos that might turn away customers or, worse yet, might bring the violence into the business. Out of desperation, the women helped organize and raise funds for a tortilla factory that could employ these young people. Today, Homeboy Industries is a multifaceted outreach program that includes a silk-screening business, a Homegirl Café, a bakery, a charter school, a solar panel training program, tattoo removal, case management, job development, mental health counseling, and a variety of other programs. Father Greg Boyle, the Jesuit priest who is largely behind these efforts, credits the women of Dolores Mission for being the founding force behind Homeboy Industries (Boyle 2010).

A community that was wracked with violence and despair suddenly had hope that there was a pathway out, a future for the youth, and that deep wounds could begin to heal. It was the women's belief that their faith was relevant to their own situation that inspired them and held them together to work on solutions. Religion provides this hope for women in cities around the globe. Particularly in inner cities of the developed world and desperately poor cities of the developing world, women find in their faith a source of strength for creating change. This chapter examines some of the ways that women in cities turn to religion as a way to transcend their struggles for existence, and it explores some of the results of this engagement. Much of the chapter focuses on work that I did as part of research teams with other faculty at the University of Southern California, primarily through the Center for Religion and Civic Culture, and therefore Los Angeles is consistently used in examples of the role of religion, particularly in the lives of immigrants.

Religious Practice in Cities

Not only do cities provide a variety of opportunities for employment, entertainment, living styles, culinary diversity, and so forth, but they also provide many options for religious engagement, a diversity of paths to spiritual and mystical presence. There is considerable freedom of choice in most cities in religious practice; even for migrants who are surrounded by a kinship or ethnic group, the cultural restraints on making choices are rarely as limiting as they were in their village or their home country. Although immigrants in Los Angeles, when interviewed, expressed concern over the dangers of such pluralism, they also noted that they relished the freedom they experienced. Women interviewed commented that in the city they can practice their religion in public ways that were proscribed in their homelands, where they had to confine their worship to the home (Miller, Miller, and Dyrness 2002).

Religious practice takes a variety of forms, and for immigrants in particular it continues to exercise a strong attraction. In my research I have found at least four major ways in which faith and its practice have been particularly relevant to the women I have worked with: (1) religion as a source for building and strengthening a sense of community; (2) religion as a source for supplying a variety of needs, from providing emergency food and clothing, to helping to find employment, to building the skills needed to flourish; (3) religion as support in time of trouble; and (4) prayer used as a coping mechanism.

A Source of Community

Churches, temples, and mosques serve as a "conduit" for people who arrive in the city. Leaving home and moving to a new location is fraught with considerable anxiety and emotion, and it is comforting to know that there is a community at the far end of the road that shares one's values and understands the challenges the newcomer faces. In the new city, "religion addresses the problem of loneliness . . . by providing entry to a familiar community with familiar beliefs and practices that give structure and meaning to life—all elements of stability that are especially important in a new environment where expectations about what to believe or think are unclear. Indeed, worship and ritual have the potential to bind people together in ways that other institutions are not equipped to do" (Miller, Miller, and Dyrness 2002: 120).

Religion in cities is a source for community with fellow immigrants and with those who come from the same traditions. The religious institution is a place where one can speak one's native tongue, eat native food, and not insignificantly, find a husband (or wife) who shares the same cultural background. A group of Hindu women told us that they didn't mind doing the cooking for the temple's activities on the weekends because it provided a welcome time for them to see their friends and talk in Gujarati, catch up on news from India, and explore the latest Indian fashions (Miller, Miller, and Dyrness 2002). The Thai temple in North Hollywood, California, has established a Thai cultural center right next to the temple to help ensure that the traditions from the homeland are not lost on the next generation. Cambodian women send their young sons to the Khemara Buddikaram in Long Beach, California, to be mentored by the priests in hopes that they will engage with Cambodian culture and resist joining the gangs in Los Angeles. Religion, therefore, welcomes the stranger, provides a community that helps replace the one left behind, and enables new generations to connect with the past of their parents.

Supplying Needs

Migrant women also rely on religion for supplying their daily needs. These needs vary across the spectrum but most often the needs relate to the children of the family, including food, health, and, especially, education. Very often the church, temple, or mosque provides food and clothing in thrift stores and food pantries, job connections, job training, and sometimes even health care. But there are also intangible ways that religion reaches down to meet the needs of the women. This does not have to happen within the temple, mosque, or church; it can also happen within the religious spaces that women set up in their homes. Andrea Dyrness relates the story of one of the mothers engaged in a struggle to reform the school that her children were attending in Oakland, California: "On her kitchen counter, Ofelia kept a votive candle to La Virgen de Guadalupe always burning.[1] Ofelia was a devotee of La Virgen de Guadalupe. She believed she had the Virgin Mother to thank for her current home." She told the story of one of the hardest years in Ofelia's life: alone, away from all her friends, apart from her husband, who was serving prison time, and living with her mother-in-law, who seemed to resent her presence. Ofelia prayed incessantly that she would be able to find her own place to live. One night the Virgin of Guadalupe appeared to her in a dream, surrounded by a pool of water. "Don't worry," she told Ofelia. "Everything is going to work out." Soon after, a kindly neighbor told her that his rental house was becoming available and offered it to Ofelia. For Ofelia there was no doubt that the Virgin Mother supplied her need for a home. To this day, she keeps a votive candle burning in her kitchen as a reminder of her debt to the Virgin (Dyrness forthcoming: 166). For migrant women the ability to turn to their religion for supplying their needs is a great source of comfort, strength, and even survival. Whatever their needs, they know that ultimately they can count on their faith and their religious community to help them get through the rough times.

Support in Time of Trouble

Religious leaders often blur the line between counselors and spiritual mentors, even when they refer their flock to specialists when they are not capable of providing all the help needed. During our study of religion and immigrants in Los Angeles in 2000, we visited the Cambodian temple Khemara Buddikaram referred to earlier. Several hundred people were gathered to pay homage to their departed relatives. As Reverend Kong Chhean burned slips of paper on which the names of the deceased were written, family units sat together on the floor sharing a meal and remembering the events that brought them to this strange city. There was a young woman in the group who, as a child, had walked through the "killing fields" over dead bodies as she and her family made their escape. At the time of our visit, there were 150 documented cases of psychosomatic blindness among women in Long Beach who had witnessed the torture of their husbands, the rape of their daughters, and the destruction of their villages. Reverend Chhean, who has training in psychology, refers his members to a local clinic for medication and treatment when they are amenable to Western styles of intervention, and otherwise he performs magical incantations to help them cope with the trauma of their past (Miller, Miller, and Dyrness 2002). It is in the temple that the women find the help they need to support them in their troubles. Reverend Chhean told us that the women firmly resisted building the temple in a contemporary, modern style, insisting that it look exactly like the temples back home. The sanctity and familiarity of the space give them the courage to remember and move on. The women at the temple also turn to Reverend Chhean and his fellow priests to give guidance and support to their children, particularly the young men, to keep them out of trouble and out of gangs. This temple and others, as well as churches and mosques, serve to provide a space where women can lay down their burdens and get support and encouragement to face their troubles.

Prayer as a Way to Cope

Personal prayers are at the core of many of the women's faith. Prayer often serves as a way to cope with the struggles that they face in the city. Whether the prayers are for their children who are engaged in violent gang activity, as in the case of the women at Dolores Mission, or for safety and protection in the insecure slum and squatter settlements in which many women live, prayer is a connection with the supernatural, the transcendent, that lifts them out of the ordinary and offers them hope of a God who can enter into their situation and provide the help they need. Ernestine Avila, in her unpublished research on transnational parenting, states that for the immigrants she interviewed prayer was the coping mechanism that cut through all of life (Avila n.d.). In the course of new migratory movements, women frequently have to leave their families behind in order to provide financially for the family. As mothers leave their children behind in the care of grandparents or other relatives, the deep sorrow of separation is a daily reminder of the world they have left behind, particularly when they are caring for the children of their employers. Thus Avila found that both mothers and fathers pray to an omnipresent God to help with their personal suffering. They also pray to God for help with the challenges related to finding work and performing their jobs so they can meet their financial obligations. Mothers ask God to watch over their children and keep them safe. In the words of one woman she interviewed, Angelina, "I pray the rosary and at times I'm praying while I work. When I'm working and can't [pray the rosary], because I have the children, I sometimes can't, but sometimes I'm praying still while I'm working. I take my time to say my prayers so that I can feel better. Prayer helps me a lot. . . . I feel God is with me. And I ask God for help. . . . I pray for my daughters. I ask God that my daughters will be safe and well back home" (Avila n.d.).

Prayer not only helps parents cope with their daily challenges as immigrant workers in the United States (and many other countries), but prayer helps to collapse the physical distance between them and their families back home. In sum, prayer is one way transnational mothers and fathers transcend the distance from their families; although the distance is still felt on many levels, it helps them cope with the separation. Furthermore, Avila says, for transnational mothers, the hope and prayer is that this separation is for an anticipated good that, in the long run, will benefit their families.

In July of 2000 the Salvadoran community in Los Angeles brought a replica of their sacred patron, El Divino Salvador del Mundo [Divine Savior of the World], to Los Angeles. As the figure was carried in the back of a truck and paraded through the streets, people crowded around, wiping away tears and beaming smiles as this transnational symbol of hope and peace came toward them (Miller, Miller, and Dyrness 2002: 102). We watched as people walked up to the image, touching it, praying to it. I saw tears stream down the cheeks of one woman. Carefully I went up to her and asked her why this was so significant. Her response provoked deep emotion in me: She had migrated from El Salvador and had not seen her mother in seventeen years. This Christ, the exact replica of the one back home, could transcend the space and bring them together again in some intangible, spiritual way. It had been kissed and blessed by her mother back in El Salvador before it embarked on the journey to Los Angeles. She could now pray, and it would unite them. In some extraordinary, mysterious way, prayer helps this woman cope with the sorrow of being so far away.

Women of Faith Serve Their Cities

For many women of faith, reaching out to others in their communities is a natural response of gratitude for what God has done for them. It is their response to a mandate that they should love their neighbor, however differently they might define who their neighbor is. Women engage in multiple ways of service to those who are needy: feeding the hungry, teaching marketable skills, healing the sick, educating the children, caring for the elderly, and so many others. The following are the stories of three women of faith who have reached out to their communities in different ways. Like these women, many others are quietly and faithfully transforming their communities. The stories illustrate how a single person, inspired by her faith, can have a broad impact on her city through serving others. The three women came into their service by different roads: one through a vision, one through the urging of her colleagues, and the other through a personal calling, but all three came into service out of a deep compassion for the very poor.

Training to Heal

Working among the Masaii tribe in southern Kenya as a medical doctor in 1997, Florence Muindi saw a vision.[2] She and her husband were going through a period of trying to discern if and when they could go to Ethiopia to work, something she felt God had been calling her to do since 1984. As she looked out the window of her home, she saw the clouds, and in the middle of the clouds she saw a mountain in such vivid detail that she was sure it was in Ethiopia. She quickly sketched it in her Bible with all of its detail, including rocks and trees growing on its side. A few weeks later, the Muindis flew to Ethiopia to assess the opportunity of service there. They arrived in a very remote area to visit a health clinic that needed Dr. Muindi's help and went to sit in the shade under some trees to get respite from the 42 degree Celsius heat (nearly 108 degrees Fahrenheit). As they sat on some benches, Florence looked out across the valley. She says, "I nearly fainted. Right there before us was a replica of the very image God had showed me earlier. I ran back into the tent and poured out the contents of my bag, looking for my Bible. When I saw it, I opened to the first page where I had drawn the image. Sitting there we compared the details. It was indeed the exact reproduction of the image I had seen in the vision. Our God is amazing! Now I knew! God had put up a clear road sign. The decision was made" (Muindi 2008: 73).

Dr. Florence Muindi began her work among the people of the Mekanisa slum in Addis Ababa, Ethiopia, in 1999. She started with a colleague doing a required health screening exercise, and what she found was shocking: Over 80 percent of the children were sick, and more than 50 percent of the sick children had at least two active diseases. Most of these illnesses were caused by lack of health education and basic hygiene. These findings served as the baseline data from which Dr. Muindi developed her strategy: She would train members of the little local church in a basic health curriculum that she had developed based on her experience among the Masaii as well as other materials she found. One health agent was selected and trained for every ten homes targeted. The main goal was to bring health knowledge to the homes, with the desire to change attitudes and practices and thereby improve people's health. After six months, when Dr. Muindi and her team did a second screening, they saw a big reduction in disease rates. Encouraged by this result, the divided the community into clusters of forty families each and focused on changing behavior patterns and mobilizing people to do something about their own health needs; this empowerment helped the families begin to address other needs as well.

Today this model has expanded into several other communities in Ethiopia, Kenya, southern and northern Sudan, Djibouti, and Cairo. To oversee this expansion, Dr. Muindi has established a nongovernmental organization, Life in Abundance International (LIA). As of 2008, LIA had teams and national boards in seven countries and over seventy full-time staff (Muindi 2008: 109). Dr. Muindi clearly sees all of this as the work of her God. She believes that God is in the business of guiding his people, and she takes to heart passages of Scripture such as one from Psalms 32:8—"I will instruct you and teach you in the way you should go; I will counsel you and watch over you" (Muindi 2008: 108). Faith motivates, inspires, and guides her. She is transforming one slum community after another as she lives out her faith. The vision that propelled her to Ethiopia has sustained her and enabled her to continue her work.

Caring for Vulnerable Children

Over 2.5 million people live in slum settlements in Nairobi, Kenya, representing 60 percent of the total population of the city. Approximately 1 million of these live in Kibera, the largest slum in Africa. The United Nations Office for the Coordination of Humanitarian Affairs estimates that there are approximately 60,000 street children in Nairobi alone (IRIN 2010a), a good portion of them living in Kibera. Praxedes Mozilla is a woman living in Kibera who is caring for 500 of these children. Her story begins when she was a teacher in the local elementary school. On her way to school she often observed children sleeping under the tables of street vendors. She felt compassion but did not feel it was her responsibility to respond, until the day some of her colleagues asked her to go with them to see two of these children. Praxedes was stunned: Here were twin toddlers, severely malnourished, who had been abandoned by their mother. Her colleagues urged her to do something about this because, they said, she was the one who had a heart. Filled with compassion, Praxedes found the mother and discovered that she had acted on a tribal custom that requires a single mother to abandon her babies if they are twins. Praxedes helped the mother re-connect with her babies and promised to help her care for them, but the whole situation caused a crisis in her faith. A devout Roman Catholic, she was angry with God: Why should all of these children suffer? Is God loving them? Unable to answer those questions, she began feeding some of the children, who now followed her on her way to school. For two years she fed twenty-five street children every day. She began to identify with the feelings of abandonment that these children had; she herself had been abandoned by her husband and left with two small children. But after two years, Praxedes could not continue, as she had no resources to draw on, and she told the children she could no longer help them. To her surprise, the children responded by saying, "Just stay with us and when God gives to you, you can give to us" (Mozilla 2010). Deeply touched, Praxedes prayed and told God that she would carry this cross but he must help her. In the middle of the Kibera slum, this woman of faith started a school with twenty-five children in 1998, Baraka za Ibrahim [Blessing of Abraham]. Today, more than 500 children are in her care, some of whom live on site at the school and others on a farm just outside Nairobi. She has received training in trauma counseling and business management. Together, she and the children grow vegetables for consumption and for sale in order to sustain the school. The surrounding community has responded by helping out, but women have also asked Praxedes for training in group savings and loan programs and business development. This has resulted in the formation of twenty groups of fifteen to twenty-five women each, who were trained by Praxedes and became empowered to bring change to their own families. Praxedes never dreamed that starting her little school would have such an impact on the whole community!

When violence erupted in Kenya in 2009 as a result of the presidential elections, Kibera was at its center. As fires raged around the neighborhood and houses were destroyed, Praxedes tried to drown out the screams by giving the children musical instruments to play so they would not hear what was happening outside. These children have since formed a marching band with uniforms that is known throughout the slum and plays regularly at special occasions. During the violence, Baraka za Ibrahim was protected by the women in the surrounding community who would not allow it to be burned. For Praxedes Mozilla the words that keep her going are from God: "Where there is darkness I will go to bring light" (Mozilla 2010). These words energize and sustain her, even in the midst of crisis. She, like Florence Muindi, is inspired by her faith, and she is transforming her community in Kibera as a result.

Empowering Through Skills Training

When I was a little girl, my mother would take me with her to the very poor, marginalized communities of San Jose, Costa Rica, where we lived. Mother brought together women who were skilled in sewing to teach other women a skill that could earn them some income and thus move them out of intense poverty. Mother would say to me: "*Dios entra por los dedos y transforma la vida de las mujeres*" [God enters through the fingers and transforms the lives of the women]. In my research around the world, I have found many examples of such women who, inspired and motivated by their faith, reach out to provide skills for marginalized, poor women and in so doing begin a transformation that goes beyond their own expectations or imagination.

The World Economic Forum lists five important dimensions of female empowerment and opportunity that are ways of measuring global patterns of inequality between men and women; the top two are economic participation and economic opportunity (the others are political empowerment, educational attainment, and health and well-being) (Lopez-Claros and Zahidi 2005: 2). Economic opportunity concerns the *quality* of women's economic involvement, a serious problem even in developed countries, where women are often in jobs that are characterized by the absence of upward mobility and opportunity. In developing countries large numbers of women participate in the informal sector of the economy, and in some parts of the world women provide about 70 percent of agricultural labor and produce over 90 percent of the food yet are not represented in the budget deliberations of their countries (Lopez-Claros and Zahidi 2005: 3). The World Economic Forum's report on women's empowerment states that "the term 'feminization of poverty' is often used to illustrate the fact that the majority of the 1.5 billion people living on US$1 a day or less are women and that the gap between women and men caught in the cycle of poverty has not lessened, but may well have widened in the past decade" (Lopez-Claros and Zahidi 2005: 4). There is much to be said about women's empowerment through economic opportunity, but it is beyond the scope of this chapter. However, in the cities of the developing world the situation is so dire for women that this issue has become central to the work of some nonprofit organizations in particular, many of which have been established by women moved with compassion for their sisters in poverty. Such is the case of Lucy Engjadim, who lives in the city of Guwahati, Assam, India.

Guwahati is a major city in eastern India and one of the country's fastest growing cities with a population of more than 800,000 as of 2001 (Bhattacharyya 2010). Lucy lives in the heart of this city. A migrant to Guwahati in 1997, Lucy feels privileged, as she has a husband with a good, steady job. Around her, people struggle for their daily existence. Eighty percent of the families in Guwahati rely on a single, often fluctuating, income brought in by the father or husband, who is usually a rickshaw puller or daily laborer. Lucy observed that the women she sees and meets are suffering the most from this harsh life; as she put it, the women are caught in "an unending struggle to stretch their meager resources so the family does not starve. . . . In such conditions, their self-respect and integrity are very low" (Engjadim 2009: 11). Lucy tells how she was moved with compassion for these women but felt helpless to do anything: "What can an ordinary woman do? I do not even know the local language. I am just an ordinary woman" (Engjadim 2009: 12). She felt frustrated by her inability to help these women. With no resources, training, experience, or affiliation to any organization, she felt limited and felt that the problems were bigger than she could handle.

Shortly after arriving in the city in 1997, Lucy was invited to attend the World Micro-Credit Conference in Washington, D.C. There she heard testimonials and sharing of experiences by different people from many countries of the world where it seemed as though miracles were being achieved "out of nothing." It was at the conference that she realized she had been too focused on her own limitations and not trusting her God to supply what she needed. "Out of nothing," she said, "God can work miracles" (Engjadim 2009: 13).

Returning to Guwahati, Lucy secured a loan to buy five sewing machines. A church in the city offered her space, and she began teaching women a skill that would provide a future for them. In 1997 Lucy founded the Priscilla Centre, where participants selected by the community are provided with one year of free training in vocational skills (stitching and embroidery to start with) and also receive counseling and personal development training. Part of the innovative aspect of the program is that the women must participate in a compulsory savings program so that by the time they graduate they can purchase their own sewing machines. The Priscilla Centre operates on a fair-trade basis, striving to ensure that weavers, designers, and tailors get fair wages. Today, there are ten Priscilla Centres in various communities. As Lucy says, "This work was entrusted to me not because of a clever plan and abundant resources, or that I had business experience or that the infrastructure was available, but because of the need and the faith we had in God to help us, and so we took the first faltering step" (Engjadim 2009: 23).

A vision, the urging of a group of colleagues, and a personal call—three responses from women who because of their faith have been able to transform communities in the cities where they live.

Women of Faith Mobilize for Civic Engagement

Religion is also an arena for mobilization, civic participation, and solidarity. The cases discussed in the previous section are based on an individual response to faith and religion. In many of the more evangelical Christian traditions this response is essential and part of the expectation for participation in the religion.[3] However, many women are engaged in religious institutional efforts within their communities, and while their participation may be an individual response to action, it is within or at the very least under the leadership of the religious institutions and does not arise as an independent action. Richard Wood, in his study on faith-based community organizing (Wood 2002), makes a point that institutions matter to democratic life, and that political action depends crucially upon cultural work done outside the political arena. In the United States, the hard work of organizing and building community where all voices are heard is often done within churches, synagogues, mosques, and other houses of worship (Wood 2002: 262). "Religious culture matters," Wood states, "because it is taken seriously by large numbers of people—and thus orients their lives either toward or away from political engagement and the habits of the heart that can sustain it" (Wood 2002: 263).

Religion provides a means for immigrants to transform their new surroundings into meaningful spiritual, cultural, and sometimes political places that facilitate their societal integration and yet help them maintain and nurture their distinct cultural identities as immigrants. Pierrette Hondagneu-Sotelo identified at least four critical factors to consider as a way of understanding what religion has to offer political and social movements: (1) It can provide social movement actors with moral justification and motivation for action; (2) it can provide immigrants and their political supporters with resources—social networks and concrete items—necessary for successful mobilization; (3) it offers legitimacy to unpopular causes because "religious authority, faith-based morality, and the 'higher law' of God and the scriptures may be used to persuade others of the need to remedy injustices in secular institutions"; and (4) it offers ritual and shared cultural practices that serve to hold people together and evoke feelings of excitement and togetherness (Hondagneu-Sotelo 2008: 19–21).

These multiple roles of religion are evident in Los Angeles. Many organizing groups engage clergy and religious leaders into their network in order to effectively promote their agenda. There are numerous examples, such as Faith Communities for Families and Children, which advocates for the rights of foster children; the Interfaith Coalition for Immigrant Rights; and Interfaith Communities United for Justice and Peace, both of which advocate against violence and war. These organizations, in some form or another, use religion in the ways outlined by Hondagneu-Sotelo. In a later section of this chapter I describe the work of one of these organizations, Clergy and Laity United for Economic Justice (CLUE), which has had a powerful impact on promoting worker justice. First, however, the broader topic of religion and social justice is discussed to show how religion can be used as a tool for social justice and how this role can be usurped into oppression and violence against women.

Religion and Social Justice

Although religion does provide support for social justice, my colleagues and I have discovered that, for better or worse, religion can also play a disruptive role in the community. Los Angeles's high tolerance for religious variety and salience of religious practices does not necessarily indicate that all segments of the city embrace these new religious communities. Whereas some people passively tolerate these incursions, others exhibit prejudice against these "foreign" religions or "foreign" expressions of religiosity particularly when they become aware of plans to build a temple, shrine, synagogue, church, or mosque, or when they have to share their congregational spaces and rituals with immigrant groups. Opposition can take the same NIMBY (Not in My Backyard) form that, for example, a homeless shelter might encounter, accompanied by complaints about a threat to "our way of life." Prejudice against immigrant communities and their religions or religious expressions is also expressed in violent forms at times, as some Muslims (and those mistaken for Muslims) have learned in the period following September 11, 2001, and as some Latina/os have faced with the rise of an anti-illegal immigration climate in the United States. In Los Angeles, for example, Reverend Frank Alton, previously senior pastor of Immanuel Presbyterian Church, was the recipient of hate mail and antagonistic voice messages in 2007 after a radio program announced nationally that a pro-immigrant march would begin in front of the church's doorstep.

For women, religion can be a roadblock to empowerment. The Scriptures from the Christian, Jewish, and Islamic faith traditions, for example, contain passages that condone violence and male domination over women. It is beyond the scope of this chapter to document those passages; however, they have been used to justify and support the use of control and domination. One need only look at the way some denominations within the Christian tradition have determined issues on birth control and abortion, or the way in which fundamentalism within Islam in the form of the Taliban, for example, determines that girls and women cannot receive an education.

The National Resource Center on Domestic Violence (NRCDV) in Harrisburg, Pennsylvania, has worked to provide understanding about the roadblocks and resources that religion provides for women. Scholars at the NRCDV have demonstrated that specific passages in the

Scriptures that might seem to condone violence need to be understood within a much larger context of the sacred Scriptures as a whole. The selective use of a text to justify actions distorts and does not represent the whole story. The NRCDV has produced resource materials to help provide insight into the seemingly contradictory positions. As noted in one of these resources, "Tragically, a critical look at the history of much of our collective religious teaching makes clear that religious institutions have explicitly or implicitly shaped the context of values which have tolerated violence against women. Indeed, examples of violence against and the silencing of women appear in many places in authoritative texts of our religious traditions. Yet there also exist persistent sources within our various traditions which, when explored and given voice, offer powerful resources for strength and courage, as well as compassion and justice, for those who have been harmed by the acts of another in the community" (Fortune and Enger 2006: 3). These are the sources that have provided the courage and strength to the women that I have studied in my research and especially for those I have described in this chapter.

Clergy and Laity United for Economic Justice

When religious institutions are positive forces for social justice, migrant and marginalized women find within them a place of security and support, and an arena for seeking justice in their own situations. CLUE illustrates this in a way that is particularly effective for women workers.

Located in Los Angeles, California, CLUE is one of the strongest religious-based labor support organizations in the country (Hondagneu-Sotelo 2008: 76). Organized in 1996 by the Los Angeles Alliance for a New Economy (LAANE) as a means of gaining the support of clergy and religious leaders for its struggles of economic justice, CLUE's mission is to educate, organize, and mobilize the faith community to walk with workers and their families in their struggle for good jobs and dignity in the workplace. CLUE's unique contribution to the worker justice movement is that it organizes religious leaders in the struggle, thus providing three important additions to the movement: (1) engaging the religious community, often the only functioning community in depressed areas, which brings people together across wide divides as equal members in one congregation; (2) providing inspiration and support, where clergy and leaders act as "chaplains" encouraging workers to remember their deepest values and providing emotional/spiritual support; and (3) breaking down community barriers, since religious leaders call on their moral authority to raise questions of justice that affect the quality of the whole community (CLUE 2010).

Although CLUE does not devote itself exclusively to the struggles for economic justice of immigrant workers, in Los Angeles the majority of workers in low-wage, marginalized jobs are Latino immigrants and many of these are women. One of CLUE's most successful campaigns has been in support of hotel workers, those invisible people who provide all the services for the fine hotels of the city and who are in many ways the backbone of the global economy (Sassen 1991). According to CLUE, 44 percent of these workers are women. Few people know the level of work it takes to maintain a comfortable and hospitable space in Los Angeles's expensive luxury hotels, or the human cost of that luxury. Luxury hotel workers are susceptible to high rates of injury because of crippling workloads. They often make poverty wages and are denied respect on the job. Without a union or community support, workers who are fighting for change are easily fired or otherwise discriminated against. Through CLUE's efforts, religious leaders across Los Angeles have brought prophetic witness to this struggle, offering workers chaplaincy when they are retaliated against by management, visiting management and asking for a process for unionization, and otherwise advocating for the workers. They employ the ancient symbols of their faith, performing foot washing and healing services in the street, and they speak at city council and other venues to help ensure a better future for the people who create a home away from home for Los Angeles's guests. After an outpouring of support from religious and community leaders and workers, the Los Angeles County Board of Supervisors passed a historic living wage law in the fall of 1999 requiring tourism industry corporations to meet a fair standard for wages and benefits. Enacted for the purpose of both economic justice and community improvement, the law was implemented after a yearlong court battle. The City of Los Angeles followed suit by passing a living wage law in 2006. The struggle continues with the hotels, as religious leaders work with immigrant and community organizations to secure better contracts for the workers that include benefits, particularly health insurance coverage.

Francisca, a hotel worker, described how hotel managers had forced workers to meet clandestinely. Hotel security guards threatened the workers, and many feared losing their jobs. But Francisca stood up in a meeting with religious leaders and said, "I'm here to ask all of the priests to support us in this campaign. I know that once our coworkers see the church is behind us, they will join our union. Right now, they are too frightened. . . . *Sacerdotes* [priests, ministers], we need you to support us . . . and accompany us on our march" (Hondagneu-Sotelo 2008: 94).

Clergy are deeply transformed by testimonials such as this one. Their participation greatly strengthens the movement, as workers feel more confident and safe with their presence on the front line (Figure 11.1).

224 Grace R. Dyrness

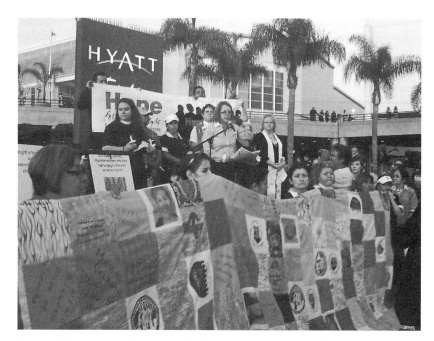

Figure 11.1. Clergy and religious leaders gather to advocate for hotel workers in Los Angeles. (Photo courtesy of Clergy and Laity United for Economic Justice [CLUE-LA], www.cluela.org.)

Maria (name has been changed to protect her identity) told me that she felt she could join the struggle for justice because of all the priests and pastors that have come out to support the workers. She trusts them. They have made a difference for her and over 1,000 other hotel workers.

Faith-based community organizing provides a voice for people at the margins, empowering them to get engaged in working for change, in making a difference in their communities. It is particularly important for women. A young Latina woman we interviewed in our research on the Active Citizenship Campaign of the Industrial Areas Foundation told us that the community organizing process and the support from her congregation provided her with the space and place to develop her own potential. She said she suddenly was given a voice as an advocate for her people (Miller, Miller, and Dyrness 2002: 124). In an interview with Richard Wood, Judy Reyes, a leader in another faith-based organizing group, was asked how the experience in community organizing had affected her life. She responded, "That's what we do, we get people engaged in things they never used to think made a difference. Before, I never did and I had no sense of power, of being able to affect anything in the political realm. . . . It's really hard, especially for women. We don't get a lot of opportunities to be leaders in society. Just to call myself a leader is a huge thing. I take a great deal of pride in it because I've always had these abilities and I've tried to use them. But before I'd never found the place where they were valued. I was always shut out or shut down. . . . Here the more I put into this the more I got. I saw results" (Wood 2002: 279–80).

Conclusion

Not all women experience religion as a positive force in their lives. Indeed, it can be a means of oppression and a roadblock to women's empowerment, particularly within the home. Domestic abuse is one issue that appears to transcend religions and cultures. Violence against women has reached epidemic proportions, and faith does not always eliminate this violence. A survey of 500 clergy and lay workers conducted by the Methodist Church in Britain in 2000-2002 found that one in four women in church-going homes has experienced or witnessed family violence as a child or adult, which mirrors the experience of British women in the general population (Radford and Cappel 2002). The report finds that many faith traditions can be harmful when interpretations of their sacred scriptures are twisted to support the violence. This can leave a woman of faith in turmoil: When she is abused, her domestic violence crisis is a spiritual crisis as well because she will question "Why me? Why am I being hurt like this? Why am I suffering? Where is God? Is God listening to me and hearing my cries of pain and hurt and suffering?" These are theological questions that require theological answers. Nevertheless, it is encouraging to note that there are numerous attempts from within the religious community to address these twisted interpretations of scriptures. For example, Jewish Women International has provided a resource guide for rabbis on domestic violence, the Presbyterian Church U.S.A. formed a task force on healing domestic violence, and the World Evangelical Fellowship's Commission on Women's Concerns has formed a task force to educate evangelical clergy, support efforts that would reduce violence, and offer avenues of healing to offenders (Radford and Cappel 2002). In Los Angeles, one of the important efforts for Muslim women in this regard has come from the Muslim Women's League, which is training women to read Arabic so that they can read the Qur'an on their own and thus be empowered to speak out against twisted interpretations.

Religion, however, is most often a source of support and empowerment for women, particularly in cities where diversity and pluralism open the door to alternatives to oppressive systems. Religion provides a community that welcomes the stranger, it supplies many of the needs of its members, and it comes alongside them in times of trouble, providing emotional and spiritual guidance. This community of faith surrounds many women, some of whom, inspired by their faith, take it upon themselves to respond to the needs they see in the city out of a personal conviction and calling. In addition to working on their own to meet the needs they find, they often establish organizations that can multiply their efforts. Other women choose to work within already established religious institutions or groups. The women whose stories I have told in this chapter bear witness to the impact women can have when they exercise their faith. No matter the path that they choose, or the way in which they come to that path, these women care deeply about their families, their neighbors, and their communities, and they are motivated and inspired by their faith to do all they can to respond to the needs they see around them. These stories show the impact that women can have working for change, finding resources, building networks, joining coalitions, and in myriad ways responding to the hardship around them, sustained by their religious beliefs.

Chapter 12

Accessibility to Health Care in Urban Environments

Francisca M. Mwangangi

The World Health Organization (WHO) defines health as a state of complete physical, mental, and social well-being and not merely the absence of disease or infirmity. The WHO has further elaborated that "the health of all the people is fundamental to the attainment of peace and security and is dependent upon the fullest co-operation of individuals and states" and that "the enjoyment of the highest attainable standards of health" is one of the fundamental rights of every human being (WHO 2000).

A population's health and productivity are directly linked. This relationship has been demonstrated in industrialized countries, which are now benefiting from years of investment in health services (Schultz and Tansel 1993). Provision of good health services satisfies a basic human need and contributes significantly toward maintaining and enhancing the productive potential of the people.

Improving health services reduces production losses caused by worker illnesses, permits the use of national funds otherwise totally or nearly inaccessible because of disease, and increases children's enrollment in school and their ability to learn (Mwabu et al. 2004). Therefore, increasing consumption of health-care services in the population should be a priority in all countries. Increasing access is the most effective way to increase the utilization of health-care services.

In its simplest sense, access refers to entry into or use of the health-care system. When health care is accessible, the health of every member of society improves because people are able to obtain care when necessary without facing obstacles. When health care is not accessible, mortality rates will be high and many people will be debilitated by disease. Access is one of the fundamental goals of every health-care system.

A major responsibility of every government is to provide effective and accessible health care to all of its citizens.

For the majority, the term "access" refers to health-care services that are within reach. The term goes beyond the availability of health-care services to refer to the elimination of personal, organizational, and financial barriers to service utilization. Obrist and colleagues have identified three aspects of accessible health care: availability, acceptability, and affordability (Obrist et al. 2007). Lack of access to health care results when any one of these three aspects of accessibility is missing.

"Availability" means that existing health services and goods meet clients' needs. Services and goods should be offered by an adequate number of skilled personnel. Supplies should cover demand. Health-care facilities should be within reach geographically. Health-care services should be organized in a manner that meets patients' needs: For example, hours of operation should be based around clients' schedules, taking into account, for instance, the daily work schedule of the small-scale business person or farmer. The health-care facilities should be clean and well kept.

"Affordability" means that the price of health care fits clients' income and ability to pay. Both direct and indirect costs of health care should be within a client's ability to pay; for example, a client should be able to pay for the consultation fee, the cost of drugs, and transportation to the health facility.

Last, "acceptability" of health care means that the information, explanations, and treatments provided take into account the clients' cultural and social values. Patients should feel welcome and cared for and have trust in the competence and personality of their health-care providers.

Differences in access to health care can have far-reaching consequences, with those denied access to basic health care living shorter and more constrained lives. Writing in 1990, Amartya Sen estimated that 100 million more women would have been alive, primarily in China, South Asia, and North Africa, if women and girls had equal access to health care and nutrition across the globe (Sen 1990). Equal access to health care is therefore a prerequisite for equality of opportunity in society.

In developing countries, health care can be accessed from such facilities as the following:

1. Hospitals, health centers, and clinics run by the central government
2. Municipality or city council-controlled facilities

3. Facilities run by faith-based organizations
4. Private sector facilities—both for-profit and nonprofit

Access to Health Care in Urban Settings: Issues, Challenges, and Opportunities

As earlier chapters have described, a lack of basic services—including safe water, sanitation, and good shelter—in rapidly expanding, poor, urban areas creates health problems that, in turn, create an enormous need for health care among those living in these areas. However, the urban poor face the greatest barriers to accessing health care. An understanding of these barriers is critical to improving health-care access for all.

Challenges stem from both the demand and supply side of health care. From the demand side, access and utilization of services can be influenced by personal, family, and community factors and the perceived benefits of the health-care system. On the supply side, the government influences the provision of health-care services. Government policies on staff distribution and allocation of medical resources affect how and where health care will be provided. In Kenya, for example, urban slums are predominantly served by privately owned and unlicensed health facilities with limited skilled staff and equipment; most of the formal health facilities are located outside of the slums (Fotso et al. 2009). Essentially, the slum dwellers are struggling to pay for inferior health care.

Another challenge to improving access to health care is the dearth of good research on urban health in developing countries. This lack of information affects planning and resource allocation for the urban poor. Data specific to the health of urban populations often suffers from at least one weakness: Most often, health data are aggregated to provide an average for all urban residents—wealthy and poor, men and women—rather than disaggregated by income or gender. The data thus mask the health conditions of the urban poor and of urban women. A multisectoral approach that involves different players—the ministries or departments of housing, environment, water and sanitation, public health, finance, and planning, among others—in collecting data on the urban poor is necessary to paint a true picture of this population's state of health.

Rapid population growth has made it especially difficult to improve urban conditions and poses enormous challenges for governments in providing health care, as governments are overwhelmed by demands on local economies, public services, and infrastructures. This problem is compounded by poor planning and scarce resources, which have resulted in overcrowded health-care facilities with long waits and lack of access to even the most basic services. A good example of this is Kenya, whose national-referral hospital—Kenyatta National Hospital in Nairobi—is often overstretched, with patients often waiting for days or weeks to get a bed. The waiting list for nonemergency surgery is just as long. Health-care facilities that were built for smaller populations can no longer cope with the demands of an ever-growing populace. Governments will have to allocate a substantial portion of their budgets to health care if the trend is to be reversed.

Government policies can also hinder access to medical services and obstruct the care of chronic conditions among poor urban dwellers. According to research conducted by the African Population and Health Research Centre (APHRC) in Nairobi—the capital city of Kenya—17 percent of people living in urban slums suffer from diabetes or hypertension and cannot get screening services or drugs; this is partly due to government policies that restrict delivery of these services to doctors operating at the district hospital level or above. Lower-level health facilities—those that are within reach of the slum population—are not equipped with the necessary equipment for screening conditions such as diabetes and hypertension; the medical staff in these facilities are not even trained in caring for patients with these conditions.

Making health care "acceptable" can be another challenge. Previous experience with medical care can determine whether one will go back to the health facility for continued care: Women have been known to refuse to go to providers for health-care services because they had bad experiences in the past with those providers. In addition, a health provider's approach may hinder women from accessing health-care services (Khan et al. 2009). For example, lack of respect for local customs by health-care providers may discourage women from seeking health services. Health workers who demonstrate respect for local customs are more likely to gain acceptance from the people they serve.

Making health care "affordable" is another challenge; with urban poverty growing, the question of affordability will only become more urgent. Growing urban poverty is a major international concern. About 30 percent of the poor now live in urban areas. By 2035 the proportion is projected to reach 50 percent. Most of the urban poor live in slums and squatter settlements without adequate access to clean water, sanitation, and health care. While health and child survival rates are better on average in urban than in rural areas, they often are worse for the poor than for other urban residents. So, not only do the poor suffer worse health, but they are also less likely to be able to afford the care necessary to address their health problems.

The urban poor might not be in a position to afford health-care services unless better methods of health-care financing are deployed (as discussed further later in this chapter). This problem with affordability is especially apparent when patients must pay fees for service. Most of the urban poor lack the purchasing power for health-care services.

Women face unique challenges in accessing health care. Of all population groups women suffer disproportionately from the barrier of lack of affordability in health care. In general, of the 1.3 billion poorest people in the world, 70 percent are women (Harcourt 2001). Women's poverty affects their health needs and their ability to use health services. Within households, women bear an inequitable burden in providing food, health care, and shelter for themselves and their families. Women also face social and physical barriers to accessing health-care services, especially due to their disproportionate need for reproductive health care. Social and physical barriers include the long distances and poor transportation networks to health-care facilities, which are especially challenging for pregnant women and those with small babies. Another difficulty is the discrimination suffered by women and girls, which often limits their opportunities to participate in decision-making. Because many societies are patriarchal and women are excluded from financial decision-making, women often have difficulty accessing basic medical care. As a result, they are at increased risk for various reproductive, communicable, and noncommunicable diseases. The Millennium Development Goals (MDGs) attempt to reduce the unacceptably high levels of maternal and child morbidity and mortality by drawing attention to the urgency of this situation as well as by pressing for increased funding and policy development to address this situation.

Lack of access to resources and to equal decision-making power means that when poor women face out-of-pocket health-care costs such as user fees, they may be unable to afford them (Nanda 2002). Much of the literature and debates on user fees and health-care access neglect the ways in which user fees are regressive in regard to gender. The overall lack of gender-disaggregated data in the studies on user fees exemplifies the problem (Standing 1997).

For poor women in both rural and urban areas, user fees have direct and obvious links to whether these women can afford health care. Where women are struggling to make ends meet, they have little to save for contingencies, which include sickness and injuries. Poor women may forgo health care in order to purchase food or fuel; alternately, they may seek lower-cost traditional health care that does not address their health needs adequately (Gilson 1997). Further, women in subsistence economies may not have the cash income necessary to pay user fees, and even if they do have the income available, men may have control over their earnings. Poverty has driven a worrying number of urban women to engage in commercial sex work in pursuit of the cash they need to meet their, and often their families', health-care and other needs. This work puts them on a dangerous pedestal of exposure to diseases and poor access to health.

Increasing Access to Health Care in Urban Environments

Since health is a basic human right, it is important to look at access to health care from a human rights perspective.

A critical analysis of the health-care system in developing countries reveals that the huge burden of disease suffered by the deprived majority in both urban and rural areas is not just an unfortunate accident. Rather, it results from deep, structural injustices and the systematic denial of healthy lifestyles to the most vulnerable. These issues should be addressed within a human rights framework that should empower each person to demand health care as a right (Dreze and Sen 2002).

For the vast majority of the poor population, the key barrier to good health is not a lack of technology within the health system; rather, inequity effectively denies a vast majority of the population their human rights to health. Poverty, a manifestation of social inequity, leads to large sections of the population being denied adequate nutrition, clean drinking water and sanitation, basic education, good-quality housing, and a healthy local environment, which are all determinants of health. At the same time, highly inequitable health systems deny quality health care to those who cannot afford it. Even in public hospitals, health care is not free, as users are expected to share the costs.

Strengthening the human rights of women, children, and marginalized groups is an important first step in addressing accessibility. For a variety of economic, social, and cultural reasons, the human rights of such groups have been eroded in most urban areas by the very institutions that are expected to protect them.

These groups are disproportionately affected by HIV/AIDS and have more limited capacity and access to resources to prevent and treat infection. Women in particular not only face a double burden of communicable and noncommunicable diseases but also have the added responsibility of looking after sick family members. Cancer, diabetes, and heart diseases are now leading the list of noncommunicable diseases in women.

In a climate of discrimination, people are less likely to seek preventive screening and so do not get treatment, care, and support when ill. This in turn hinders efforts by health-care institutions to control disease.

The right to health care should be made a legally enforceable entitlement. Realizing the core right to health care will require the development of national health policies with comprehensive plans and timetables. Additionally, health infrastructure essential to the treatment of cancer and other noncommunicable diseases will have to be developed, as it is currently unavailable. These changes will require money and political will: Investing sufficient resources in health care and allocating these funds in a cost-effective and fair manner will be critical, as will lobbying and educating politicians.

Other measures include adopting a comprehensive strategy based on a gender perspective so as to overcome inequalities in women's access to health facilities and making screening for cancer and lifestyle diseases a component of reproductive health. Such a strategy will entail empowering women to know what to demand and expect from the health-care system.

The catchphrase "Prevention Is Better Than Cure" (and certainly cheaper) has been used without paying due consideration to the difference its application could make in developing countries. Considering that most deaths in these countries occur from preventable diseases, increasing the consumption of preventive services will reduce mortality from these diseases. Several studies conducted in low- and medium-income countries (African Medical and Research Foundation 2004; Nyamwaya 2008; Obrist et al. 2007) have shown that the utilization of preventive-care services can promote healthier lifestyles, provide early detection of illnesses, and reduce the need for subsequent inpatient care. On a more individual level, a low-cost approach that can rapidly be implemented entails empowering the population—from schoolchildren to villagers to slum dwellers—to take responsibility for disease prevention through such simple interventions as hand washing and using latrines.

To improve access to health care, demand—the willingness and the ability to purchase services or goods—for preventive health care must be increased. In developing countries whose health systems are overloaded and whose resources are limited, preventive services are definitely more cost-effective than curative services and, in addition, reduce the burden of both communicable diseases (e.g., AIDS, malaria, and tuberculosis) and noncommunicable diseases (e.g., heart disease, cancer, and diabetes). In Kenya, for example, as in many African countries, women seen for breast cancer often present with late-stage cancer. An unpublished survey done in 2009 identified causes of delay in seeking care: lack of access to mammograms, a knowledge deficit, fear and denial, and a strong belief in traditional medicine. These findings are in keeping with a number of studies done in developing countries focusing on the problem of late diagnosis. Increasing the demand for preventive services will reduce disease burden and many other complications associated with late diagnosis among the urban population. Educating the general population and target groups about health can increase demand for preventive and promotive services such as lifestyle adjustments to prevent lifestyle diseases, including some cancers. Treatment of early disease is cheaper than treatment of advanced disease; thus if the population seeks help early, the cost of treatment will be far less.

A lack of knowledge about what health-care services exist and a lack of awareness about the importance of these services limit health-care access. By making people aware of how to maintain good health and avoid disease, health promotion furthers good personal health as well as good community health. In a study on access to maternal care among the urban poor in Nairobi, Kenya, Tenambergen (1994) found that health promotion (i.e., being advised during antenatal-care visits) influenced the likelihood that a women would deliver in a health-care facility; this influence was significantly higher among the poorest women than among other women in the study. Health education can improve women's perception of the benefits of the health-care system, which, as discussed earlier, factors into the system's accessibility. Print and electronic media, as well as community outreach by health workers and local leaders, can be used effectively to disseminate health information.

Another way to increase the consumption of preventive services is to make them "public goods" rather than "private goods." In contrast to private goods, no one can be effectively excluded from using public goods. By eliminating cost of these goods to the consumer, the issue of economic access is addressed.

Nongovernmental organizations (NGOs) play an important role in increasing access to health-care services in urban areas, though their contribution has not been fully recognized. Through its focus on the health of Kenyans who reside in informal urban settlements in Nairobi, Jhpiego exemplifies the importance of NGOs in increasing access to health care. Jhpiego improves access to health-care services in these communities by educating and empowering clients and the community, training and preparing service providers, and equipping health-care facilities. By working with health-care providers and slum residents to identify and address residents' needs, this NGO has energized these communities to actively seek to improve the quality and accessibility of health care and especially the uptake of family planning, which in most places was lagging behind.

Financing Health Care

To make health care affordable, better ways of financing health care must be embraced. User fees have been implemented in many countries since the 1980s. The large body of empirical evidence on the impact of user fees on the utilization of health-care services, however, suggests that user fees are regressive and inequitable, in that poor people pay a greater proportion of their incomes out-of-pocket for health care than those who are better off. Many consider insurance a better way of cushioning people when they fall sick.

Insurance is defined as "the means by which risks or uncertain events are shared between many people" (Akin 1987). The insurer or its agent collects premiums, which are then used to compensate insured individuals for financial losses resulting from an insured event. Health insurance is an institutional and financial mechanism that helps households and private individuals set aside financial resources to meet the costs of medical care in the event of illness (Wang'ombe 1994).

Health insurance is based on the principle of pooling funds among a large, heterogeneous group of members and entrusting a third party to manage these funds to pay for the health care of members who contribute to the pool. In this way, risks are averaged among the members contributing to the pool, reducing the variability in risk for any one member. Because everybody pays a premium irrespective of whether he or she falls sick, insurance schemes have a high potential for cost recovery (Tenambergen 1994; Shaw and Ainsworth 1995).

Without such risk pooling, individuals often undergo severe and unexpected economic hardships when faced with medical expenditures, especially hospitalization. These economic hardships may be especially severe when one episode of illness leads to several rounds of care seeking. The reasons may vary from inadequate treatment of the primary problem to emergence of new problems. These hardships can be avoided or alleviated if a system, such as health insurance, exists to smooth out these economic shocks.

Health insurance can help to defer, delay, reduce, or altogether eliminate payment for health care incurred by individuals and households. Any system that creates financial protection against the cost of illness by spreading the risk is in a way a "health insurance" system, including subsidized care from the government.

Because both common but expensive illness and catastrophic, unexpected illness are costly, individuals, households, and organizations need health insurance (Wang'ombe 1994). By pooling the risk of large health-care expenditures among many people, health insurance can make necessary health care affordable to all (Cholletta and Leuris 1997). In addition, people with insurance can be reasonably assured of treatment in a health facility when they decide to seek it (Wang'ombe 1994).

Social health insurance can reduce inequities in health-care financing. Since the health-care burden resulting from out-of-pocket expenses falls more on those least able to pay, social health insurance is seen as way of meeting the equity objective of a functioning health-care system.

No matter how poor people may be, they are often better equipped to cope with certain risks as a group or as a collective rather than as isolated individuals. That is why social health insurance is a powerful weapon to buffer the poor from the vulnerability a health crisis could trigger.

When it comes to financing, the costs of providing adequate health care to cover people's "reasonable" expectations are not currently met with sufficient funds. Often the poor are required to make high direct payments, which they often cannot do. Solidarity mechanisms, such as social health insurance, have the potential to reduce the financial and social burden of disease mainly for the people who are the worst off. As stated in the International Labour Organization's Constitution: "Poverty anywhere constitutes a danger to prosperity everywhere."

Community insurance schemes are one form of insurance that helps protect the urban poor financially. Though this form of health insurance has been deployed mostly in rural areas, I believe it can also work in urban areas. Though urban areas have a wide diversity of people from different communities with diverse values, they have strong and cohesive groups and networks formed to help them face economic challenges.

Innovations in Health Promotion: Partnering with Retail Outlets

Nyamwaya (2008) argues that the primary challenge facing health promotion in African cities is the fact that most health programs are mainly planned, managed, and controlled by health professionals whose concept of health is based on the clinical model, where the focus is curative rather than preventive services. This model provides for only very passive participation by women in health promotion. Some countries, such as Kenya, South Africa, Mauritius, Uganda, Guinea, and Niger, are adopting broad concepts of health that encourage the involvement of multiple stakeholders including women (Nyamwaya 2008).

The problem of widespread ill health in both rural and urban Kenya is not primarily a technical-medical issue. The fact that the rich enjoy reasonably good health implies that the technical means to achieve good health do exist in Kenya today. However, these need to be better adapted to the social, cultural, and economic circumstances of the wider populace. The key requirement to meeting the health-care needs of urban dwellers is not newer medical technologies, more sophisticated vaccines, or more advanced diagnostic techniques; rather, culturally acceptable, cost-effective, and innovative health-care delivery systems are needed.

One model that has proven useful is a partnership between health-care facilities and private commercial entities. The model was first used in Kenya by the private hospitals in Nairobi to create breast cancer awareness among urban women.

These private hospitals seek to deliver all-inclusive health care by working with governments, private individuals, corporate entities, and communities to ensure that all citizens can access world-class health care at an affordable cost.

Breast cancer is one of the leading cancers among women in developing countries. The Nairobi Cancer Registry (2004) reports that breast cancer accounts for more than 20 percent of all cancers among Kenyan women. The disease as seen in Kenya is predominantly premenopausal, with a peak age of 35 to 44 years. This differs from its presentation in North America and Europe, where it is mainly postmenopausal. In Kenya, the majority of women with breast cancer present with advanced disease, with no realistic chance of a cure. Early detection of breast cancer entails both early diagnosis in symptomatic women and screening in asymptomatic women. Key prerequisites for early detection are ensuring that women are supported in seeking care and that they have access to appropriate, affordable diagnostic tests and treatment. Breast health awareness appears to be a pragmatic method for achieving early detection and is the focus of breast cancer awareness campaigns. The campaigns give women an opportunity to get an appraisal of their breast health, training in breast self-examination (BSE), and health education, and to undergo a cervical cancer screening. Though the campaigns are done in retail outlets, they can be carried out in other suitable premises, such as churches. Women who have been taught and who practice BSE are more likely to detect breast cancers and other breast problems at an earlier stage than are women who do not practice BSE (Thomas et al. 2002).

The breast and cervical cancer early-detection program offered by the private hospitals in Nairobi in partnership with retail outlets was created in 2007. The objective was to ensure that women across the socioeconomic spectrum had equal access to community-based cancer screening, outreach, and referral services. This ongoing program is expected to increase early detection of breast and cervical cancers and to improve treatment outcomes.

The program delivery model is simple. Target locations are identified based on a community's social and economic characteristics as well as the availability of health-care facilities. Local retail outlets, usually supermarkets or shopping malls, are then asked to provide a screening venue and related logistical support. The venues chosen are mainly within areas where health facilities are few and far apart. The venues benefit by having a chance to give back to the community through their corporate social responsibility programs. Supermarkets and shopping malls, which are not as impersonal and intimidating as hospitals, provide a more women-friendly environment than traditional health-care facilities. The hospital doing the campaign and the partner retail outlet jointly publicize the program. Print and electronic media are used to hype the event. Leaders in churches, mosques, and other places of worship are engaged early to help in mobilizing their followers.

The hospital provides the required supplies, resources, and personnel. The nurses and doctors undergo a short training to empower them with skills and knowledge to address breast and other health issues afflicting women. Since the health-care professionals come from varied backgrounds, the aim of the training is to ensure uniformity and consistency in the messages given to the women.

To date, nearly 10,000 screening clinical breast examinations have been provided, mainly to underserved women. Approximately 25 to 30 percent of these women had either major breast problems (such as fixed lumps, fungating wounds, pain, or bloody nipple discharges) or precancerous cervical lesions. However, this program reaches only a small fraction of eligible women within a narrow geographical radius because many needy women living in the city outskirts cannot afford the $1 round-trip fare to the program sites. Although this program is free of charge, a large challenge is in finding funding to pay for further diagnostic investigations and treatments for the very poor who require them. The costs for full diagnostics, treatment (including surgery and chemotherapy), and follow-up for a typical breast cancer patient range from US$1,000 to US$5,000 or more: far above what most Kenyans can afford. Some private hospitals have set up a welfare fund to underwrite the cost of treatment for some of the patients. Funding to widen the reach of this welfare program and to make it sustainable has been very challenging, with needs far exceeding financial resources. The welfare programs are primarily funded by private citizens and corporate entities.

These campaigns demonstrate the vital role played by the private sector in mobilizing resources to make health care accessible to all.

Conclusion

Urban areas face a myriad of health challenges from rapid population growth, pollution, unplanned settlements, and an increase in both communicable and noncommunicable diseases. Multiple factors, especially social, cultural, and economic, make women the most vulnerable in the unfolding epidemic of communicable and noncommunicable diseases. Poor government investment in health care further compounds the problem. There is an urgent need for health planners, policymakers, and other stakeholders to engage and involve communities in designing new, innovative, and cost-effective health-care delivery models for promotive, preventive, and curative services. The breast and cervical cancer education, awareness, and screening campaign, which is a private-sector initiative, is one such model that can be replicated to address all health problems, not only in women but in the entire urban population. This model of partnering with retail outlets in the provision of services underscores the important role the private sector plays in health-care delivery to urban populations.

As the world continues to become more urbanized, with resultant health challenges, it is the responsibility of government, civil society, ordinary people, policymakers, and researchers to make cities healthy. On World Health Day 2010, the World Health Organization recommended the following actions to achieve this goal.

1. Improve urban living conditions.
2. Ensure participatory urban governance.
3. Promote urban planning for healthy behaviors and safety.
4. Make urban areas resilient to emergencies and disasters.
5. Build inclusive cities that are accessible and age friendly.

Though these calls to action do not exclusively address women's health, the aspects they cover will have a big impact on women's health. Fortunately these action areas do not require additional funding, though political will is vital to distribute resources to priority interventions.

Chapter 13

Mobilizing Communities to Prevent Violence Against Women and HIV in Kampala, Uganda

Tina C. Musuya

Kampala, the capital city of Uganda, is a home to approximately 1,420,200 people, predominantly Baganda but also others originating from different tribes and parts of the country (Uganda Bureau of Statistics 2008). As in many places in sub-Saharan Africa, gender inequity is the norm with many believing that male supremacy is a natural and "God-given" privilege. In this view, women are considered men's property and therefore have limited power over their own lives and bodies, a factor that increases their vulnerability to HIV and a range of reproductive health problems. In addition, women are often victims of violence including sexual assault, physical violence, and verbal and emotional abuse (Uganda Law Reform Commission 2006). A 2008 study of 1,585 community members in Makindye and Rubaga Divisions in Kampala by the London School of Hygiene and Tropical Medicine, Makerere University, and Raising Voices (a Kampala-based nongovernmental organization working to prevent violence against women and children) revealed the following: Almost half of the women (49 percent) who were currently married or were in an intimate relationship had experienced physical and/or sexual violence from a partner. Many women reported both physical and sexual violence. Almost a third of the women (31 percent) reported experiencing physical or sexual violence from a partner in the last year. Three quarters of the women (75 percent) said that their partners had used one or more forms of controlling behavior in the past twelve months. When men were asked the same questions, 50 percent reported using one or more controlling behaviors with their partners in the past twelve months (Watts et al. 2010).

Many women and young girls in Makindye and Rubaga Divisions (two of the administrative zones of the city of Kampala) attest that violence is part of their lives, revealing that they are always under the control of their partners and live in fear of physical violence. In addition, many women depend entirely on their partners to provide for their basic needs because the men prohibit them from seeking any form of employment. Finally, many do not have power to decide when and how to have sex because their male partners make these decisions. Many women in intimate relationships are resigned to their situations. Talking about prevention of HIV during a community outreach activity, one middle-aged woman reflected the views of the group:

> What can we do? You know very well that our men never have one partner and yet they do not accept to use protection with us their wives, so we are doomed to get the infection any time. We survive by the grace of God. (a middle-aged woman in a Nakulabye market)

Hope Turyasingura, a long-time activist for women's rights, explained gender perceptions and customs in the community as follows:

> There is a widespread practice in the community that condones male infidelity. Many community members expect the wife to tolerate it as long as the husband is discreet about his numerous relationships.

Although the Constitution of the Republic of Uganda (1995) recognizes women's rights and the government is party to the Convention on the Elimination of All Forms of Discrimination Against Women and the Declaration on the Elimination of Violence Against Women, violence against women still occurs in Uganda at alarming rates. While many advances have been made in the promotion and protection of girls' and women's rights in the public arena in Uganda, critical policy areas that undermine women's right to safety still remain. Violence against women (VAW) is deeply rooted in the unequal relations between men and women because the Ugandan society has developed a social hierarchy that accords men a higher status than women and permits men to use VAW as a way of imposing their will. Preventing violence calls for a change in these norms. Notably, addressing VAW is a means of preventing HIV because VAW is both a cause and a consequence of HIV (Michau et al. 2009).

Mobilizing Communities to Prevent Domestic Violence and Associated Health Problems

One response to preventing VAW and associated health problems comes from the Center for Domestic Violence Prevention (CEDOVIP), a non-governmental organization formed in 2003 and supported by American

Jewish World Service, the Elton John AIDS Foundation, the Foundation for Open Society Institute, Irish Aid, the United Nations Development Programme, and Raising Voices. CEDOVIP originated from a partnership between Raising Voices, the National Association of Women's Organizations in Uganda (NAWOU), and ActionAid Uganda. From 2000 to 2002 these groups operated the Domestic Violence Prevention Project. By 2003, this effort was so successful that the partners created CEDOVIP.

CEDOVIP's first program drew from the Raising Voices programmatic tool *Mobilizing Communities to Prevent Domestic Violence: A Resource Guide for Organizations in East and Southern Africa* (Michau and Naker 2003). The program had three interrelated, mutually reinforcing parts: (1) the Domestic Violence Prevention Demonstration Project, (2) the National Domestic Violence Prevention Initiative, and (3) the National Advocacy Program. The lessons learned from the Domestic Violence Prevention Demonstration Project informed the development of SASA!

Developed by Raising Voices, SASA! is a systematic approach to mobilizing communities to change attitudes and practices that perpetuate VAW. CEDOVIP uses SASA!, which is described more fully in the remaining sections of this chapter, in its efforts to mobilize communities to prevent VAW. When CEDOVIP began its work, many community members were not aware of the connection between VAW and HIV. Even more worrying was that many did not see men's widely accepted infidelity as the problem but instead blamed women as the source of infection. Two quotations from community members are emblematic of this sentiment:

> Women and young girls love money, [and] in their pursuit for money they get infected with HIV from men. (a male participant in an impromptu discussion at a carpentry workshop in Bwaise-Kawempe)

> If a man does not provide for his wife, she may get another man who will provide for her needs in exchange for sex and she will get infected with HIV. (a woman met during a door-to-door visit in Kasubi parish)

SASA! Mobilizing Communities to Prevent Violence Against Women and HIV

Sasa means "now" (now is the time to prevent violence against women and HIV) in Swahili, the common language in eastern Africa. SASA! is also an acronym for a four-phased approach to community mobilization to prevent VAW and HIV: Start, Awareness, Support, and Action. The start phase begins by engaging communities to start thinking about VAW and HIV as interconnected issues and fostering power *within* communities to address these issues. The awareness phase follows and features raising awareness about how communities' acceptance of men's use of *power over* women fuels the dual pandemics of VAW and HIV. The support phase supports the women, men, young people, and activists affected by and confronting issues of power, violence, and HIV by encouraging the community to join their *power with* others to collectively address the problem. The action phase occurs as the participants take action by using *power to* prevent VAW. SASA! generates much-needed momentum to create new community norms to support a balance of power between women and men.

In implementing SASA! CEDOVIP uses the ecological model of community mobilization (Heise, Ellsberg, and Gottenmoeller 1999). It works with individuals, including both men and women living in the targeted communities, and engages families, neighbors, friends, relatives, and in-laws. Next, it involves local leaders, community groups, police, health-care providers, nongovernmental organizations, religious leaders, business owners, and cultural groups. Finally, it works with the media and also engages in national-level policy advocacy and law formulation processes. Working across the social spectrum enables CEDO-VIP to reach the critical mass needed to set the pace for social change in norms and behaviors.

SASA! in Action

SASA! began in the Rubaga and Makindye Divisions using lessons learned from CEDOVIP's earlier work in the Kawempe Division. The Rubaga Division, with an estimated population of 344,752, accommodates the seat of the Buganda Kingdom and the Christian missions' headquarters. The Makindye Division, with an estimated population of 350,800, accommodates the largest police barracks and training school in the country. Located on the edge of Kampala, both are densely populated, low-income, peri-urban communities that are characterized by widespread poverty, unemployment, congested settlement patterns, and an unsupportive law enforcement and social services environment. The residents of these divisions typically live on less than US$1 per day (Kampala City Council 2002). Many refer to these communities as slums because they lack basic infrastructure, services such as water, sanitation, and electricity, and lack permanent housing structures.

Members of these communities tend to interact with their neighbors frequently, since the houses are close together and because community members commonly share resources such as common water sources and shared toilets. Community members depend on one another for information, belong to common village savings groups, and work together to address problems within their communities. Because community members tended to know one another and had a history of working together, these communities were well suited to the SASA! community mobilization approach to preventing VAW.

As mentioned earlier, the CEDOVIP model employs different levels of engagement: fostering local activism coordinated with strategic communications and engagement in national media and advocacy campaigns. To use and build local activism, CEDOVIP promotes community drama, community conversations, soap operas, quick chats, and films. These efforts come to life through the work of a sixty-two-member team (half men and half women) recruited to be community activists (CAs). Carefully selected and trained through skill-building workshops and bimonthly meetings, they spearhead a variety of activities to enable dialogue about VAW, HIV, and female-male power relationships. (Although the activities are the same throughout the four phases, their content changes to focus on each phase's theme.) Raising Voices developed the *SASA! Activist Kit*, which details the work. CEDOVIP and the CAs translate and, if needed, adapt the activities to fit the context. The following are general descriptions of the activities.

Community Drama

Six drama troupes (each with approximately five men and five women) trained by CEDOVIP perform short, participatory dramas in open places to engage community members in dialogue on preventing VAW; Figure 13.1 depicts a well-attended performance in Nakulabye. During intervals, the CAs ask the audience questions about violence and HIV. The discussion helps to shift attention from entertainment to raising awareness, building support, and taking action to prevent VAW and HIV. Many community members speak out about VAW in their communities during these shows, and often local leaders make commitments to take action against VAW.

Community Conversations

CEDOVIP provides CAs with a set of pictures related to VAW, which are designed to begin conversations among small groups of people at sports grounds, places of worship, shops, men's or women's groups, and around the water sources. The CA chooses a picture, asks some leading questions, and encourages everyone to participate in the ensuing conversation. Having community conversations is an excellent way to intro-

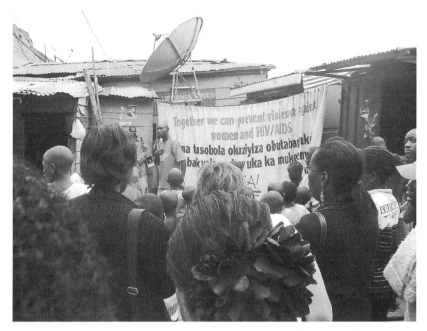

Figure 13.1. A community drama troupe performs in Nakulabye. (Photo courtesy of CEDOVIP.)

duce new ideas and to stimulate reflective discussions and debates about how to promote change in attitudes and behaviors related to gender roles. In these situations, some community members are very conservative while others are less so. The following are examples of community members' differing attitudes regarding who should do domestic chores:

> I always help my wife to wash dishes and cook food because my father told me that is one thing that will keep you close to your wife and kids. (local council leader, Nakulabye)

> If you try doing domestic chores, then the women will start ordering you around. You will become the laughing-stock of the village. Many people will say that you have become a woman. (young man in Kasubi)

Such dialogue enables community members to reflect on some of the issues that many take for granted. Some men said that they began by doing domestic chores behind the scenes, and later, as they gained confidence and the community appreciated their efforts, they started to do them more openly. Kisembo, one of the male community activists, said that his participation in domestic chores has created new warmth in his family, and he encourages men to do domestic chores more often.

Soap Operas

CEDOVIP also provides the CAs with audio soap operas featuring short skits followed by mini–talk shows about HIV and VAW. Small groups of people listen to a recording and, with a CA's guidance, discuss the themes. This is a popular activity with young men at the trading centers and drinking joints. The mini–talk show at the end of a drama helps the participants reflect on VAW, on men's use of power over women as the root cause of VAW, and on how VAW increases women's vulnerability to HIV infection. In two of these soap opera discussion groups, one in Kibuye parish and one in Salama parish, an elderly woman and a middle-aged man made the following comments:

> Many men in my village always control and intimidate their wives and are also unfaithful just like Musa [character in the soap opera]. Do you really think that women in such relationships can negotiate for safe sex? People, let us embrace SASA! to make difference. (elderly woman in Kibuye parish)

> I am just learning that controlling and coercing your wife into sex is also VAW. I feel bad that I have done this many times thinking that I was being a man. So what should we do? (middle-aged man in Salama parish)

With the support of CEDOVIP staff and CAs, community members make the connections between VAW and HIV, are encouraged to seek more information, and receive tips on negotiating for safe sex and respecting others in intimate relationships. Often, CEDOVIP refers community members to the team of Sengas (traditional marriage counselors trained by CEDOVIP) for one-on-one support to guide them through their long journey of behavior change.

Quick Chats

CEDOVIP trains the CAs to begin brief, impromptu discussions with community members about VAW and HIV, providing the CAs with simple topic guides and suggestions for how to open up a chat with another person. The CAs use this tool with people who are in transit or are very busy, such as people waiting at a bus stop, riding a hired motorbike taxi (i.e., *boda boda* men), or shopping at the market. Here is a typical comment:

> I first heard about balancing power in intimate relationship at the *boda boda* stage. Since then every time I want to tell my partner to do things for

me as her husband, I wonder whether I am using my power over her. This makes me ask for her opinion about things. It is not easy, but I think I am beginning to balance power. (a man in a Nakulabye market)

Often, those who have been introduced to ideas through the quick chats seek more information from the CAs. The quick chats are an effective way to get people to start questioning their own behavior and beliefs regarding VAW, women, and power.

The SASA! Film

The SASA! film relates the stories of two women, Mama Joyce and Josephine, who experience violence and HIV infection. Available for viewing at home, in open places such as barber shops, canteens, and saloons, or in larger places such as in churches, the film has played in more than 100 video halls in Rubaga and Makindye and has attracted large crowds. After showing the film, CAs, provided with questions by CEDOVIP, probe the audience on the connection between VAW and HIV and the nature of male-female relationships. The film has been especially useful in reaching out to men—more than 5,000 have seen it. One viewer, a man in Nakinyuguzi, observed:

> I always thought that women sleep around [and] that is why they are vulnerable to HIV. SASA! has made me learn that women's lack of power over their sexuality is the risk for their increased HIV infection. We must start to address this problem.

The film offers community members insights about women's realities and provides an urgent rationale for addressing men's use of power over women, showing how it is a means to reverse the current trends of HIV infection. A word of caution, however: Some conservative community members hardly pay attention to key issues raised in the film and focus instead on things such as Mama Joyce treating her co-wife with respect as something that women in polygamous relationships should emulate.

All the activities that have been described introduce new ideas, prompting community members to reflect on many things in their everyday lives and to start asking the most important "why," "how," and "for what" questions about women and men's lives and realities.

Communication Materials

A second strategy in the SASA! program is to disseminate fun and creative communication materials. As with the activities, use of these materials—including posters, comic strips, and card and other games—evolves over the phases of community mobilization. So while a poster might be used in each phase, its content changes to focus on the key themes: *power over* (awareness phase), *power with* (support phase), and *power to* (action phase).

The communication materials aim to expose people continuously to information that is thought provoking and appealing without portraying violent scenes. The materials show VAW as an urgent injustice that is everyone's responsibility to address. Most important, they do not contain threatening or blaming messages. Instead, they focus on more neutral topics such as the benefits of nonviolence in relationships, sharing domestic chores between men and women, negotiation of condom use, and safe sex. Community members often hang materials in such strategic places as on the doors of their retail shops, walls of their living rooms, and walls in busy marketplaces.

Posters and Comic Strips

CEDOVIP employs posters and comic strips to expose community members to VAW and HIV prevention ideas and to illustrate the types of VAW, causes of VAW, and connection between VAW and HIV. CAs and staff use the posters and comic strips to open up dialogue with small groups of between ten to twenty people, often leading to heated debates. Figure 13.2 shows Teo, a community activist in Kasubi parish, facilitating a conversation on power, VAW, and HIV. CAs also distribute the posters and comic strips to the participants, who later hang them up in open spaces in their communities or on the walls in their houses. These messaging activities occur in neighborhoods, in women's savings groups, at the carpentries and garages where men congregate, and within places of worship. Because the posters do not explicitly show scenes of VAW, both men and women easily identify with the ideas. One woman in Kibuye said:

> It was difficult to talk about VAW or improving my relationship with my partner. He never turns up in these activities. I hung one poster in the living room and put the comic strip in the bedroom—I found him reading, and he started to ask questions about balancing power. We now talk about these things and he talks to his friends too.

The CAs find them useful as well, as indicated by the following two quotations:

> I shared the comic strip with the imam of the mosque in Kitebi, [and] he now asks the congregation to spend thirty minutes after the Friday prayers

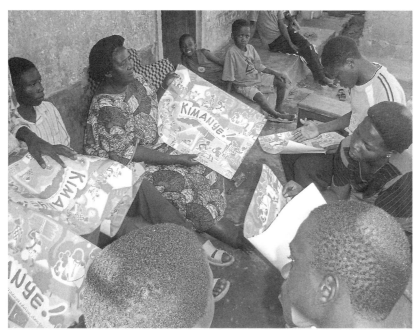

Figure 13.2. A community activist in Kasubi parish uses a poster to facilitate a discussion on power, violence against women, and HIV. (Photo courtesy of CEDOVIP.)

to talk about VAW with our support. The imam encourages the people to work with activists to prevent VAW. (a CA in Mutundwe parish)

These stickers and comic strips made it easy for me to talk with my peers about VAW. They always ask me to lead discussions about women's rights, which they say are their problems. (a CA in Nakulabye)

While the colorful posters are quite popular with community members and leaders, people sometimes pull them down to use for making paper beads for sale, and some highly political communities avoid using posters that have colors similar to the different political party colors. CEDOVIP takes care not to use any political party colors in order to avoid situations related to partisan politics that would cause the community members to disregard VAW prevention.

Card Games

The card game is both an activity and a communications strategy. With a different set of cards for each SASA! phase, a CA guides participants to take turns saying what they know (awareness phase), what they would say (support phase), or what they would do (action phase) about the various scenarios portrayed on the cards about rights, gender, power, and VAW. When one participant answers the question, others can decide if that answer is right. Each participant reflects on what this means to his or her life and community. Many commit to something very specific that they will do in their daily lives to address VAW. The game is played in homes and with men and youth at the video halls, pork joints, and other places of recreation. One middle-aged woman said that the card game enabled her to recognize that what she had experienced and assumed was "normal" were actually different forms of VAW. She committed to bring both her sons and daughters to learn about VAW and how to prevent it. Focusing a dialogue with the card game calls for tact on the part of the CA, as the conversation can easily go off track to other community problems.

Guiding questions on the back of each card help to enable in-depth chats about types of VAW, its root causes, its consequences, and what a person can do to address it, given his or her means and situation. Through such discussion, the materials are used as tools to help people feel responsible for addressing VAW in their everyday lives.

When continuously implemented, the SASA! strategies create ripple effects, with messages diffused throughout the community by word of mouth to reach a critical mass. This is important, as a critical mass is essential to undoing inequitable norms, effecting social change, and calling for nonviolence.

Media and Advocacy

In addition to working with local activism and communication materials, CEDOVIP has developed a national media campaign. It spreads provocative facts and stories about VAW and HIV in print and across the air waves, linking the messages to countrywide advocacy efforts in order to press political leaders and policymakers to take small and big actions to halt the VAW and HIV epidemics. CEDOVIP has conducted the activity through information and sensitivity training as well as media campaigns, among other means.

Information and Sensitivity Training

CEDOVIP works with journalists and editors to improve the quality of their reporting by building skills in objective writing on VAW issues. As a result, the media fraternity play an important role in public aware-ness-raising and advocacy as they attract and maintain attention to the prevention of VAW through their free coverage of VAW issues. How-ever, since most of the Ugandan media houses are profit-making insti-tutions, editors' concerns about the bottom line cause them be torn between publishing "sexy and sensational" stories and publishing more reasoned accounts about women and VAW. To address these concerns, CEDOVIP encourages the media to report on VAW as a human rights and public health problem by sharing story ideas and facts that connect VAW to HIV, political participation, economic growth, maternal health, and women's empowerment. Though some of the journalists and edi-tors claim that they have a right to present their views (even if they are stereotypical views about women) without embedding their stories in a human rights framework, the CEDOVIP effort is slowly transforming media coverage, as writers are now seeking more information regarding VAW, questioning the legitimacy of VAW, and calling for more account-ability on the part of government and policymakers. This level of sup-port is very important in the prevention of VAW. A colleague from the media observed:

> Before the engagement with CEDOVIP, we always wanted to get a selling story and oftentimes sensationalized stories on VAW. We had no idea that this puts the victim in further danger and worst of all popularizes the use of VAW. We now try to care about the safety and dignity of the victim and do all that is possible to report objectively. (journalist in the Parliamen-tary Press Association, Uganda)

CEDOVIP's Media Campaign

The bond between the media and CEDOVIP is based on recognizing each other's contributions, supporting each other in the promotion of human rights, and giving constructive feedback in areas that need to be strengthened. CEDOVIP keeps track of print media reports and shows its appreciation of objective reports by giving writers green cards for promoting the rights of women. It gives red cards to those who write biased, negative, or sensationalized reports. Though some journalists are offended when they receive red cards, this recognition program and the other collaborations have led journalists to begin to observe the ethics code of the International Federation of Journalists when report-ing on VAW. One media house with a popular daily newspaper, FM station, and TV station has recently adopted a policy to prevent sensa-tionalism of VAW stories and to protect the survivors' identity. Other media houses are beginning to emulate this action by putting similar policies in place.

CEDOVIP increases media coverage of VAW by holding press conferences, conducting radio and TV talk shows, issuing press releases, and supporting newspaper publications. At the forefront in articulating feminist analysis of gender relationships and VAW in Uganda, CEDOVIP uses these media spaces strategically. It clarifies myths and stereotypes regarding women. It persuasively and provocatively frames appeals to end VAW to the government, the public, religious institutions, and individuals. In the talk show environment, some participants' reject the idea of equity between men and women as a Western phenomenon, but others have increasingly recognized that VAW is an intolerable injustice. Clearly espousing the latter viewpoint, a caller from Entebbe said:

> My brothers, using violence against women is an embarrassment—it is a sign that you are not worth being called a man and you ought to be ashamed. The problem is with you, and you must start to take steps to change this behavior.

Advocacy for Law Reform

CEDOVIP's media work feeds into advocacy on VAW prevention at the local and national levels. CEDOVIP builds on grassroots connections to ensure that community voices inform the law-making processes. For example, in 2007, CEDOVIP inspired the Kawempe community and the local authorities to outlaw domestic violence through passage of the first domestic violence bylaw in Uganda. It used this bylaw to demonstrate to national policymakers that communities were ready for legislation against domestic violence. CEDOVIP then coordinated a coalition of twenty-two civil and women's rights organizations and built alliances with media groups and policymaking bodies to advocate for a domestic violence act. In addition, CEDOVIP helped draft the law. In 2009, parliament passed the bill, and in March 2010 the president assented to it. For the next four years, CEDOVIP is committed to coordinating the coalition's advocacy for the government's implementation of the Domestic Violence Act.

Coalition-building is challenging, requiring major organizing efforts and perseverance. In the example of the national Domestic Violence Act, some coalition members were discouraged by the length of the process—four years; others thought that CEDOVIP was asking them to do "CEDOVIP's work"; and some thought that they did not have time for lobbying because they had to run their everyday programs. In addition, at times during the process, members of the government law-making bodies did not prioritize the domestic violence law—claiming that since Uganda was a poor country, commercial laws were more urgently needed or that VAW was a family matter not to be handled by the courts of law, police, or local leaders.

SASA! Trainings

VAW is a problem rooted in behaviors, beliefs, and practices. Working to prevent VAW requires both tact and skills to enable community members to unlearn the values they consider "normal." Training can inspire participants to start looking at VAW as an injustice and to recognize that men's use of power over women has severe negative consequences for everyone.

SASA! trainings are personal events that move beyond information-giving to help participants—who include practitioners, community activists, cultural, religious and local leaders, media groups, police, and health-care providers—explore their own values, assumptions, and actions. The SASA! trainings are modular, structured, interactive, and thought-provoking exercises. The sessions enable personal reflections and allow questions from participants about their concerns or hesitations about VAW. CEDOVIP also provides special training for health-care providers and local leaders.

Why SASA! Engages Men and Not Only Women

VAW is a community problem: It happens because everyone in the community allows it to happen. Prevention requires a change in social norms, which cannot occur without the concurrent engagement of men and women to rethink and reorient their perceptions about women, gender, violence, and power. Therefore, men and women must be part and parcel of mobilizing communities to prevent VAW. CEDOVIP's work involves men as well as women throughout all SASA! phases.

Bringing men on board alongside women at the onset of SASA! reduces male backlash because it enables both men and women to be on the same footing in their understanding of VAW as an injustice and in recognizing the need for deliberate action in its prevention. Men become confident and less defensive when they recognize that the work is aimed at improving their relationships with their partners and at creating safe and healthy homes for everyone. It is of critical importance to have men stand against VAW; this ultimately increases safety for women and the success in changing social norms.

SASA! recognizes that men need support to unlearn many aspects of the masculine identity that perpetuates abusive practices. SASA! promotes dialogue on power, on how men use their power with others (particularly their partners), on sharing roles at home, on talking about sex, on collective decision-making, and on the intentions of some of the norms that maintain rigid gender roles and identities. During a discussion held for men from the communities of Makindye and Rubaga on what balancing power with their partners could look like or mean in their relationships, one young man commented:

> My position in the house is a given: A man is the head and that is how it has always been. A good wife is one who will always obey me as her husband. She has to have sex with me whenever I want . . . no need for me to talk with her about sex because the topic is embarrassing. It is easier to talk with men about sex.

A contrasting view was expressed by another man, a middle-aged cobbler, during a card game in Kabawo zone, Mutundwe parish:

> Involving your wife in decision-making is a good thing because you plan together for your family. My participation in these SASA! activities has challenged and inspired me to talk about sex with my partner, something I had never imagined before. Let these community activists give you tips on how to negotiate for sex and condoms with your partner.

Men tend to resist gender equality ideas when only women promote them. When other men are involved, the dynamic changes dramatically. Surprisingly, many men fear reaching out to their peers on these matters, fearing ridicule or desiring to maintain the status quo. Thus, despite the challenges, it is essential to get men on board to promote women's rights. Half of CEDOVIP's team of CAs are men whose role is to reach out directly to men. While SASA! creates space for men to create new norms to change unequal power dynamics with their partners, this work is neither quick nor easy. It takes support, time, and alternatives—but it is possible. One man in Nakulabye parish remarked that SASA! enabled him to talk about sex with his long-time partner:

> Brothers, now I talk about sex and balancing power with my partner—I feel really free and more like a man because I believe and know that we are both enjoying it [sex]. My wife is beaming once again, and I just can't wait to get home to my wife. That is why I am seen rarely at the place we used to spend our evenings.

In shaping SASA!, CEDOVIP learned that most men do not turn up for organized activities. They claim to be too busy working or socializing with their peers. However, the male CAs know where to find them and devise ways to engage them, selecting venues that are convenient to men rather than to the organization. They reach out to men through the radio, at their work or leisure places, at trading centers, and at sporting events. They employ continuous engagement, using short persuasive dialogue to build men's interests and involve them in alternatives to violence. In this way, the men feel respected, and many become activists. For CAs, reaching out to men for the first time can be very intimidating because many men dismiss ideas about women's rights, thinking that this topic does not concern them. Some demand payment for their time. Others ask the CA to speak to their wives or to women's groups.

In this work, CEDOVIP avoids using threatening and blaming language, instead using a benefits-based approach that enables men to link women's lack of power in relationships with their own experiences of lack of power in other spheres of life, such as the workplace. In so doing, the dialogue avoids the common pitfall of men versus women but rather focuses on VAW as an injustice that hurts both men and women. This way, men get to connect to what abuse is and to the feelings of powerlessness, which helps get on board to prevent VAW. One man in Makindye said:

> I had no idea that preventing VAW means promoting respect, fairness, safety, and dignity for women and men. SASA! has made this clear to us, and I will always support SASA! by bringing more men on board.

CEDOVIP has seen results in this work with men. Increasingly, men who have been reached by the male CAs seek support from CEDOVIP to change. Some men develop simple codes of conduct that suit their peer groups; these may include treating their wives and children with respect and avoiding the use of violence. The young men of "Boda boda" Riders' Association in Kibuye remarked:

> We [members of the "Boda boda" Riders Association] want to make a difference by proving that men can be very loving and caring—we feel ashamed that some men have made their homes the most unsafe places for their wives and children . . . we commit to proving to the world that men can prevent VAW.

Building men's confidence to promote women's rights helps to keep men deeply engaged in creating new norms because, with this confidence, they do not feel threatened that they have to give away their power. Though some men are resistant to balancing power with their partners, many men feel that this is a worthwhile and long overdue cause and commit to do everything possible to create an environment for women to live free of violence.

A Final Note on Terminology

In places where people have limited opportunity to analyze power and the implications of the imbalance between men and women, it is essential to provide space for this—and to do so on the community's terms. Terminology is critical. Some programs use the expression "gender-based violence," as is commonly employed in the international development community. But this terminology can be confusing, alienating, and often does not translate well into local languages. "Gender" to most community members in Uganda means "women and men." Therefore, if the term gender-based violence is used, a fundamental misunderstanding occurs: Community members interpret it as violence that happens to women or men. When CEDOVIP unpacks VAW/HIV issues and contextualizes them at the community level, it translates the concept of gender-based violence into common, everyday language and experiences understandable to community members. This helps people focus and clarifies the discourse.

Conclusion

In Uganda, as in many places, the belief in men's use of power over women as natural is widespread. This attitude leads to resistance to promoting gender equality and preventing VAW, which makes working to prevent VAW a long-term process. The process requires changing people's beliefs and practices by enabling them to create new values. It involves raising awareness to increase knowledge. But this process does not stop there. Social change requires moving beyond raising awareness to helping community members build skills and commitment to prevent VAW in their own relationships and in their communities. It calls for encouraging them to use their power collectively and individually to create norms that support a culture that refuses to tolerate violence.

To achieve this, it is important to avoid using rhetoric such as "eliminate or stop violence now." If you heard that, would you automatically know what to do? Probably not, yet these types of admonitions are repeatedly used in communities—with poor results. There is an urgent need to go further if men and women are to unlearn many things and find replacements for what they have always known.

Programs to change social norms need to be both practical and inspiring. They can help men explore what a loving husband is *and* how to be one; they can help men explore the benefits of partners making joint decisions *and* how to do that. They can share tips for anger management, for talking about sex, *and* for figuring out how to negotiate sex with a partner without coercion. They can support changes in gender roles at home *and* what that means in practice—helping with domestic chores and care-giving for their children. This challenges men to try out new ways of relating to women and it also frees some from the guilt of trying to play the "macho" stereotype all the time as they create new identities in which they are respected and appreciated.

Community mobilization to prevent VAW takes time and requires stamina, and it requires commitment from the lead organization, from community activists, and from community members, but it can ultimately have effective and sustainable results.

Many thanks to the management of CEDOVIP for their inspirational leadership and to Lori Michau, Hope Turyasingura, Olive Nabisubi, Paul Buzibwa, Josephine Kamisya, Yvette Alal, Deus Kiwanuka, Brenda Kugonza, and Janet Nakuti for their support in compiling information for this chapter and their untiring commitment to promoting the rights of women.

Chapter 14

Philanthropy and Its Impact on Urban Women's Health

Katherina M. Rosqueta and Carol A. McLaughlin

If I had a million dollars to spend philanthropically, how could I spend these funds to make the greatest social impact? For impact-focused donors, this is the central question. Though straightforward to pose, it is a difficult question to answer in a way that is both informed by the evidence and actionable. Yet if philanthropists and the organizations they support are to achieve the social impact both seek, answering this million-dollar question is critical.

Philanthropy in Urban Women's Health

Each year billions of dollars of philanthropic funding go to address issues related to health in the United States and other developed countries and in developing countries worldwide. In the United States, health represents approximately 7 percent of charitable gifts domestically, totaling $22.46 billion dollars in 2009 (Giving USA Foundation 2010). U.S.-based foundations also donated more than half of the $4.5 billion given worldwide to address health issues in developing countries in 2008 (The Foundation Center 2010a). That year, approximately 80 percent of all U.S. foundation giving to global health came from the Gates Foundation, which awarded an estimated $2 billion in global health grants (The Foundation Center 2010c). A quick scan of the top fifty global health gifts made by U.S. foundations reveals that twelve of those grants, or over $361 million, made explicit reference to women or urban health issues, with all of those grants given by the Gates Foundation (The Foundation Center 2010d).

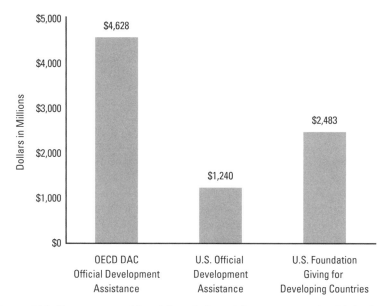

Figure 14.1. Government aid and foundation giving to support health in developing countries, 2008. OECD DAC, Organisation for Economic Co-operation and Development, Development Assistance Committee.
Source: The Foundation Center 2010b. Copyright © 2010 The Foundation Center. Used by permission.

While many philanthropists share the same aspirations for impact, few can match the Gates Foundation's capacity to give. However, compared with aid from government and multilateral and bilateral aid organizations, even Gates funding can seem small (Figure 14.1). The aspirations of philanthropists and the relative size of their funding make it even more important that they spend their funds wisely to have lasting impact on women's lives.

Philanthropy's Potential for Impact

Much is at stake. Recent analysis estimates that each year 358,000 women (or one woman every 1.5 seconds) die in pregnancy and childbirth, often from causes that are treatable and preventable (WHO, UNICEF, UNFPA, and the World Bank 2010). In addition, earlier studies estimate that 10 million women each year suffer from illnesses and lifelong disabilities due to complications in pregnancy and childbirth (The White Ribbon Alliance n.d.).

The disparities between rich and poor countries are great. For example, a woman's lifetime risk of dying in pregnancy and childbirth in Niger is 1 in 7; in the United States, the risk is 1 in 4,800 (UNICEF 2010a, 2010b). Even within cities in wealthy countries such as the United States, great disparities exist. For example, poor people living in U.S. urban communities have disproportionately high rates of HIV. A recent study by the Centers for Disease Control and Prevention (2010: para. 10) found that "within the low income urban areas included in the study, individuals living below the poverty line were at greater risk for HIV than those living above it (2.4 percent prevalence vs. 1.2 percent), though the prevalence for both groups was far higher than the national average (0.45 percent)."

The stakes are great not only for these women but also for their children, their countries, and the global community. Since women are children's main caregivers, their health is critical to children's health, well-being, and future prospects (Figure 14.2). Children up to 10 years of age whose mothers die are three to ten times more likely to

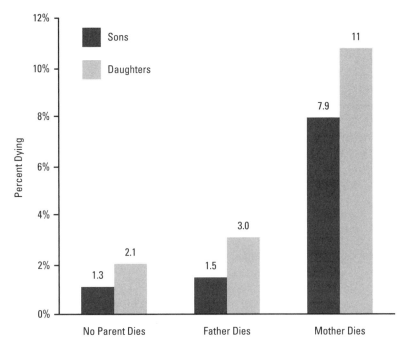

Figure 14.2. Child deaths when a parent dies.
Source: Strong 1992.

die within two years than children whose mothers are still alive. Children whose mothers die are less likely to be immunized, less likely to complete schooling, and more likely to suffer malnutrition and stunted growth. Globally, each year an estimated $15.5 billion in potential productivity is lost when mothers and newborns die (The White Ribbon Alliance n.d.).

For poor, urban women, philanthropy plays an essential role in addressing health needs. Unlike aid from governments or bilateral and multilateral aid organizations, private philanthropy is less beholden to the political, cultural, and economic interests that can prevent public investments in urban women's health despite mounting evidence of the tremendous social and economic return such investments have (The White Ribbon Alliance n.d.). What's more, the relative lack of public accountability for private philanthropists also means that such donors can act more nimbly and assume greater risk than is tolerated by public taxpayers, government agencies, or even the communities in which these poor, urban women live.

This lack of accountability has a clear downside as well. While it can isolate donors from criticism, it can also isolate them from the information and people that can help them craft successful philanthropic strategies. For those private donors seeking to achieve impact, philanthropy can become a frustrating endeavor.

Frustrated Philanthropists

In the spring of 2006, a small group of Wharton alumni made an anonymous gift that launched the Center for High Impact Philanthropy at the University of Pennsylvania's School of Social Policy & Practice. Unlike some private donors, they were not interested in getting their names on a building. Nor were they inclined to engage in the kind of social gala events that characterize many philanthropic activities. Instead, they were trying to understand how to spend their philanthropic funds so that those funds made the greatest difference in improving the lives of others. In other words, they were impact-driven donors. Like other impact-driven donors around the world, they were frustrated by the lack of resources available to them to make wise decisions.

This frustration is justified. The most broadly accessible information on nonprofit organizations continues to be expense ratios (e.g., percent of overhead). While nonprofit organizations frequently tout these percentages to attract donors, these ratios are crude measures, easily manipulated, and often out-of-date. Most important, they offer little insight into impact. A McKinsey report commissioned by the William and Flora Hewlett Foundation (2008: 15) described how current-ratings Web sites "can tell you which groups have the lowest overhead ratios, but they can't tell you which have the most impact." The *Rating the Raters* report (National Council of Nonprofits and the National Human Services Assembly 2005: 2) noted that in the wake of the Pacific tsunami "percent and ratios reported by charity watchdogs were frequently cited in the media. However, few news reports or the ratings they cited indicated *how effective* the nonprofit organizations were at delivering services." One high net-worth philanthropist commented, "Somebody needs to pay for the overhead in order for [the organization] to provide their services, so why shouldn't it be us? And if we believe in the organization, why shouldn't we pay for the overhead?" (Noonan and Rosqueta 2008: 10). Another indicated, "The whole issue of overhead expenses as a percentage of your total budget is . . . not regular. It seems like the wrong way to think about it" (Noonan and Rosqueta 2008: 10).

In other words, even if such ratios were made accurate, standardized, and up-to-date, they wouldn't tell a philanthropist how well the money is spent improving the lives of others. Unfortunately, information that could provide insight on impact is all too often locked up in silos. The McKinsey/Hewlett report (The William and Flora Hewlett Foundation 2008: 32) states that "foundations routinely uncover great nonprofits and ideas that they pass up for funding because they don't fit their own strategy; they could pass on these leads to other donors." Not only do many foundations not pass on these leads, they often fail to share the very mistakes and lessons learned that could be most instructive to those seeking impact (Giloth and Gewirtz 2009).

Even when impact-related information is made physically accessible to donors, the language, metrics, and complexity of social issues can limit the usefulness of that information. In the Center for High Impact Philanthropy's *I'm Not Rockefeller* report, participating donors bemoaned the lack of useful information. One donor summed things up this way: "Maybe it exists and I just don't know it. I wish I could get research reports that are readable, that aren't bureaucratic I-had-to-fill-a-hundred-pages [reports]" (Noonan and Rosqueta 2008: 15).

The lack of common measures also contributes to the difficulty in developing better resources for donors. Lynn Karoly (2008: 77), a researcher at the RAND Corporation, noted, "Even programs that have a common objective (e.g., early childhood intervention) do not necessarily incorporate common measures into the evaluations" and, without such common measures, as Karoly indicated in her response to Melinda Tuan (Tuan 2008: 19), "you can't make the argument that you should invest in program x vs. program y because the outcomes are different. It's really a problem of apples to oranges."

Brian Trelstad (2008), CIO of the Acumen Fund, suggested in a report by Melinda Tuan that there are cultural barriers as well: "As Trelstad noted, 'There is a fear of failure in the social sector' . . . [and] *if* the social sector is able to generate high quality data to allow analyses and comparisons of organizations or programs based on their cost-effectiveness 'there will be clear "winners" and "losers" based on these analyses'" (Tuan 2008: 21).

Given these obstacles, how can impact-driven donors achieve the impact they seek?

Rethinking Evidence for Philanthropists

Multiple disciplines examine the issues affecting the health of urban women in the developing world as well as in the United States and other developed countries. Urban planners, demographers, educators, epidemiologists, public health professionals, economic development specialists—each of these fields has its own framework, language, approach, and professional bias. Each discipline offers a piece of the answer to the philanthropist's million-dollar question. Breaking down silos between and among these disciplines is a first step in understanding where to spend philanthropic funds to improve urban women's health.

In addition, connections need to be made between researchers, practitioners, and other informed players. These different players offer different insights into how to achieve impact when addressing the needs of poor, urban women. The work of researchers and academics can help donors understand the causes of sickness and death. However, their work often cannot answer questions such as, "Will this work in the community I want to help?" or "What should I consider before funding this program?" Nonprofit/nongovernmental organization staff, clinicians, and other practitioners in the field often *do* possess exactly this kind of practical knowledge necessary for impact but rarely discussed in the more rigorous research. Program staff and practitioners in the field can provide insight into what has worked and failed in the past, who the key opinion leaders are, and how to adapt best practices to a particular context.

Further, people and agencies whose jobs require them to aggregate and synthesize information for resource allocation can offer a different perspective. While their decision-making considerations may not be identical to those of a high net-worth donor or a private foundation,

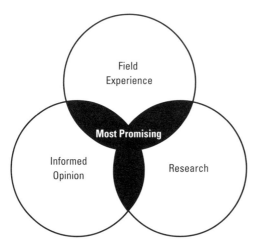

Field Experience
- Practitioner insights
- Performance assessments
- In-depth case studies

Informed Opinion
- Expert opinion
- Stakeholder input
- Policy analyses

Research
- Randomized controlled trials and quasi-experimental studies
- Modeled analyses (e.g., cost-effectiveness)

Figure 14.3. Center for High Impact Philanthropy's sources of information.
Source: Rhodes 2008.

these policymakers, think tanks, and aid organizations have knowledge that can also yield valuable insight.

Philanthropists—and the organizations they support—require a broad definition of evidence. This broad definition of evidence leverages the unique knowledge of different players and disciplines while mitigating their respective limitations. With a mandate to provide guidance that is both actionable and informed by the evidence, the Center for High Impact Philanthropy has adopted a broad definition of evidence that synthesizes the best available information from three domains: research, informed opinion, and field experience. The Center believes that the most promising philanthropic opportunities exist where the recommendations of these three domains overlap (Figure 14.3).

A Checklist for Donors

Armed with a broader definition of evidence, philanthropists—and the organizations they support—will have a greater capacity for developing a philanthropic strategy focused on impact. The rest of this chapter provides a checklist of questions for impact-driven donors to ask in designing effective philanthropic strategies to address women's health in cities. These are the key questions that drive the Center for High Impact Philanthropy's work.

What Is the Impact I Seek (and Is It a Meaningful One)?

While decreases in morbidity, decreases in mortality, and increases in quality of life may be relevant to all global health philanthropists, framing a donor's perspective around cities and women's health highlights specific philanthropic opportunities for impact.

Many of the factors that affect poor, urban women also affect poor, urban men. However, understanding the differences in gender roles can help donors understand what specific changes to target when trying to improve the health of women. For example, women, not men, do the majority of household cooking. Many in developing countries use solid fuels for cooking. Such cooking techniques, coupled with the crowding and poor ventilation that characterize urban slums, cause chronic lung problems in mothers and their children. In addition, women face a higher risk of intimate partner violence than do men. Safer cooking practices and protection from sexual violence represent meaningful impacts for a philanthropist concerned with addressing the needs of poor, urban women.

Understanding differences in rural versus urban life can further help philanthropists identify opportunities to improve the health of women in cities. While urban areas have a higher concentration of economic opportunities than found in rural areas, cities also concentrate the many risks to women's health. For women in both the developing and the developed world, these risks include air and water pollution, traffic injuries, infectious diseases, and chronic noncommunicable diseases from tobacco use, alcohol consumption, poor diets, and physical inactivity. In addition, although big hospitals tend to be located in urban areas, women in urban slums often have less access to basic health services than their rural counterparts do. For example, in Bangladesh, health indicators are worse for urban poor than rural poor due to the lack of prenatal care and skilled birth attendants available to the poor women living in urban slums (The International Centre for Diarrhoeal Disease Research, Bangladesh 2002–2010). The same is true of some urban communities in the United States. Philanthropists who can remove any one of these hazards can make a meaningful difference in the life of poor, urban women. Changes across multiple risk factors can have a transformative effect.

What Has Worked? What Hasn't?

The key to spending philanthropic funds wisely is to build on previous success and not waste money either reinventing the wheel or making mistakes that others have made before. For those donors who are entrepreneurially minded, understanding what has worked and what hasn't also helps focus innovation where innovation is most needed.

Specific case examples can be especially helpful to philanthropists seeking high-impact strategies. The work of Manoshi, in the Dhaka slums of Bangladesh, offers important lessons.

Case Example: Manoshi, Dhaka, Bangladesh

Like many other developing countries, Bangladesh has a high maternal death ratio: 570 maternal deaths per 100,000 live births compared to 11 per 100,000 live births in the United States (UNICEF 2010c). Approximately 80 percent of all deliveries in the urban slums of Bangladesh are conducted at home by unskilled friends or relatives (The International Centre for Diarrhoeal Disease Research, Bangladesh 2002–2010).

Understanding the importance of antenatal care and the use of skilled birth attendants on maternal and newborn health, the non-profit BRAC started an urban maternal and newborn health program called Manoshi in 2007 in the Dhaka slums. The project delivers proven maternal health interventions through an integrated package of essential health services.

Through Manoshi, BRAC has adapted to the urban setting its Essential Care Program model, which had been highly successful in rural Bangladesh. Key components include the use of community health workers and skilled birth attendants who make care accessible to women close to where they live. Community health workers identify and follow all pregnant women no matter where they go for medical care. They encourage women to give birth at a BRAC birthing hut where skilled birth attendants and clean conditions are available. Community health services are also linked with referral services to preselected quality health facilities for women who need a higher level of care during childbirth (e.g., cesarean section for obstructed labor) (The International Centre for Diarrhoeal Disease Research, Bangladesh 2009).

In addition, a key part of Manoshi's implementation strategy is community empowerment through the support of women's groups—a key success factor learned from BRAC's decades of health and development work in rural Bangladesh.

Most important, there is already evidence of impact: In the three years since the project's launch, Manoshi has seen a marked shift in where urban slum-dwelling women are delivering their babies. At project baseline, 86 percent of women delivered in their homes. In 2009, that number dropped to 25 percent. Of those who were not delivering in their homes, 33 percent were giving birth in BRAC delivery centers and 42 percent were delivering in hospitals (BRAC Blog 2010). Evidence from many countries shows that skilled birth attendants represent one of the most important interventions for decreasing maternal death and ensuring the health of newborns (WHO 2010c).

When There Has Been Success, How Much Did It Cost?

Linking considerations of cost and impact is at the heart of high-impact philanthropy. Too often philanthropic conversations focus only on costs (e.g., "Look at our low overhead ratios!") or only on impact (e.g., "Look what good we've done!"). For a philanthropist seeking to make the greatest difference in improving the lives of others, understanding the relationship between cost and impact serves many purposes. It can help set realistic expectations, particularly in a fundraising world where philanthropic opportunities can be pitched on the promise of outsized results for the money requested. It can provide meaningful benchmarks for performance management. It can help identify well-earned efficiencies as well as opportunities to do more good with the same resources (Rosqueta 2010).

Again, a case example illustrates how philanthropists can link considerations of cost and impact.

Case Example: Nurse-Family Partnerships, United States

Low-income mothers pregnant with their first child represent a vulnerable population, even in wealthy countries such as the United States. The nonprofit Nurse-Family Partnership (NFP) targets such women. NFP identifies an expectant mother early in her pregnancy and partners her with a registered nurse who provides in-home support and guidance to that woman until the woman's child reaches his or her second birthday. Early in the mother's pregnancy, the registered nurse will teach the woman and her family about healthy practices such as having regular and early prenatal checkups, good nutrition, and the importance of not smoking or drinking during pregnancy. After the baby is born, support can take the form of coaching the mother on infant and toddler care, family planning, and helping the mother develop skills to reach educational and employment goals.

Participating registered nurses receive over sixty hours of training. The program maintains high standards of care through regular and ongoing supervision of participating nurses and case conferences where nurses meet in teams to share experiences and learn from one another.

As with Manoshi, earlier implementations of the model were conducted in rural settings. However, a pivotal study focused specifically on the effectiveness of the model among inner-city black families in

Memphis, where rates of infant mortality and morbidity were among the highest in the nation. This study, along with other randomized controlled trials, has demonstrated the program's impressive impact on both the participating women and their children (Goodman 2006). The women visited by the nurses had

- 23 percent fewer hypertensive disorders in pregnancy than did women in the control group
- 25 percent reduction in cigarette smoking during pregnancy
- 83 percent increase in workforce participation by low-income unmarried mothers by the time the child was 4 years old

Their children had

- 56 percent fewer doctor and hospital visits due to childhood injuries through age 2
- 48 percent less incidence of child abuse and neglect
- 69 percent fewer convictions by age 15

NFP's impact is especially impressive given its relative cost. A 2005 RAND study found that for every one U.S. dollar invested, the program returned $5.70, providing a net benefit to society of over $34,148 per high-risk family served (Karoly, Kilburn, and Cannon 2005) (Figure 14.4).

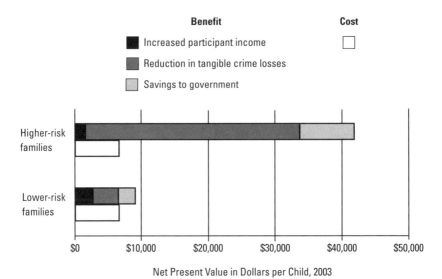

Figure 14.4. Nurse-Family Partnership's monetary benefits to society.
Source: Data from Karoly et al. 2005. Graphic courtesy of Nurse-Family Partnership.

NFP's consideration of both cost and impact significantly affected its design, leading it to test modifications to its models to look for improved efficiencies. In the mid-1990s similar home-visiting programs had been developed using paraprofessionals instead of registered nurses. Some suggested that using such paraprofessionals might be an effective way to reduce the program's cost. NFP undertook a controlled study examining this question. Their findings, published in *Pediatrics* in 2002, revealed that there were virtually no differences between paraprofessional-visited mothers and the control group. Paraprofessionals were indeed cheaper, but they also showed no evidence of meaningful, positive impact (Goodman 2006).

What Organizations Are Best Positioned to Deliver the Impact I Seek?

Ultimately, philanthropists achieve impact through the work of organizations on the ground. To achieve that impact, philanthropists need to know how to assess a potential partner or project. BRAC's Manoshi and Nurse-Family Partnerships provide two good examples of what to look for in organizations on the ground. Both had the following capacities:

- Preventive care and treatment that reached women where they lived. In Manoshi's case, community health workers and skilled birth attendants worked with women in the slums of Dhaka. In the NFP model, registered nurses were deployed to provide support in women's homes in the United States.
- Links to a referral system. In Manoshi's case, referrals were made to BRAC birthing huts and preselected quality health facilities. In the case of NFP, the existence of a clear and simple referral network in Memphis was one of the reasons the nonprofit decided to conduct a major study and implementation there. For the inner-city, low-income women who participated in Memphis, a single clinic existed for prenatal care. From that clinic, women could be referred to neighborhood health centers and a local hospital for delivery.
- Partnerships and networks that address the root causes of ill health. In Manoshi's case, support groups fostered community empowerment and links to social services, health education, and economic opportunity. In the case of NFP, nurses made necessary referrals to human service agencies, educational opportunities, medical care for mother and baby, and job training.
- A large learning component not only to improve the program's performance, but also to develop generalizable knowledge for

others working to achieve similar change. In collaboration with the Research and Evaluation Division (RED) of BRAC, the International Centre for Diarrhoeal Disease Research, Bangladesh (ICDDR,B), and the Bill & Melinda Gates Foundation, Manoshi developed a research framework with five components: formative research, impact survey, system performance research, cost-effectiveness research, and scaling-up research. Throughout the thirty-year development of its model, NFP's founder, David Olds, insisted that the model be "evidence based" (Goodman 2006: 6). More than once, he refused public financing to scale up because he felt it was premature given what was then known about the model's effectiveness.

How Can My Funding Help?

Private philanthropy played an essential role in enabling the remarkable impact that Manoshi and Nurse-Family Partnerships achieved in addressing health outcomes for poor, urban women. These projects serve as examples of how such funding—along with bilateral, multilateral, and public financing—can make a difference in the lives of women in cities.

Interestingly, in both cases, private philanthropic funding from U.S.-based foundations was especially instrumental in testing and refining the model. In other words, philanthropic funding provided crucial research and development financing to the nonprofits working to improve the health of these poor, urban women. In Manoshi's case, that funding was in the form of over $25 million dollars over five years provided by the Gates Foundation "to demonstrate an effective and transferable program model for improving maternal, newborn and child health, especially around delivery, in poor urban communities of developing countries" (Bill & Melinda Gates Foundation 2007: under "Purpose").

In the case of Nurse-Family Partnerships, that funding was in the form of grants at key stages in the model's development. In 1979 the Robert Wood Johnson Foundation supported the continuation of a study initially funded by the U.S. Public Health Service that provided the first test of David Olds's original model. Olds recounted, "That initial Johnson grant was a god-send that solidified everything we have done since" (Goodman 2006: 9). Carnegie Corporation, Pew Charitable Trusts, and W. T. Grant Foundation, along with Robert Wood Johnson, funded the pilot study with inner-city black communities in Memphis. Other foundations, including Edna McConnell Clark, Gates, Google

Grants, Kellogg, Picower, and Kresge, would help replicate the model nationwide.

Conclusion

In both the developing and the developed world, philanthropic funding is relatively small compared to public financing and bilateral and multilateral aid. Yet it has played a critical role in addressing the health of women in cities. Manoshi in Bangladesh and Nurse-Family Partnerships in the United States are two examples of how philanthropists have funded solutions that are making a measurable and meaningful improvement in the health of poor, urban women and their children. In particular, both illustrate the powerful role that philanthropic funding can play in testing and refining solutions to some of the most important, and difficult, public health issues facing women in cities.

Given the many factors that influence the health of women in cities, philanthropists seeking impact must employ a broad definition of evidence to inform their strategies. By focusing on impact, understanding what has worked and what hasn't, linking considerations of cost and impact, and identifying what capacities are required of good nonprofit/nongovernmental organization partners, today's philanthropists will be well positioned to make the improvements in women's health that they seek. Given the role of women in families and society, such improvements will have tremendous impact not just for these women and their children, but for the entire global community.

Afterword

Susan M. Wachter

Global urbanization is a revolutionary force, easily one of the most important transformations in human history. It is, at once, responsible for both an unprecedented increase in the standard of living for many and also systemic inequality. The dual nature of this transformation and the resulting need to assure that the life chances of the most vulnerable, including women and children, improve, present a global challenge.

The development and market forces driving global urbanization can be placed in a larger frame. Picture the world before capitalism. Workers produce almost everything necessary for survival—and, if possible, a bit of recreation—but do not specialize in one task or career. It is a world of subsistence. Only a few are privileged to own their own land. In many countries, the majority of the population serve as feudal serfs to the landlords, in exchange for which they receive protection from outside dangers and a minimal share of the land's yield.

It is also a world that does not move forward. According to the renowned classical economist Thomas Robert Malthus, increases in the standard of living are unsustainable: If a community's income per capita increases, families use that extra money to feed more mouths. The population grows until income per capita falls back to its original level (Malthus 1789).

Now imagine the upheaval this world experiences with the potential of economic growth. Within firms, each worker specializes in part of the production process, and together they create more valuable products than they did by themselves. Technological progress allows income to grow faster than the population.

This transition occurs in cities. Families migrate from rural to urban regions because they want the chance of work and a standard of living beyond subsistence. But in fact, while economic development occurs, the rural-to-urban migration overwhelms the city's ability to provide even basic services for its new residents. Indeed, urban unemployment is high, and a large underclass fills the new slums. Women and children are particularly at risk.

Collective action is needed to address the underside that accompanies urban economic growth. Having many people in one place increases vulnerability to the spread of disease and to natural disasters. Massive urban migration requires public services for the corresponding increase in the numbers of urban poor. Inadequate housing, malnourishment, lack of potable water or sanitation, and lack of other basic services are for too many the unfortunate reality of global urbanization. In the next decades, more than a billion more people will migrate to cities.

Viewed through this lens, alleviating global poverty, improving public health, and achieving gender equality are daunting challenges, in both size and complexity. These challenges are not, as some observers contend, mere by-products of corrupt officials or lawless states, nor are they caused by inferior industrialization or cultural deficiencies. The problems discussed in this book are systemic and market driven.

Recent efforts to solve these problems have come up woefully short. In September 2010, the United Nations held a summit to review progress on the Millennium Development Goals, which include eradicating extreme poverty and hunger, promoting gender equality and empowering women, and improving maternal health. Jeffrey Sachs, the economist leading these efforts, specified women and health as "major gaps" in this progress (Commonwealth News and Information Service 2010).

These underwhelming results should not come as a surprise. As William Easterly has documented exhaustively, the capitalist world has been trying to "aid" the "backward" world since colonial days, with little to show for it (Easterly 2001, 2006). But even Easterly does not deny that targeted programs have strong track records.

The chapters in this book have documented proven methods to close those gaps:

Chapter 1. Julio Frenk and Octavio Gómez-Dantés use Mexico's recent health reforms as an illustration of how developing nations can improve their citizens' well-being simply by changing the organizational priorities and increasing insurance coverage.

Chapter 2. Ruth Levine illustrates that we have the tools to prepare for the demographic, epidemiologic, environmental, and economic trends in the developing world and to take appropriate near-term policy action to invest in women.

Chapter 3. Varina Tjon-A-Ten, Brad Kerner, Shweta Shukla, and Anne Hochwalt explain how critical compulsory education is to female health and development and how third parties can encourage female education in the developing world by offering free health products, especially related to reproductive issues.

Chapter 4. Claudia Garcia-Moreno and Manupreet Chawla show how cultures and institutions allow violence against women and how improved access to hospital care; safer, more affordable, and reliable public transportation; and increased information and awareness can reduce this danger.

Chapter 5. Eugenie L. Birch describes urban designs, neighborhood features, and transportation networks that would improve the health of the environment and the women living in it.

Chapter 6. Sheela Patel identifies community programs and public policies that have helped and could help street dwellers in India and how political power is necessary for the underclass to penetrate the caste system.

Chapter 7. Rosaly Correa-de-Araujo documents the barriers that prevent women from sharing fully in the economic growth of developing nations and the resources needed to overcome those barriers.

Chapter 8. DeAnne K. Hilfinger Messias sheds light on rural-to-urban migration and immigrant policies—both good and bad—that affect this process.

Chapter 9. Vivian W. Pinn and Nida H. Corry highlight research programs that have found innovative ways to improve women's health and identify where research funds need to be focused going forward.

Chapter 10. Diane Cornman-Levy, Grace Dyrness, Jane Golden, David Gouverneur, and Jeane Ann Grisso profile grassroots efforts in Philadelphia, Manila, Medellín, and Mantua that have turned regions of disparate individuals into safer, healthier, more attractive, more sustainable communities.

Chapter 11. Grace R. Dyrness illustrates religious programs that reduce violence, increase social bonds, improve mental health, and enhance education for women in low-income communities across the globe.

Chapter 12. Francisca Mwangangi points to the importance of medical care delivery in urban environments and models for improvement despite lackluster government performance.

Chapter 13. Tina C. Musuya details a program in Kampala, Uganda, that is successfully reducing violence and HIV/AIDS through awareness, education, and open dialogue.

Chapter 14. Katherina Rosqueta and Carol A. McLaughlin drive to the heart of William Easterly's concern and hopefully the United

Nation's new attitude: investing in programs that have the most impact per dollar donated.

These specific investigations go deeper into the factors that affect women's health and urban development than any other book you will find. They are a ray of optimism in a dark world of research that all too often has implied that we are helpless before the complexity of economic growth and the powers that control it.

Since Douglass North began his Nobel Prize-winning research in the 1970s, economists and historians have become increasingly convinced that legal and political institutions determine a country's growth path (North 1990). Empirical work from Daron Acemoglu, Simon Johnson, and James Robinson seemed to confirm that finding over the past decade (Acemoglu, Johnson, and Robinson 2001, 2002). Only in the past few years have we begun to understand that markets rely on far more than property rights and democracy to function properly. Edward Glaeser, Rafael La Porta, Florencio Lopez-de-Silanes, and Andrei Shleifer, for instance, have plumbed the New Institutionalists's regressions and found that human capital has more explanatory power than laws or governance, though they too are important (Glaeser et al. 2004). Now the experts in this book have contributed a wealth of examples to support this proposition: Despite geopolitical constraints, we *can* improve the education, health, and economic opportunities of the global poor and we can do so in such a way that women can participate fully, safely, and without exploitation.

Despite the slow manifestation of international efforts, some women have shown remarkable resiliency in their willingness to rise above the toxic and malnourished circumstances in which they find themselves. The organization and partnership of the Society for the Promotion of Area Resource Centres, the National Slum Dwellers Federation, and Mahila Milan described in Sheela Patel's chapter clearly illustrate this urban resolve. In this alliance, women of slum communities and neighborhood collectives have created a mobilized identity and voice, a support system, as well as a vehicle to swiftly spread and integrate new solutions across all stakeholders. These women are not waiting; they continue to effectively leverage the limited resources around them to improve their lives and engineer change. With effective public collective action, in education and public health, there is hope that the standard of living will be raised for all.

Notes

Chapter 3

1. Recently, however, others have suggested that in some communities provision of adequate menstrual protection may not affect school attendance (Oster and Thornton 2011; Lloyd forthcoming).

2. Prior to conducting the research, the author expected to find gaps in girls' knowledge about what was happening in their maturing bodies, along with a potential gap in knowledge about how to manage their menstruation in potentially "girl-unfriendly" school settings. The research was designed to collect girls' own perceptions of the challenges they face and to help develop appropriate solutions. This summary focuses on the data that were used to develop a girls' puberty book project in Tanzania (Sommer 2009b).

Chapter 5

1. Asian urban population is bi-modal: 46 percent (868 million) live in the smallest cities (under 500,000) and another 22 percent (418 million) live in cities with 1 to 5 million people.

2. Substandard sanitation includes openly defecating (7 percent of the total), using an unimproved facility (20 percent), or using a shared facility (8 percent).

3. Substandard drinking water is that from an unprotected dug well or spring, from a cart with a small tank/drum, from surface water (river, stream, pond, lake), or bottled water.

4. The informal sector is defined as the unregulated nonformal portion of the market economy that produces goods and services for sale or for other forms of remuneration. It includes those who work in homes, as independent contractors, as street vendors, and as seasonal workers.

5. These figures include agricultural and nonagricultural work.

Chapter 7

1. The Convention on the Elimination of All Forms of Discrimination Against Women (CEDAW), adopted in 1979 by the United Nations General Assembly, is often described as an international bill of rights for women (CEDAW 1979: article 12). It identifies what constitutes discrimination against women and sets up an agenda for national action to end such discrimination. The convention

defines discrimination against women as "any distinction, exclusion or restriction made on the basis of sex which has the effect or purpose of impairing or nullifying the recognition, enjoyment or exercise by women, irrespective of their marital status, on a basis of equality of men and women, of human rights and fundamental freedoms in the political, economic, social, cultural, civil or any other field." The convention provides a firm basis for bringing about equality between women and men through ensuring women's equal access to, and equal opportunities in, political and public life—including the right to vote and to stand for election—as well as education, health, and employment. Under this convention, States agreed to take all the necessary steps, including legislation or temporary measures, for women to benefit from all their human rights and fundamental freedoms.

2. The International Conference on Population and Development, coordinated by the United Nations and held in Cairo, Egypt, in 1994, with delegates from various governments, United Nations agencies, and nongovernmental organizations, achieved consensus around universal education, reduction of infant and child mortality, reduction of maternal mortality, and access to reproductive and sexual health services including family planning (The International Conference on Population and Development 1994).

3. The 1995 Fourth World Conference on Women adopted the Beijing Platform for Action, which consolidated the recommendations of seven previous conferences and reaffirmed the commitment to the empowerment and advancement of women including the right to freedom of thought, conscience, religion, and belief, thus contributing to the moral, ethical, spiritual, and intellectual needs of women and men, individually or in community with others, and thereby guaranteeing them the possibility of realizing their full potential in society and shaping their lives in accordance with their own aspirations (Beijing Platform for Action 1995: paragraph 12).

4. In 2000, the United Nations established eight Millennium Development Goals to address the world's main development challenges. Each goal has elements that can be enhanced through gender and urbanization (The Millennium Development Goals 2000). For example, the first goal on halving extreme poverty and hunger by 2015 requires considerable attention to impoverished women in slums to help them overcome the extra barriers they face in securing rewarding employment. In its third goal, gender equality and women's empowerment are clearly emphasized. The seventh goal refers to ensuring environmental sustainability, which directly relates to gender equality and sustainable urbanization. In addition, this goal targets the improvement of the lives of at least 100 million slum dwellers by 2020. For this purpose, data collection is needed to support the analysis of sex/gender-disaggregated data to identify the interrelationship between slum life, urban poverty, gender, and disability status.

Chapter 9

1. The Global Health Working Group co-chairs were Kirsten Bibbins-Domingo, M.D., Ph.D., M.A.S. (UCSF); Warner Greene, M.D., Ph.D. (Gladstone/UCSF); F. Gray Handley, M.S.P.H. (NIAID); Amy Levi, Ph.D., C.N.M. (UCSF); Paula Tavrow, Ph.D. (UCLA); and Linda Wright, M.D. (NICHD).

2. The Understudied and Underrepresented Populations Working Group co-chairs were Vickie M. Mays, Ph.D., M.S.P.H. (overall co-chair, UCLA); Gloria

Sarto, M.D., Ph.D. (overall co-chair, University of Wisconsin–Madison); Pamela K. Brown, M.P.A. (West Virginia University); Rebecca L. Clark, Ph.D. (NICHD); Naomi Lynn Gerber, M.D. (George Mason University); Celia J. Maxwell, MD (Howard University Hospital); Anne E. Sumner, MD (NIDDK); and Derrick Tabor, Ph.D. (NCMHD).

3. The Women's Health and the Environment Working Group co-chairs were Tracey J. Woodruff, Ph.D., M.P.H. (UCSF); Lawrence H. Kushi, Sc.D. (Kaiser Permanente); Eveline Shen, M.P.H. (Reproductive Justice); Kris Thayer, Ph.D. (NIEHS); Estella Parrott, M.D., M.P.H. (NICHD); and Deborah Winn, Ph.D. (NCI).

Chapter 11

1. La Virgen de Guadalupe is the Patron Saint of the Americas. Latinos from around the world make pilgrimages to Our Lady of Guadalupe in Mexico City, where, according to Catholic teaching, the Virgin first appeared to an indigenous man. La Virgen de Guadalupe has become highly significant in Latino Catholic identity.

2. The meaning of vision in this discussion is, as defined by the *American Heritage Dictionary of the English Language* (Boston: Houghton Mifflin, 1978), "the mystical experience of seeing as if with the eyes the supernatural or a supernatural being." In the Hebrew Scriptures a vision is explained as a revelation of knowledge, an experience that points to a special awareness of God (Marshall et al. 1996: 1227).

3. For more on this differentiation see *Tongues of Fire: The Explosion of Protestantism in Latin America* (Martin 1990), in which David Martin explores the difference between an individual or internal motivation of faith and an institutional motivation of faith.

References

AC Nielsen Project Parivartan Research. 2010. Field work conducted in March 2010 to understand the impact of sanitary napkins.

Acemoglu, Daron, Simon Johnson, and James Robinson. 2001. The Colonial Origins of Comparative Development: An Empirical Investigation. *American Economic Review* 41(5): 1361–401.

Acemoglu, Daron, Simon Johnson, and James Robinson. 2002. Reversal of Fortune: Geography and Institutions in the Making of the Modern World Income Distribution. *Quarterly Journal of Economics* 68(4): 1231–79.

Active Design Guidelines, Promoting Physical Activity and Health in Design. 2010. New York: New York City Departments of Design and Construction, Health and Mental Hygiene, Transportation and City Planning.

Adeyi, O., O. Smith, and S. Robles. 2007. *Public Policy and the Challenge of Chronic Noncommunicable Diseases.* Washington, D.C.: World Bank.

African Medical and Research Foundation (AMREF). 2004. Together in Hope: Health Promotion and Health Education in the Anglophone African Sub-Region (report of an intercountry workshop, Nairobi).

Agustín, Laura M. 2003. A Migrant World of Services. *Social Politics* 10(3): 377–96.

Ahmad, Fauzia, Tariq Modood, and Stephen Lissenburgh. 2003. *South Asian Women and Employment in Britain: The Interaction of Gender and Ethnicity.* London: Policy Studies Institute.

Akin, J. 1987. *Financing Health Services in Developing Countries: An Agenda for Reform (A World Bank Policy Study).* Washington, D.C.: World Bank, 40–43.

Alaggia, Ramona, Cheryl Regehr, and Giselle Rishchynski. 2009. Intimate Partner Violence and Immigration Laws in Canada: How Far Have We Come? *International Journal of Law and Psychiatry* 32: 335–41.

Alliance for Cervical Cancer Prevention. 2010. http://www.alliance-cxca.org/index.html.

Alliance of Indian Wastepickers. 2010. *Livelihoods with Dignity.* Pune, India.

Almeida-Filho, N., J. Lucélia Magalhães, M. Aráujo, E. Acquino, S. James, and I. Kawachi. 2004. Social Inequality and Depressive Disorders in Bahia, Brazil: Interactions of Gender, Ethnicity, and Social Class. *Social Science and Medicine* 59(7): 1339–53.

AMDD (Averting Maternal Death and Disability). 2010. http://www.amddprogram.org/?gclid=CPXe2I2Z1J8CFQJinAodfBFIaQ.

American Planning Association. 2006. *Planning and Urban Design Standards.* Chicago: APA Planners Press.

Anderson, Joan, and S. Reimer Kirkham. 1998. Constructing Nation: The Gendering and Racializing of the Canadian Health Care System. In *Painting the*

Maple: Essays on Race, Gender, and the Construction of Canada, eds. V. Strong-Boag, S. Grace, A. Eisenberg, and J. Anderson. Vancouver: University of British Columbia Press, 242–61.

Annan, Kofi. 2000. "The first step is for societies to recognize that educating girls is not an option; it is a necessity." Statement made by the former United Nations Secretary General at the Dakar World Education Forum. http://www.unis.unvienna.org/unis/pressrels/2000/soc338.html.

Asakura, Takashi, and Alice K. Murata. 2006. Demography, Immigration Background, Difficulties with Living in Japan, and Psychological Distress Among Japanese Brazilians in Japan. *Journal of Immigrant Health* 8: 325–38.

Austen, Jane. 1814. *Mansfield Park*. London: Thomas Egerton.

Avila, Ernestine. n.d. Unpublished manuscript on transnational parenting. Used by permission.

Backman, G., P. Hunt, R. Khosla, C. Jaramillo-Strouss, B. M. Fikre, and C. Rumble. 2008. Health Systems and the Right to Care. An Assessment of 194 Countries. *Lancet* 372: 2047–85.

Barrington, Clare, DeAnne K. Hilfinger Messias, and Lynn Weber. (In review.) Exploring the Implications of Racial/Ethnic Dynamics for Health and Well-being Among Latinos: A Case Study of West Columbia, South Carolina. *Latino Studies*.

Bartlett, S. 2002. The Problem of Children's Injuries in Low-Income Countries: A Review. *Health Policy and Planning* 17(1): 1–13.

Baumann, Andrea, and Jennifer Blythe. 2008, May 31. Globalization of Higher Education in Nursing. *OJIN: The Online Journal of Issues in Nursing* 13(2), manuscript 4. http://www.nursingworld.org/MainMenuCategories/ANAMarketplace/ANAPeriodicals/OJIN/TableofContents/vol132008/No2May08/GlobalizationofHigherEducation.aspx.

Beijing Platform for Action. 1995. http://www.un.org/womenwatch/daw/beijing/pdf/BDPfA%20E.pdf.

Benschop, M. 2004. *Women's Rights to Land and Property*. London: UN-HABITAT.

Bharadwaj, Sowmyaa, and Archana Patkar. 2004. Menstrual Hygiene and Management in Developing Countries: Taking Stock. *The Museum of Menstruation and Women's Health*. http://www.mum.org/menhydev.htm.

Bhattacharyya, Jay. 2010. *Guwahati—The City*. http://www.docstoc.com/docs/8713630/Guwahati-The-City.

Bill & Melinda Gates Foundation. 2007. *Grants 2007: BRAC*. http://www.gatesfoundation.org/Grants-2007/Pages/BRAC-OPP41956.aspx.

Birch, E., and S. Wachter. 2008. *Growing Greener Cities, Urban Sustainability in the 21st Century*. Philadelphia: University of Pennsylvania Press.

Birch, E., and S. Wachter. 2011. *Global Urbanization*. Philadelphia: University of Pennsylvania Press.

Blanco, C., and H. Kobayashi. 2009. Urban Transformation in Slum Districts Through Space Generation and Cable Transportation at Northeastern Area: Medellín, Colombia. *Journal of International Social Research*. 2(8): 75–90.

Blank Noise Blog. 2009, May 13. http://blog.blanknoise.org/

Blankespoor, Brian, Susmita Dasgupta, Benoit Laplante, and David Wheeler. 2010. *The Economics of Adaptation to Extreme Weather Events in Developing Countries*. Center for Global Development Working Paper No. 199. Washington, D.C.: Center for Global Development.

Boneham, M. A., and J. A. Sixsmith. 2006. The Voices of Older Women in a Disadvantaged Community: Issues of Health and Social Capital. *Social Science & Medicine* 69(2): 269–79.

Bottorff, Joan L., Joy L. Johnson, and Lisa J. Venables. 2001. Voices of Immigrant South Asian Women: Expressions of Health Concerns. *Journal of Health Care for the Poor and Underserved* 12(4): 392–403.

Boyle, Gregory S. J. 2010. *Tattoos on the Heart: The Power of Boundless Compassion.* New York: Simon & Schuster.

BRAC Blog. 2010, May 25. *BRAC's Kaosar Afsana Presents Outstanding Maternal Health Program Results at Gates Foundation.* Seattle. http://blog.bracusa. org/2010/05/ bracs-kaosar-afsana-presents.html.

Bradshaw, Della. 2010, January 25. Resolving a Taboo. *Financial Times.*

Breast Health Global Initiative. 2008. Guidelines for International Breast Health and Cancer Control—Implementation. *Cancer* 113(S8): 2215–371.

Brocklehurst, C., and J. Bartram. 2010. Swimming Upstream: Why Sanitation, Hygiene and Water Are So Important to Mothers and Their Daughters. *Bulletin of the WHO* 88: 482.

Burgel, Barbara J., Nan Lashuay, Leslie Israel, and Robert Harrison. 2004. Garment Workers in California: Health Outcomes of the Asian Immigrant Women Workers Clinic. *American Association of Occupational Health Nurses Journal* 52(11): 465–75.

Burgess, G. 2008. Planning and the Gender Equality Duty—Why Does Gender Matter? *People, Place and Policy Online* 2/3: 112–21.

Buvinić, M., A. Médici, E. Fernández, and A. C. Torres. 2006. Gender Differentials in Health. In *Disease Control Priorities in Developing Countries*, 2nd ed., eds. D. T. Jamison, J. G. Breman, A. R. Measham, G. Alleyne, M. Claeson, D. B. Evans, et al. New York: Oxford University Press.

Byrne, C. 1996. Breast. In *Cancer Rates and Risks*, 4th ed., eds. A. Harris, B. K. Edwards, W. J. Blot, and L. A. G. Ries. Washington, D.C.: U.S. Department of Health and Human Services, 120–23.

Campbell, J. 2002. Health Consequences of Intimate Partner Violence. *Lancet* 359: 1331–36.

Campbell, T., and A. Campbell. 2007. Emerging Disease Burdens and the Poor in Cities of the Developing World. *Journal of Urban Health* 84(1): i54–i64.

Carling, Jørgen. 2005. *Gender Dimensions of International Migration.* Geneva: Global Commission on International Migration. http://www.gcim.org/mm/ File/GMP%20No%2035.pdf.

Castles, Stephen. 2004. The Factors That Make and Unmake Migration Policies. *International Migration Review* 38(3): 852–84.

Cavanagh, S. 1998. *Making Safer Places: A Resource Book for Neighbourhood Safety Audits.* London: Women's Design Service.

Centers for Disease Control and Prevention. 2010, July 19. *Press Release. New CDC Analysis Reveals Strong Link Between Poverty and HIV Infection: New Study in Low-Income Heterosexuals in America's Inner Cities Reveals High HIV Rates.* http://www.cdc.gov/nchhstp/newsroom/povertyandhivpressrelease. html.

Central Intelligence Agency. n.d. *World Factbook, 2007.* https://www.cia.gov/ library/publications/the-world-factbook/geos/et.html.

Central Intelligence Agency. n.d. *World Factbook, 2010.* https://www.cia.gov/ library/publications/the-world-factbook/geos/et.html.

Centro de Intercambio y Servicios Cono Sur, Argentina (CISCSA); UNIFEM; Spanish Agency for International Cooperation (AECI). 2005. *Tools for the Promotion of Safe Cities from the Gender Perspective*, trans. Laura Hunt. Cordoba: CISCSA.

Chen, M., J. Vanek, F. Lund, and J. Heintz. 2005. *Progress of the World's Women 2005: Women, Work, and Poverty.* New York: United Nations Development Fund for Women.

Cholletta, D., and M. Leuris. 1997. *Private Insurance Principles and Practices.* World Bank Discussion Paper 365. Washington, D.C.: World Bank, 77–112.

Clark, Lauren. 2002. Mexican-Origin Mothers' Experiences Using Children's Health Care Services. *Western Journal of Nursing Research* 24: 159–79.

CLUE (Clergy and Laity United for Economic Justice). 2010, June 30. http://cluela.org.

Cohen, J. 2002. World Population in 2050: Assessing the Projections. In *Seismic Shifts: The Economic Impact of Demographic Change,* eds. J. Little and R. J. Triest. Boston: The Federal Reserve Bank of Boston.

Cohen, J. 2011. Human Population Grows Up. In *Global Urbanization,* eds. E. Birch and S. Wachter. Philadelphia: University of Pennsylvania Press.

Collins, F. 2009. *NIH All-Hands Town Meeting with Dr. Collins—Inaugural Address.* http://videocast.nih.gov/Summary.asp?File=15247.

Commission on Social Determinants of Health. 2008. *Closing the Gap in a Generation: Health Equity Through Action on the Social Determinants of Health.* Geneva: World Health Organization.

Commonwealth News and Information Service. 2010. *Jeffrey Sachs Charts the Way Forward for MDGs Ahead of UN Summit. London, UK.* http://allafrica.com/stories/201008250896.html.

Convention on the Elimination of All Forms of Discrimination Against Women (CEDAW). 1979. http://www.un.org/womenwatch/daw/cedaw/text/econvention.htm#article12.

Coogan, P. F., L. F. White, J. A. Thomas, K. M. Hathaway, J. R. Palmer, and L. Rosenberg. 2009. Prospective Study of Urban Form and Physical Activity in the Black Women's Health Study. *American Journal of Epidemiology Advance Access* 170(9): 1105–17.

Costello, A., M. Abbas, A. Allen, S. Ball, S. Bell, R. Bellamy, et al. 2009. Managing the Health Effects of Climate Change: Lancet and University College London Institute for Global Health Commission. *Lancet* 373(9676): 1693–733.

Cowichan Women Against Violence Society. 2002. *Women and Community Safety: A Resource Book on Planning for Safer Communities.* Duncan, Canada: Cowichan Women Against Violence Society.

Day, K. 2006. Active Living and Social Justice. *Journal of the American Planning Association* 72(1): 88–99.

De Jesus, Maria. 2009. The Importance of Social Context in Understanding and Promoting Low-Income Immigrant Women's Health. *Journal of Health Care for the Poor and Underserved* 20(1): 90–97.

Dean, J. 2002. Safety Audits and Beyond: Round Table (First International Seminar on Women's Safety—Making the Links, Montreal).

DeJaeghere, Joan. 2004, September 8–11. Quality Education and Gender Equality (Background Paper, Workshop I, International Conference on Education, 47th Session, UNICEF, Geneva).

Demick, Barbara. 2010, July 12 and 19. Letter from Yanji: Nothing Left. Is North Korea Finally Facing Collapse? *New Yorker,* 44–49.

Depouy, L. (Special Rapporteur of the Sub-Commission on Prevention of Discrimination and Protection of Minorities). 1988. *Human Rights and Disabled Persons.* Human Rights Studies Series, no. 6. United Nations Publication No. E.92.XIV.4, paragraph 140. Geneva: Centre for Human Rights.

DiabeDiario. 2009. http://201.116.23.233:81/nuestrosprogramas/Paginas/telecomunicaciones.aspx.

Divi, C., R. G. Koss, S. P. Schmaltz, and J. M. Loeb. 2007. Language Proficiency and Adverse Events in US Hospitals: A Pilot Study. *International Journal for Quality in Health Care* 19: 60–67.

Dollar, David, and Roberta Gatti. 1999. *Gender Inequality, Income, and Growth. Are Good Times Good for Women?* Policy Research Report on Gender and Development, Working Paper Series, no. 1. Washington, D.C.: World Bank.

Donnelly, Tam Truong. 2006. Living "In-Between"—Vietnamese Canadian Women's Experiences: Implications for Health Care Practice. *Health Care for Women International* 27: 695–708.

Dossal, Mariam. 1991. *Imperial Designs and Indian Realities: The Planning of Bombay City, 1845–1875.* Delhi: Oxford University Press, 143–44.

Doyal, L. 2004. Women, Health, and Global Restructuring: Setting the Scene. *Development* 47(2): 18–23.

Doyle, S., A. Kelly-Schwartz, M. Schlossberg, and J. Stockard. 2006. Active Community Environments and Health. *Journal of the American Planning Association* 72(1): 19–31.

Dreze, J., and A. Sen. 2002. *India: Development and Participation.* Oxford: Oxford University Press.

Drusine, H. 2002. Claiming the Night. *Habitat Debate, 8*(4). http://www.unhabitat.org/hd/hdv8n4/forum6.asp.

Dufour, Darna L., and B. A. Piperata. 2004. Rural-to-Urban Migration in Latin America: An Update and Thoughts on the Model. *American Journal of Human Biology* 16: 395–404.

Dupas, Pascaline, and Jonathan Robinson. 2009. *Savings Constraints and Microenterprise Development: Evidence from a Field Experiment in Kenya.* NBER Working Paper No. 14693. Cambridge, Mass.: National Bureau of Economic Research.

Dyrness, Andrea. (Forthcoming.) *Mothers United: An Immigrant Struggle for Socially Just Education.* Minneapolis: University of Minnesota Press.

Dyrness, Grace R. 1978. A comparative study on the activities of relocated low income women (Master's thesis, Ateneo de Manila University).

Dyson, T. 2003. HIV/AIDS and urbanization. *Population and Development Review* 29: 427–42.

Easterly, William. 2001. *The Elusive Quest for Growth: Economists' Adventures and Misadventures in the Tropics.* Cambridge, Mass.: MIT Press.

Easterly, William. 2006. *The White Man's Burden: Why the West's Efforts to Aid the Rest Have Done So Much Ill and So Little Good.* New York: Penguin Books.

Echeverri, Alejandro. 2008, February. Verbal account. Lecture for students and faculty of the University of Pennsylvania in Medellín.

Echeverria, Sandra E., and Olveen Carrasquillo. 2006. The Roles of Citizenship Status, Acculturation, and Health Insurance in Breast and Cervical Cancer Screening Among Immigrant Women. *Medical Care* 44(8): 788–92.

ECLAC. 2008. *Statistical Yearbook for Latin America and the Caribbean, 2007.* http://websie.eclac.cl/anuario_estadistico/anuario_2008/docs/ANUARIO2008.pdf.

Ehrenreich, Barbara, and Arlie Russell Hochschild. 2002. Introduction. In *Global Woman: Nannies, Maids and Sex Workers in the New Economy,* eds. Arlie Hochschild and Barbara Ehrenreich. New York: Owl Books, 1–14.

Ellsberg, Mary C., A. F. M. Jansen Henrica, L. Heise, C. Watts, and C. Garcia-Moreno, on behalf of the WHO Multi-country Study on Women's Health and Domestic Violence Against Women Study Team. 2008. Intimate Partner Violence and Women's Physical and Mental Health in the WHO Multi-country Study on Women's Health and Domestic Violence: An Observational Study. *Lancet* 371: 1165–72.

Engjadim, Lucy. 2009. *The Priscilla Story.* Guwahati, Assam: Priscilla Centre.

Ethiopian Ministry of Health. 2007. *National Adolescent and Youth Reproductive Health Strategy, 2007–2025.* Addis Ababa: Ethiopian Ministry of Health.

EUROSTAT. 2001. *Disability and Social Participation in Europe.* Luxembourg: European Commission.

Evans, F., and T. Dame. 1999. *Cowichan Valley Safety Audit Guide.* Duncan, Canada: Cowichan Women Against Violence Society.

Evans, J. 1987. Introduction: Migration and Health. *International Migration Review* 21: v–xiv.

Falconer A., E. Crisp, C. Warwick, and F. Day-Strik. 2009. Scaling Up Human Resources for Women's Health. *BJOG* 116(Suppl. 1): 11–14.

Falú, A. 2007. Presentation in UNIFEM Cuadernos de Dialogos. Regional Programme, Cities Without Violence Against Women, Safe Cities for All.

Farmer, P, J. Frenk, F. M. Knaul, L. N. Shulman, G. Alleyne, L. Armstrong, et al. 2010. *Expansion of Cancer Care and Control in Countries of Low and Middle Income: A Call to Action.* http://www.thelancet.com/journals/lancet/article/PIIS0140-6736(10)61152-X/fulltext.

FAWE Uganda. 2004. Sexual maturation in relation to education of girls in Uganda: documenting good practices in girls' education. Unpublished report. Kampala: FAWE U.

Fay, M. 2005. *The Urban Poor in Latin America.* Washington, D.C.: World Bank.

Federation of Neighborhood Centers. 2009. Unpublished survey of fifteen community centers.

Fekete, Liz. 2009. *Suitable Enemy: Racism, Migration and Islamophobia in Europe.* London: Pluto Press.

Fikree, F, R. Gray, W. Berendes, and M. Karim. 1994. A Community-Based Nested Case-Control Study of Maternal Mortality. *International Journal of Gynecology & Obstetrics* 47: 247–55.

Flores, Glenn. 2005. The Impact of Medical Interpreter Services on the Quality of Health Care: A Systematic Review. *Medical Care Research and Review* 62(3): 255–99.

Ford, P. 2010, June 28. In China, Prosperous Lawyer Liu Pifeng Aids Migrant Workers. His Ultimate Goal: Fix a Faulty Legal System. *Christian Science Monitor,* 7.

Fortune, Marie, and C. Enger. 2006, March. *Violence Against Women and the Role of Religion.* Harrisburg: VAWnet, a project of the National Resource Center on Domestic Violence/Pennsylvania Coalition Against Domestic Violence. http://new.vawnet.org.

For Want of a Drink: A Special Report on Water (Special issue). 2010, May 22. *The Economist.*

Fotso, Jean-Christophe, Alex Ezeh, Nyovani Madise, Abdhallah Ziraba, and Reuben Ogollah. 2009. What Does Access to Maternal Care Mean Among the Urban Poor? Factors Associated with Use of Appropriate Maternal Health Services in the Slum Settlements of Nairobi, Kenya. *Maternal and Child Health Journal* 13(1): 130–37.

The Foundation Center. 2010a. *Global Philanthropy: Giving by U.S. Foundations for Global Health, 2008.* http://foundationcenter.org/gpf/health/chart-giving.html.

The Foundation Center. 2010b. *Government Aid and Foundation Giving to Support Health in Developing Countries, 2008.* http://foundationcenter.org/gpf/health/chart-oecd.html.

The Foundation Center. 2010c. *Top 25 Foundations Awarding International Grants for Global Health, Circa 2008.* http://foundationcenter.org/gpf/health/tables/3-F_Health_Intl_2008.pdf.

The Foundation Center. 2010d. *Top 50 International Grants Awarded by Foundations for Global Health.* http://foundationcenter.org/gpf/health/tables/1-Top_50_Grants_Health_Intl_2008.

Frenk, J. 2009. Reinventing Primary Health Care: The Need for Systems Integration. *Lancet* 374: 170–73.

Frenk, J., O. Gómez-Dantés, and F. M. Knaul. 2009. The Democratization of Health in Mexico: Financial Innovations for Universal Coverage. *Bulletin of the WHO* 87: 542–48.

Frenk, J., E. González-Pier, O. Gómez-Dantés, M. A. Lezana, and F. M. Knaul. 2006. Comprehensive Reform to Improve Health System Performance in Mexico. *Lancet* 368: 1525–34.

Fry, Richard. 2006. *Gender and Migration.* Pew Hispanic Center Report. Washington, D.C.: Pew Hispanic Center. http://pewhispanic.org/files/reports/64.pdf.

Frye, V., S. Putman, and P. O'Campo. 2008. Whither Gender in Urban Health? *Health and Place* 14: 616–22.

Garau, P., and E. Sclar. 2005. *A Home in the City.* London: Earthscan.

Garcia, M., A. Jemal, E. M. Ward, M. M. Center, Y. Hao, R. L. Siegel, et al. 2007. *Global Cancer Facts and Figures 2007.* Atlanta: American Cancer Society.

Garcia-Moreno, C., and H. Stoeckl. 2009. Protection of Sexual and Reproductive Health Rights: Addressing Violence Against Women. *International Journal of Gynecology and Obstetrics* 106(2): 144–47.

Gathoni, Peninnah. 2009, June 12. High Cost of Sanitary Towels Cause School Absenteeism. *The New Times.*

Giloth, Robert, and Susan Gewirtz. 2009. Philanthropy and Mistakes: An Untapped Resource. *Foundation View* 1(1): 115–24. Also available online at http://www.aecf.org/news/fes/mar2009/pdf/TFRIssue1-Philanthropy_and_Mistakes.pdf.

Gilroy, Goss. 2005. *Retention and Integration of Immigrants in Newfoundland and Labrador—Are We Ready? Final Report.* http://www.nlimmigration.ca/media/2854/immigrationstudyfinal.pdf.

Gilson, L. 1997. The Lessons of User Fee Experience in Africa. *Health Policy and Planning* 12(4): 273–85.

Giving USA Foundation. 2010. *Giving USA 2010: The Annual Report on Philanthropy for the Year 2009.* Glenview, Ill.: Giving USA Foundation.

Glaeser, Edward L., Rafael La Porta, Florencio Lopez-de-Silanes, and Andrei Shleifer. 2004. Do Institutions Cause Growth? *Journal of Economic Growth* 9(3): 271–303.

Global Campaign for Education. 2004. *Learning to Survive: How Education for All Would Save Millions of Young People from HIV/AIDS.* Brussels: Global Campaign for Education Briefing.

Global Migration Group. 2008. *International Migration and Human Rights: Challenges and Opportunities on the Threshold of the 60th Anniversary of the Universal Declaration of Human Rights.* http://www.globalmigrationgroup.org/pdf/Int_Migration_Human_Rights.pdf.

Goebel, A., B. Dodson, and T. Hill. 2010. Urban Advantage or Urban Penalty? A Case Study of Female-Headed Households in a South African City. *Health and Place* 16(3): 573–80.

Goetz, A. 2008. *Who Answers to Women? Gender and Accountability, Progress of the World's Women Report.* New York: United Nations Development Fund for Women.

Goodman, Andy. 2006. *The Story of David Olds and the Nurse Home Visiting Program.* Grants Results Special Report, Robert Wood Johnson Foundation. http://www.rwjf.org/files/publications/other/DavidOldsSpecialReport0606.pdf.

Government of India, Ministry of Home Affairs. 2010. *Indian Government Census Data.* www.censusindia.gov.in.

Gozdziak, Elzbieta. 2008. On Challenges, Dilemmas, and Opportunities in Studying Trafficked Children. *Anthropological Quarterly* 81(4): 903–23.

Greed, C. 2005. An Investigation of the Effectiveness of Gender Mainstreaming as a Means of Integrating the Needs of Women and Men into Spatial Planning in the United Kingdom. *Progress in Planning* 64: 243–321.

Greed, C. 2007. *A Place for Everyone? Gender Equality and Urban Planning.* Oxford, UK: Oxfam.

Grewal, Sukhdev, Joan L. Bottorff, and B. Ann Hilton. 2005. The Influence of Family on Immigrant South Asian Women's Health. *Journal of Family Nursing* 11(3): 242–63.

Grown, C., G. R. Gupta, and R. Pande. 2005. Taking Action to Improve Women's Health Through Gender Equality and Women's Empowerment. *Lancet* 365(9458): 541–43.

Guruge, Sepali, JoAnne Hunter, Keegan Barker, Mary Jane McNally, and Lilian Magalhães. 2010. Immigrant Women's Experiences of Receiving Care in a Mobile Health Clinic. *Journal of Advanced Nursing* 66(2): 350–59.

GWE-PRA. 2001. *Policy Brief: Menarche and Its Implications for Educational Policy in Peru.* Girls' and Women's Education Policy Research Activity. www.worlded.org/docs/Policy_brief.pdf.

Hack, G., E. Birch, P. Sedway, and M. Silver. 2009. *Local Planning: Contemporary Principles and Practice.* Washington, D.C.: International City/County Association.

Hamlin, C. 2009. The History and Development of Public Health in Developed Countries. In *Oxford Textbook of Public Health,* eds. R. Detels, R. Beaglehole, M. A. Lansang, and M. Gulliford. New York: Oxford University Press, 20–38.

Haniff-Cleofas, R., and R. Khedr. 2005a. *Women with Disabilities and the Environment.* http://www.nnewh.org/images/upload/attach/2668Women%20with%20Disabilities%20EN.pdf.

Haniff-Cleofas, R., and R. Khedr. 2005b. *Women with Disabilities and the Urban Environment.* Toronto: National Network on Environments and Women's Health (NNEWH) and Toronto Women's Call to Action (TWCA).

Harcourt, W. 2001. *Women, Health and Globalization.* Rome: Society for International Development.

Harpham, T. 2009. Urban Health in Developing Countries: What Do We Know and Where Do We Go? *Health and Place* 15(1): 107–16.

Harrison, Mark. 1994. *Public Health in British India: Anglo-Indian Preventive Medicine 1859–1914.* New Delhi: Cambridge University Press, 120.

Hassouneh-Phillips, D. 2005. Understanding Abuse of Women with Physical Disabilities: An Overview of the Abuse Pathways Model. *Advances in Nursing Science* 28(1): 70–80.

Hazarika, I. 2010. Women's Reproductive Health in Slum Populations in India: Evidence from NFHS-3. *Journal of Urban Health* 87(2): 264–77.

Heise, L., M. Ellsberg, and M. Gottenmoeller. 1999. *Ending Violence Against Women*. Population Reports, series L, no. 11. Baltimore: Johns Hopkins University School of Public Health, Populations Information Program.

Herz, Barbara, K. Subbarao, Masooma Habib, and Laura Raney. 1991. *Letting Girls Learn: Promising Approaches in Primary and Secondary Education/No 133*. Washington, D.C.: World Bank.

Híjar, M., J. Trostle, and M. Bronfman. 2003. Pedestrian Injuries in Mexico: A Multi-Method Approach. *Social Science and Medicine* 57(11): 2149–59.

The HMS Mobile Swine Flu App keeps you armed against this deadly disease. 2009. http://www.ismashphone.com/2009/10/the-hms-mobile-swine-flu-app-keeps-you-armed-against-this-deadly-disease.html.

Hochschild, Arlie Russell. 2002. Love and Gold. In *Global Woman: Nannies, Maids and Sex Workers in the New Economy*, eds. Arlie Hochschild and Barbara Ehrenreich. New York: Owl Books, 15–30.

Hogan, M. C., K. J. Foreman, M. Naghavi, S. Y. Ahn, M. Wang, S. M. Makela, et al. 2010. Maternal Mortality for 181 Countries, 1980–2008: A Systematic Analysis of Progress Towards Millennium Development Goal 5. *Lancet* 375(9726): 1609–23.

Hondagneu-Sotelo, Pierrette. 2008. *God's Heart Has No Borders: How Religious Activists Are Working for Immigrant Rights*. Berkeley: University of California Press.

Hsieh, C. H., C. Y. Wang, M. McCubbin, S. Zhang, and J. Inouye. 2008. Factors Influencing Osteoporosis Preventive Behaviours: Testing a Path Model. *Journal of Advanced Nursing* 62(3): 336–45.

Hunt, L. 2007. *Inventing Human Rights. A History*. New York: W.W. Norton.

Hutchinson, R. N., M. A. Putt, L. T. Dean, J. A. Long, C. A. Montagnet, and K. Armstrong. 2009. Neighborhood Racial Composition, Social Capital and Black All-Cause Mortality in Philadelphia. *Social Science and Medicine* 68: 1859–65.

Institute of Medicine (IOM). 2009. *The U.S. Commitment to Global Health: Recommendations for the Public and Private Sectors*. Washington, D.C.: The National Academies Press.

The International Centre for Diarrhoeal Disease Research, Bangladesh. 2002–2010. *Manoshi*. http://centre.icddrb.org/activity/?typeOfActivity=Manoshi.

The International Centre for Diarrhoeal Disease Research, Bangladesh. 2009. *Manoshi: Research Brief* (February, Issue 1). http://www.icddrb.org/uploads/originaluploads/Manoshi-Resbrief_Issue-1-Feb09.pdf.

The International Conference on Population and Development. 1994. http://www.un.org/popin/icpd2.htm.

International Disability Rights Monitor. 2004. *Regional Report of the Americas*. http://www.dpi.org/lang-en/resources/topics_detail?page=316.

IRIN. 2010a. KENYA: *Nairobi's Street Children: Hope for Kenya's Future Generation*. http://www.irinnews.org/InDepthMain.aspx?InDepthId=28&ReportId=69987&Country=Yes.

IRIN. 2010b. NEPAL: *Menstruating Girls Miss Out on School*. www.irinnews.org/report.aspx?ReportID=88992.

ISTED. 2010. *Urbanization in Developing Countries*. http://www.isted.com/pole-ville/urban_cooperation/coop_ch1.pdf.

Jacobs, J. 1961. *The Death and Life of Great American Cities*. New York: Random House.

Jagori. 2007. *Is This Our City? Mapping Safety for Women in Delhi.* Delhi: Jagori.

Jargowsky, P. 2003. *Stunning Progress, Hidden Problems: The Dramatic Decline of Concentrated Poverty in the 1990s.* Washington, D.C.: The Brookings Institution.

Johnson, Joy L., Joan L. Bottorff, Annette J. Browne, Sukhdev Grewal, B. Ann Hilton, and Heather Clarke. 2004. Othering and Being Othered in the Context of Health Care Services. *Health Communication* 16(2): 253–71.

Jordans, F. 2009. *World's Poor Drive Growth in Global Cell Phone Use.* http://abcnews.go.com/Technology/wireStory?id=6986939.

Kaiser Family Foundation. 2010. *Global Health Facts.* http://www.globalhealthfacts.org/topic.jsp?i=31.

Kampala City Council, Makindye and Rubaga Headquarters. 2002. *Sub-County Summary.*

Karim, Q. A., S.S.A. Karim, J. A. Frohlich, A. C. Grobler, C. Baxter, L. E. Mansoor, et al., on behalf of the CAPRISA 004 Trial Group. 2010. Effectiveness and Safety of Tenofovir Gel, an Antiretroviral Microbicide, for the Prevention of HIV Infection in Women. *Science* 329(5996): 1168–74. doi: 10.1126/science.1193748.

Kariuki, W. 2003.The Impact of Institutional Management of Menstruation: A Case Study. In *What's (Not) Happening in Our Schools*, eds. P. Mutunga and J. Stewart. Harare, Zimbabwe: Weaver Press.

Karn, Sunil Kumar, Shigeo Shikura, and Hideki Harada. 2003, August 23. Living Environment and Health of Urban Poor: A Study in Mumbai. *Economic and Political Weekly.*

Karoly, Lynn A. 2008. *Valuing Benefits in Benefit-Cost Studies of Social Programs.* Santa Monica, Calif.: RAND Corporation. Quoted in Tuan, Melinda. 2008. *Measuring and /or Estimating Social Value Creation: Insights into Eight Integrated Cost Approaches.* Bill & Melinda Gates Foundation, Impact Planning and Improvement, 19. http://www.gatesfoundation.org/learning/documents/wwl-report-measuring-estimating-social-value-creation.pdf.http://www.gatesfoundation.org/learning/documents/wwl-report-measuring-estimating-social-value-creation.pdf.

Karoly, Lynn A., M. Rebecca Kilburn, and Jill S. Cannon. 2005. *Early Childhood Interventions: Proven Results, Future Promise.* Santa Monica, Calif.: RAND Corporation. http://www.rand.org/pubs/monographs/2005/RAND_MG341.pdf.

Kern, J. 1997. Across Boundaries: The Emergence of an International Movement of Women with Disabilities. *Hastings Women's Law Journal* 8: 233, 244.

Kessler, R. C., and T. B. Ustun, eds. 2008. *The WHO World Mental Health Surveys: Global Perspective on the Epidemiology of Mental Disorders.* New York: Cambridge University Press.

Kettel, B. 1996. Women, Health, and the Environment. *Social Sciences & Medicine* 42(10): 1367–79.

Khan, Z., S. Mehnaz, M. A. Ansari, N. Khalique, and A. R. Siddiqui. 2009. Existing Practices and Barriers to Avail of Maternal Healthcare Services in Two Slums of Aligarh. *Health and Population: Perspectives and Issues* 32(3): 113–23.

Khosla, P. 2005. *Gendered Cities: Built and Physical Environments. Women and Urban Environments.* http://www.cawi-ivtf.org/pdf/Gendered_Cities_-_Built_and_Physical_Environments.pdf.

King, Elizabeth, and Andrew Mason. 2001. *Engendering Development: Through Gender Equality in Rights, Resources and Voice.* Washington, D.C.: World Bank.

Kirk, J., and Marni Sommer. 2006. Menstruation and Body Awareness: Linking Girls' Health with Girls' Education. *Special on Gender and Health.* Royal Tropical Institute (KIT), Amsterdam.

Kishnor, S., and K. Johnson. 2004. *Profiling Domestic Violence: A Multi-Country Study.* Calverton, Md.: Measure DHS.

Kothari, M. 2003. *Women and Adequate Housing.* Report of the Special Rapporteur on Adequate Housing as a Component of the Right to an Adequate Standard of Living. United Nations Document E/CN.4/2003/5.

Kristof, N., and S. WuDunn. 2010. *Half the Sky, Turning Oppression into Opportunity for Women Worldwide.* New York: Random House.

Kunieda, M., and A. Gauthier. 2003. Gender and Urban Transport: Fashionable and Affordable, Module 7a. In *Sustainable Transportation: A Sourcebook for Policy-makers in Developing Cities.* Frankfurt, Germany: Deutsche Gesellschaft für Technische Zusammenarbeit (GTZ).

Lacy, Elaine. 2007. Mexican immigrants in South Carolina: A Profile. University of South Carolina. http://www.sph.sc.edu/cli/pdfs/final_final[1].pdf.

Lacy, Elaine. 2009. Cultural Enclaves and Transnational Ties: Mexican Immigration and Settlement in South Carolina. In *Latino Immigrants and the Transformation of the U.S. South*, eds. Mary E. Odem & Elaine Lacy. Athens: University of Georgia Press, 1–17.

Lambrick, M., and K. Travers. 2008. Women's safety audits: what works and where. Draft report. UN-Habitat Safer Cities Programme; Women in Cities International.

Lawson, Sandra. 2008. *Women Hold Up Half the Sky.* Goldman Sachs Global Economics Paper No. 164. New York: Goldman Sachs.

Leinaweaver, J. B. 2007. On Moving Children: The Social Implications of Andean Child Circulation. *American Ethnologist* 34(1): 163–80.

Li, Peter S. 2003. *Destination Canada: Immigration Debates and Issues.* Ontario: Oxford University Press.

Liamputtong, Pranee, and Charin Naksook. 2003. Life as Mothers in a New Land: The Experience of Motherhood Among Thai Women in Australia. *Health Care for Women International* 24: 650–68.

Lieber, M. 2002. Les marches exploratoires à Paris (Presentation, 1st International Seminar on Women's Safety, Montreal, Canada, May 9–11).

Lloyd, Cynthia. Forthcoming. *Girls Transformed: The Power of Education for Adolescent Girls.* New York: Population Council.

Lopez, A., D. Mathers, M. Ezzati, T. Jamison, and C. Murray. 2006. Global and Regional Burden of Disease and Risk Factors, 2001: Systematic Analysis of Health Data. *Lancet* 367(May): 1747–57.

Lopez-Claros, Augusto, and Saadia Zahidi. 2005. *Women's Empowerment: Measuring the Global Gender Gap.* Geneva, Switzerland: World Economic Forum.

Loukaitou-Sideris, A., with A. Bornstein, C. Fink, L. Samuels, and S. Gerami. 2009. *How to Ease Women's Fear of Transportation Environments: Case Studies and Best Practices.* San José, Calif.: Mineta Transportation Institute.

Lozano, R., H. Gómez-Dantés, S. Lewis, L. Torres-Sánchez, and L. López-Carrillo. 2009. Tendencias del cáncerde mama en América Latina y el Caribe. *Salud Pública de México* 51(Supplement 2): S147–S156.

Malthus, Thomas Robert. 1789. *An Essay on the Principle of Population.* London: J. Johnson.

Maman S., J. Campbell, M. Sweat, and A. C. Gielen. 2000. The Intersections of HIV and Violence: Directions for Future Research and Interventions. *Social Science & Medicine* 50: 459–78.

Marin, G., and R. J. Gamba. 1996. A New Measurement of Acculturation for Hispanics: The Bidimensional Acculturation Scale for Hispanics (BAS). *Hispanic Journal of Behavioral Science* 18: 297–318.

Marshall, Howard, A. R. Millard, J. I. Packer, and D. J. Wiseman, eds. 1996. *New Bible Dictionary*, 3rd ed. Downers Grove, Ill.: Inter-Varsity Press, 1227.

Marshall, Khiya J., Ximena Urrutia-Rojas, Francisco Soto Mas, and Claudia Coggin. 2005. Health Status and Access to Health Care of Documented and Undocumented Immigrant Latino Women. *Health Care for Women International* 26(10): 916–36.

Martin, David. 1990. *Tongues of Fire: The Explosion of Protestantism in Latin America.* Oxford: Blackwell.

Mati, J.K.G. 2003. A Case Study: Nairobi and Machakos District. In *What's (Not) Happening in Our Schools.* eds. P. Mutunga and J. Stewart. Harare, Zimbabwe: Weaver Press.

McGuire, Sharon. 2001. Crossing myriad borders: a dimensional analysis of the migration and health experiences of indigenous Oaxacan women (Unpublished doctoral dissertation, University of San Diego, California).

McGuire, Sharon, and Mary K. Canales. 2010. Of Migrants and Metaphors: Disrupting Discourses to Welcome the Stranger. *Advances in Nursing Science* 33(2): 126–42.

Melchiorre, Angela. 2004. *At What Age? . . . Are School-Children Employed, Married and Taken to Court?* 2nd ed. The Right to Education Project. http://unesdoc. unesco.org/images/0014/001427/142738e.pdf.

Meleis, Afaf I., Linda M. Sawyer, Eun-Ok Im, DeAnne K. Hilfinger Messias, and Karen Schumacher. 2000. Experiencing Transitions: An Emerging Middle Range Theory. *Advances in Nursing Science* 23(1): 12–28.

Menjívar, Cecilia. 1997. Immigrant Kinship Networks: Vietnamese, Salvadoreans and Mexicans in Comparative Perspective. *Journal of Comparative Family Studies* 28(1): 1–24.

Menjívar, Cecilia. 2000. *Fragmented Ties: Salvadoran Immigrant Networks in America.* Berkeley: University of California Press.

Messias, DeAnne K. Hilfinger. 2001. Transnational Perspectives on Women's Domestic Work: Experiences of Brazilian Immigrants in the United States. *Women & Health* 33: 1–20.

Messias, DeAnne K. Hilfinger. 2002. Transnational Health Resources, Practices, and Perspectives: Brazilian Immigrant Women's Narratives. *Journal of Immigrant Health* 4: 183–200.

Messias, DeAnne K. Hilfinger. 2010. Migration Transitions. In *Transitions Theory: Middle Range and Situation-Specific Theories in Nursing Research and Practice*, ed. Afaf Ibrahim Meleis. New York: Springer, 226–31.

Messias, DeAnne K. Hilfinger, Liz McDowell, and Robin Dawson Estrada. 2009. Language Interpreting as Social Justice Work: Perspectives of Formal and Informal Healthcare Interpreters. *Advances in Nursing Science* 32(2): 128–43.

Messias, DeAnne K. Hilfinger, and Mercedes Rubio. 2004. Immigration and Health. In *Annual Review of Nursing Research.* Vol. 22, eds. Antonia M. Villarruel and Cornelia P. Porter. New York: Springer, 101–34.

Metropolitan Action Committee on Violence Against Women and Children (METRAC). 2002. *Community Safety Audit Resource Kit.* Toronto: METRAC. Available in English, French, Spanish, Chinese, Punjabi, and Tamil.

Michau, L. 2007. Approaching Old Problems in New Ways: Community Mobilization as a Primary Prevention Strategy to Combat Violence Against Women. *Gender & Development* 15.1: 95–109.

Michau, L., and D. Naker. 2003. *Mobilising Communities to Prevent Domestic Violence: A Resource Guide for Organizations in East and Southern Africa.* Kampala, Uganda: Raising Voices.

Michau, Lori, Stephanie Sauve, Chanda Chevannes, Deborah Sekitoleko-Ensor, Kara McMullen, and Marjolein Moreaux. 2009. *The SASA! Activist Kit for Preventing Violence Against Women and HIV.* Kampala, Uganda: Raising Voices.

Michaud, A. 2003. *Pour un environment Urbain sécuritaire. Guide d'aménagement.* Montreal: Femmes et Villes de la Ville de Montreal.

Michaud, A., and M. Chappaz. 2001. *De la dépendance à l'autonomie—La boîte à outils du CAFSU* (From Dependence to Autonomy: CAFSU Toolkit). Montreal: Comité d'action femmes et sécurité urbaine (CAFSU).

Millennium Development Goals. 2000. http://www.unmillenniumproject.org/goals/index.htm.

Miller, Donald E., Jon Miller, and Grace Dyrness. 2002. Religious Dimensions of the Immigrant Experience in Southern California. In *Southern California and the World*, eds. Eric J. Heikkila and Rafael Pizarro. London: Praeger.

Ministry of Community Services. 2005. *Community Guide for Preventing Violence Against Women.* Victoria: Government of British Columbia.

Miranda, Jeanne, Juned Siddique, Claudia Der-Martirosian, and Thomas R. Belin. 2005. Depression Among Latina Immigrant Mothers Separated from Their Children. *Psychiatric Services* 56(7): 717–20.

Mitra, S. 2006. The Capability Approach and Disability. *Journal of Disability Policy Studies* 16(4): 236–47.

Mohl, Raymond A. 2003. Globalization, Latinization and the Nuevo New South. *Journal of American Ethnic History* 22(4): 31–65.

Montgomery, M. 2009. Urban Poverty and Health in Developing Countries. *Population Bulletin* 64(2): 1–16.

Mozilla, Praxedes. 2010, May 23. Interview by the author.

Mtani, A. 2002. The Women's Perspective: The Case of Manzese, Dar es Salaam, Tanzania (Presentation, 1st International Seminar on Women's Safety, Montreal, Canada, May 9–11).

Muindi, Florence. 2008. *The Pursuit of His Calling: Following in Purpose.* New Delhi, India: Thomson Press.

Murray, C.J.L., and J. Frenk. 2000. A Framework for Assessing the Performance of Health Systems. *Bulletin of the WHO* 78(6): 717–31.

Mwabu, G., P. Kimalu, S. Mwaura, and D. K. Manda. 2004. *A Review of the Health Sector in Kenya.* Kenya Institute for Public Policy Research and Analysis (KIPPRA), Social Sector Division, Working Paper No.11. Nairobi, Kenya: KIPPRA.

Nadeem, Erun, Jane M. Lange, Dawn Edge, Marie Fongwa, Tom Belin, and Jeanne Miranda. 2007. Does Stigma Keep Poor Young Immigrant and U.S.-Born Black and Latina Women from Seeking Mental Health Care? *Psychiatric Services* 58(12): 1547–54.

Nairobi Cancer Registry. 2004. *Annual Report.* Nairobi: Kenya Medical and Research Institute (KEMRI).

Nanda, Priya. 2002. Gender Dimensions of User Fees: Implications for Women's Utilization of Health Care. *Reproductive Health Matters* 10(20): 127–34.

Nannini, A. 2006. Patterns of sexual assault among women with and without disabilities. *Women's Health Issues* 16(6): 372–79.

National Cancer Institute, U.S. National Institutes of Health. 2010. *Surveillance Epidemiology and End Results.* http://rex.nci.nih.gov/NCI_Pub_Interface/raterisk/risks120.html.

National Human Services Assembly, National Council of Nonprofit Associations. 2005. *Rating the Raters: An Assessment of Organizations and Publications That Rate/Rank Charitable Nonprofit Organizations.* http://www.nationalassembly. org/Publications/documents/ratingtheraters.pdf.

National Science Foundation. 2009, November 4. *Press Release 09-215. Secretary Clinton Announces New Initiatives to Bolster Science and Technology Collaboration with Muslim Communities Around the World.* http://128.150.4.107/news/news_ summ.jsp?cntn_id=115900.

Noonan, B., S. Gallor, N. Hensler-McGinnis, R. Fassinger, S. Wang, and J. Goodman. 2004. Challenge and Success: A Qualitative Study of the Career Development of Highly Achieving Women with Physical and Sensory Disabilities. *Journal of Counseling Psychology 51*(1): 68–80.

Noonan, Kathleen, and Katherina Rosqueta. 2008. *I'm Not Rockefeller: 33 High Net Worth Philanthrophists Discuss Their Approach to Giving.* Philadelphia: The Center for High Impact Philanthropy, School of Social Policy & Practice, University of Pennsylvania. http://www.impact.upenn.edu/images/uploads/ UPenn_CHIP_HNWP_Study.pdf.

North, Douglass C. 1990. *Institutions, Institutional Change and Economic Performance.* New York: Cambridge University Press.

Nosek, M. A., C. C. Foley, R. B. Hughes, and C. Howland. 2001. Vulnerabilities for Abuse Among Women with Disabilities. *Sexuality and Disability* 19: 177–89.

Nosek, M. A., R. B. Hughes, S. Robinson-Whelen, H. B. Taylor, and C. A. Howland. 2006. Physical Activity and Nutritional Behaviors of Women with Physical Disabilities: Physical, Psychological, Social, and Environmental Influences. *Women's Health Issues* 16(6): 323–33.

Nyamwaya, D. 2008. Health Promotion in Africa: Strategies, Players, Challenges and Prospects. *Health Promotion International* 18(2): 85–87.

Obrist, B., N. Iteba, C. Lengeler, A. Makemba, C. Mshana, R. Nathan, et al. 2007. Access to Health Care in Contexts of Livelihood Insecurity: A Framework for Analysis and Action. *PLos Medicine* 4(10): e308.

Office of AIDS Research, National Institutes of Health. 2010. *FY 2011 National Institutes of Health Trans-NIH AIDS Research By-Pass Budget Estimate and Trans-NIH Plan for HIV-Related Research.* Bethesda, Md.: National Institutes of Health. http://www.oar.nih.gov/strategicplan/fy2011/index.asp.

Office of Research on Women's Health (ORWH). 2009. *Report of the Advisory Committee on Research on Women's Health: Fiscal Years 2007–2008.* Bethesda, Md.: National Institutes of Health.

Olshen, E., K. H. McVeigh, R. A. Wunsch-Hitzig, and V. I. Rickert. 2007. Dating Violence, Sexual Assault, and Suicide Attempts Among Urban Teenagers. *Archives of Pediatric and Adolescent Medicine* 161: 539–45.

O'Reilly, A. 2003. Employment Barriers for Women with Disabilities. In *The Right to Decent Work of Persons with Disabilities.* IFP/Skills Working Paper No. 14. Geneva: International Labor Organization.

Oster, Emily, and Rebecca Thornton. 2011. Menstruation, Sanitary Products and School Attendance: Evidence from a Randomized Evaluation. *American Economic Journal: Applied Economics* 3(1): 91–100.

Parkar, S., J. Fernandes, and M. Weiss. 2003. Contextualizing Mental Health: Gendered Experiences in a Mumbai Slum. *Anthropology & Medicine* 10(3): 291–308.

Parra-Medina, Deborah, DeAnne K. Hilfinger Messias, Elizabeth Fore, Rachel Mayo, Denyse Petry, and Irene Prabhu Das. 2009. The Partnership for Cancer Prevention: Addressing Access to Cervical Cancer Screening Among

Latinas in South Carolina. *Journal of the South Carolina Medical Association* 105(7): 297–305.

Parreñas, Rhacel Salazar. 2001. *Servants of Globalization: Women, Migration, and Domestic Work.* Stanford, Calif.: Stanford University Press.

Parsons, T. 1975. The Sick Role and the Role of the Physician Reconsidered. *Health and Society* 53: 257–78.

Peirce, Neal R., Curtis W. Johnson, with Farley M. Peters. 2008. *Century of the City: No Time to Lose.* New York: The Rockefeller Foundation.

Peters, D. 1998. Breadwinners, Homemakers, Beasts of Burden. *Habitat Debate* 4(2).

Peters, D. 2002. Gender and Transport in Less Developed Countries: A Background Paper in Preparation for CSD-9 (background paper for the Expert Workshop "Gender Perspectives for Earth Summit 2002: Energy, Transport, Information for Decision-Making," January 10–12, 2001, Berlin, Germany).

Pfeiffer, D. 2001. The Conceptualization of Disability. In *Exploring Theories and Expanding Methodologies*, Vol. 2, eds. B. M. Altman and S. Barnartt. Oxford, U.K.: Elsevier, 29–52.

Phaure, J. 2004. *Evaluation of the Making Safer Places Project. Women's Design Service.* Online. Women's Design Service. http://www.wds.org.uk/www/projects_msp.htm.

PLAN. 2008. Paying the Price: The Economic Cost of Failing to Educate Girls. *Children in Focus.* Surrey, U.K.: Plan Ltd.

Plouffe, L., and A. Kalache. 2010. Towards Global Age-Friendly Cities: Determining Urban Features that Promote Active Aging. *Journal of Urban Health* 87(5): 733–38.

Podesta, John, and Peter Ogden. 2007. The Security Implications of Climate Change. *The Washington Quarterly* 31(1): 115–38.

Population Reference Bureau. 2008. *Data by Geography: Ethiopia: Summary.* http://www.prb.org/Datafinder/Geography/Summary.aspx?region=37&region_type=2.

Portier, C. J., T. K. Thigpen, S. R. Carter, C. H. Dilworth, A. E. Grambsch, J. Gohlke, et al. 2010. *A Human Health Perspective on Climate Change: A Report Outlining the Research Needs on the Human Health Effects of Climate Change.* Research Triangle Park, N.C: Environmental Health Perspectives/National Institute of Environmental Health Sciences. doi:10.1289/ehp.1002272. Available at www.niehs.nih.gov/climatereport.

Powers, L. E., R. B. Hughes, and E. M. Lund. 2009. *Interpersonal Violence and Women with Disabilities: A Research Update.* Harrisburg, Pa.: VAWnet, a Project of the National Resource Center on Domestic Violence/Pennsylvania Coalition Against Domestic Violence. Available at http://vawnet.org.

Pregnant women in Peru will improve their health via cell phones. 2010. http://www.iadb.org/news-releases/2010-08/english/pregnant-women-in-peru-will-improve-their-health-via-cell-phones--7708.html.

Prince, M., V. Patel, S. Saxena, M. Maj, J. Maselko, M. Phillips, et al. 2007. No Health Without Mental Health. *Lancet* 370: 859–77.

Project Masiluleke. 2009. http://www.poptech.org/project_m_press.

Psacharopoulos, George, and Harry Anthony Patrinos. 2002. *Returns to Investment in Education: A Further Update.* Policy Research Working Paper 2881. Washington, D.C.: World Bank.

Public Law 103-43. *National Institutes of Health Revitalization Act of 1993.* 42 USC 289(a)(1).

Purushothaman, S., S. Silliman, S. Basu, and P. Sanjeev. 2010. *Grassroots Women and Decentralized Governance, Change Through Partnership.* New York: Huairou Commission.

Radford, Lorraine, and C. Cappel. 2002. *Social Action Project 2000–2002: Women and Violence.* Commissioned by Southlands Methodist Centre. http://www.methodist.org.uk/index.cfm?fuseaction=churchlife.content&cmid=458.

Ramachandran, Ambady, Shobhana Ramachandran, Chamukuttan Snehalatha, Christina Augustine, Narayanasamy Murugesan, Vijay Viswanathan, et al. 2007. Increasing Expenditure on Health Care Incurred by Diabetic Subjects in a Developing Country: A Study from India. *Diabetes Care* 30(2): 252–56.

Reitmanova, S., and D. L. Gustafson. 2008. "They Can't Understand It": Maternity Health and Care Needs of Immigrant Muslim Women in St. John's, Newfoundland. *Maternal Child Health Journal* 12: 101–11.

Remennick, Larissa I. 2004. Providers, Caregivers, and Sluts: Women with a Russian Accent in Israel. *Nashim: A Journal of Jewish Women's Studies and Gender Issues* 8: 87–114.

Reuter. 2010. "Urban poor suffer water crisis as cities grow." March 22. http://in.reuters.com/article/idINIndia-47117720100322?sp=true.

Rhodes, Hilary J., Kathleen Noonan, and Katherina Rosqueta. 2008. *Pathways to Student Success: A Guide to Translating Good Intentions into Meaningful Impact.* Philadelphia: Center for High Impact Philanthropy, School of Social Policy & Practice, University of Pennsylvania. http://www.impact.upenn.edu/images/uploads/UPenn_CHIP_Pathways_Dec08.pdf.

Riverson, J., M. Kunieda, P. Roberts, N. Lewi, and W. M. Walker. 2005. An Overview of Women's Transport Issues in Developing Countries. The Challenges in Addressing Gender Dimensions of Transport in Developing Countries: Lessons from the World Bank Projects. http://siteresources.worldbank.org/INTTSR/Resources/462613-1152683444211/06-0592.pdf.

The Right to Health Care: From Rhetoric to Reality. 2008. *Lancet* 372: 2001.

Robinson, K.-S. 2004, May. For Working Women, Job Quality Elusive. *HR Magazine.* http://findarticles.com/p/articles/mi_m3495/is_5_49/ai_n6036862/.

Rodigou, M., M. Nazar, S. Pérez, and S. Monserrat. 2008. *Cuaderno de Propuestas. Más Mujeres en las calles sin miedo ni violencia* (Proposal workbook: more women in the streets without fear or violence). UNIFEM 2010. Safe Cities, *Virtual Knowledge Centre to End Violence Against Women and Girls.* http://www.endvawnow.org/?safe-cities.

Rodriguez, Anne-Line. 2007. Migration and Increased Participation in Public Life: The Case of Pakistani Women in London. *Frontiers* 28(3): 94–112.

Rosqueta, Katherina. 2010, January. Lessons Learned from Answering the Million Dollar Question. *Philadelphia Social Innovations Journal.* http://www.philasocialinnovations.org/site/index.php?option=com_content&view=article&id=105:lessons-learned-from-answering-the-million-dollar-question&catid=22:editorials&Itemid=37.

Royal Town Planning Institute. 2007. *Gender and Spatial Planning.* RPTI Good Practice Note 7. http://www.rtpi.org.uk/download/3322/GPN7.pdf.

Sai, F. T. 1993. Political and Economic Factors Influencing Contraceptive Uptake. *British Medical Bulletin* 49(1): 200–209.

Sassen, Saskia. 1991. *The Global City: New York, London, Tokyo.* Princeton, N.J.: Princeton University Press.

Sattherwaite, D. 2008. *The Transition to a Predominantly Urban World and Its Underpinnings.* London: Earthscan.

Save the Children. 2009a. *Adolescent and Reproductive Health Update*. Westport, Conn.: Save the Children.

Save the Children. 2009b. *Annual Report*. Westport, Conn.: Save the Children.

Schneider, F. 2002. Size and Measurement of the Informal Economy in 110 Countries Around the World (paper presented at Workshop of Australian National Tax Centre, ANU, Canberra, Australia, July 17).

Schultz, P. T., and A. Tansel. 1993. *Measurement of Returns to Adult Health: Living Standards Measurement Study*. Working Paper No.95. Washington, D.C.: World Bank.

Sclar, E., and M. E. Northridge. 2001. Property, Politics, and Public Health. *American Journal of Public Health* 91: 1013–15.

Secretaría de Salud. 2006. *Encuesta Nacional de Salud y Nutrición 2006*. Cuernavaca, México: Secretaría de Salud, Instituto Nacional de Salud Pública.

Secretaría de Salud. 2009. *Encuesta Nacional de Violencia contra la Mujer*. http://www.mujerysalud.gob.mx/mys/doc_pdf/encuesta.pdf.

Sen, A. 1990, December 20. More Than 100 Million Women Are Missing. *New York Review of Books* 37(20).

Sen, A. 2008. Why and How Is Health a Human Right? *Lancet* 372: 2010.

Shattell, Mona M., Ann Quinlan-Colwell, José Villalba, Nathaniel N. Ivers, and Marina Mails. 2010. A Cognitive Behavioral Group Therapy Intervention with Depressed Spanish-Speaking Mexican Women Living in an Emerging Immigrant Community in the United States. *Advances in Nursing Science* 33(2): 158–69.

Shaw, P., and M. Ainsworth. 1995. *Financing Health Care in Sub-Saharan Africa Through User Fees and Insurance*. Washington, D.C.: World Bank, 55–80.

Sistren Theatre Collective. 2009. *Tek it to dem and Rise Up wi Community*. In Sistren Theatre Collective. http://www.sistrentheatrecollective.com/tek-it-to-dem-and-rise-up-wi-community/

Smedley, B. D., A. Y. Stith, and A. R. Nelson, eds. 2003. *Unequal Treatment: Confronting Racial and Ethnic Disparities in Healthcare*. Washington, D.C.: National Academy Press.

Sokoloff, Natalie J., and Ida Dupont. 2005. Domestic Violence at the Intersections of Race, Class, and Gender: Challenges and Contributions to Understanding Violence Against Marginalized Women in Diverse Communities. *Violence Against Women* 11(1): 38–63.

Sommer, Marni. 2009a. Ideologies of Sexuality, Menstruation, and Risk: Girls' Experiences of Puberty and Schooling in Northern Tanzania. *Culture, Health and Sexuality* 11(4): 383–98.

Sommer, Marni. 2009b. Where the Education System and Women's Bodies Collide: The Social and Health Impact of Girls' Experiences of Menstruation and Schooling in Tanzania. *Journal of Adolescence* 33(4): 521–29.

Southern Poverty Law Center (SPLC). 2009. *Under Siege: Life for Low-Income Latinos in the South*. Montgomery, Ala.: SPLC.

Spence, M., P. Annez, and B. Buckley, eds. 2009. *Urbanization and Growth*. Washington, D.C.: Commission on Growth and Development, International Bank for Reconstruction and Development.

Springer, Pamela J., Mikal Black, Kim Martz, Cathy Deckys, and Terri Soelberg. 2010. Somali Bantu Refugees in Southwest Idaho: Assessment Using Participatory Research. *Advances in Nursing Science* 33(2): 170–81.

Stafford, Stephen. 2010. Caught Between "The Rock" and a Hard Place: The Native Hawaiian and Pacific Islander Struggle for Identity in Public Health. *American Journal of Public Health* 100(5): 785–89.

Standing, H. 1997. Gender and Equity in Health Sector Reform Programmes: A Review. *Health Policy and Planning* 12(1): 1–18.

Stewart, Miriam J., A. Neufeld, M. J. Harrison, D. Spitzer, K. Hughes, and E. Makwarimba. 2006. Immigrant Women Family Caregivers in Canada: Implications for Policies and Programmes in Health and Social Sectors. *Health and Social Care in the Community* 14(4): 329–40.

Stromquist, Nelly. 2007. The Gender Socialization Process in School: A Cross-National Comparison (commissioned paper by UNESCO for the *EFA Global Monitoring Report 2008*).

Strong, Michael A. 1992. The Health of Adults in the Developing World: The View from Bangladesh. *Health Transition Review* 2(2): 215–24.

Summers, Lawrence. 1994. *Investing in All the People: Educating Women in Developing Countries.* EDI Seminar Paper, No 45. Washington, D.C.: World Bank.

Tembon, Mercy, and Lucia Fort, eds. 2008. *Girls' Education in the 21st Century, Gender Equality, Empowerment, and Economic Growth.* http://siteresources. worldbank.org/EDUCATION/Resources/278200-1099079877269/ 547664-1099080014368/DID_Girls_edu.pdf.

Temin, Miriam, and Ruth Levine. 2009. *Start with a Girl: A New Agenda for Global Health.* Washington, D.C.: Center for Global Development.

Tenambergen, E. 1994. Proposal for Community Based Health Insurance in Kenya: Siaya (Financing District Health Services International Workshop, Dept. of Community Health and duetsche Gesellschft fur Techniche Zusammenarbeit Annex XV11), 1–4.

Thomas, D. B., D. L. Gao, R. M. Ray, and W. W. Wang. 2002. Randomized Trial of Breast Self-Examination in Shanghai: Final Results. *Journal of the National Cancer Institute* 94: 1445–57.

Tjon-A-Ten, Varina. 2009. *De eeuwige schaamte voorbij . . . !/Gone with the Never-Ending Shame . . . !* Amsterdam: KIT Publishers.

Torun, Benjamin, Aryeh D. Stein, Dirk Schroeder, Ruben Grajeda, Andrea Conlisk, Monica Rodriguez, et al. 2002. Rural-to-Urban Migration and Cardiovascular Disease Risk Factors in Young Guatemalan Adults. *International Journal of Epidemiology* 31: 218–26.

Touraine, A. 1992. *Critique de la modernité.* Paris: Fayard.

Trelstad, Brian. 2008. Measuring and/or Estimating Social Value Creation Meeting. Bill & Melinda Gates Foundation, Seattle, October 20–21. Quoted in Tuan, Melinda. 2008. *Measuring and/or Estimating Social Value Creation: Insights into Eight Integrated Cost Approaches.* Bill & Melinda Gates Foundation, Impact Planning and Improvement, 21. http://www.gatesfoundation. org/learning/documents/wwl-report-measuring-estimating-social-value-creation.pdf.

Tuan, Melinda. 2008. *Measuring and/or Estimating Social Value Creation: Insights into Eight Integrated Cost Approaches.* Bill & Melinda Gates Foundation, Impact Planning and Improvement. http://www.gatesfoundation. org/learning/documents/wwl-report-measuring-estimating-social-value-creation.pdf.

Uganda Bureau of Statistics (UBOS). 2008. *2008 Population Estimates of Kampala District.* http://www.citypopulation.de./Uganda.

Uganda Law Reform Commission. 2006. *A Study Report on Domestic Violence.* Kampala: Uganda Law Reform Commission.

UNAIDS, UNFPA, UNIFEM. 2010. *Women and HIV/AIDS: Confronting the Crisis.* http://www.unfpa.org/hiv/women/report/chapter1.html.

UN-HABITAT. 2002. *Survivors Speak. A Snapshot Survey on Violence Against Women in Nairobi.* Safer Cities, Series 3. Nairobi: UN-HABITAT.

UN-HABITAT. 2004a. *Preventing Gender-Based Violence in the Horn, East and Southern Africa: A Regional Dialogue.* Nairobi: UN-HABITAT.

UN-HABITAT. 2004b. *State of the World's Cities 2004/5. Globalization and Urban Culture.* London: Earthscan.

UN-HABITAT. 2006. *State of the World's Cities 2006/7.* London: Earthscan.

UN-HABITAT. 2008a. *Best Practices Database. Fair Shared City: Gender Mainstreaming Planning Strategy in Vienna.* http://www.unhabitat.org/bestpractices/2008/mainview04.asp?BPID=1806

UN-HABITAT. 2008b. *Safer Cities Programme Approaches.* Safer Cities Program.

UN-HABITAT. 2009a. *Planning Sustainable Cities: Global Report on Human Settlements 2009,* xxii. http://www.preventionweb.net/english/professional/publications/v.php?id=11308

UN-HABITAT. 2009b. *State of the World's Cities 2008/9: Harmonious Cities.* London: Earthscan. http://www.un-habitat.org/pmss/listItemDetails.aspx?publicationID=2562.

UN-HABITAT. 2010a. *Urban Indigenous Peoples and Migration: A Review of Policies, Programmes and Practices.* UN Housing Rights Programme Report No. 8. Nairobi: UN HABITAT. http://www.unhabitat.org/pmss/listItemDetails.aspx?publicationID=2916.

UN-HABITAT. 2010b. *State of the World's Cities 2010–2011––Cities for All: Bridging the Urban Divide.* London: Earthscan. http://www.unhabitat.org/content.asp?cid=8051&catid=7&typeid=46&subMenuId=0.

UNICEF. 2005. *Sanitation: The Challenge.* www.childinfo.org.

UNICEF. 2007. Women and Children: The Double Dividend of Gender Equality. *The State of the World's Children.* New York: UNICEF.

UNICEF. 2008. *State of the World's Children Report 2009.* New York: UNICEF.

UNICEF. 2010a. *At a Glance: Niger.* http://www.unicef.org/infobycountry/niger_statistics.html.

UNICEF. 2010b. *At a Glance: United States of America.* http://www.unicef.org/infobycountry/usa_statistics.html.

UNICEF. 2010c. *Bangladesh: Statistics.* http://www.unicef.org/infobycountry/bangladesh_bangladesh_statistics.html.

United Nations. 2005. *A Home in the City.* Report of the Task Force on Improving the Lives of Slum Dwellers. London: Earthscan.

United Nations. 2006. *The Millennium Development Goals Report 2006.* New York: United Nations Department of Economic and Social Affairs.

United Nations. 2008a. *State of the World Population 2007.* New York: United Nations Department of Economic and Social Affairs.

United Nations. 2008b. *World Urbanization Prospects: The 2007 Revision.* New York: United Nations Department of Economic and Social Affairs.

United Nations. 2008c. *The Millennium Development Goals Report 2008.* United Nations Department of Economic and Social Affairs.

United Nations. 2009. *Demographic Yearbook, 2007.* New York: United Nations Department of Economic and Social Affairs. http://unstats.un.org/unsd/demographic/products/dyb/dybsets/2007%20DYB.pdf.

United Nations. 2010a. *The Millennium Development Goals Report 2010.* New York: United Nations Department of Economic and Social Affairs.

United Nations. 2010b. *World Urbanization Prospects: The 2009 Revision.* New York: United Nations Department of Economic and Social Affairs.

United Nations Development Fund for Women (UNIFEM). 2003. *Making a Difference: Strategic Communications to End Violence Against Women.* New York: UNIFEM.

United Nations Development Fund for Women (UNIFEM). 2008. *Who Answers to Women?* Progress of the World's Women 2008–2009. http://www.unifem. org/progress/2008/media/POWW08_Report_Full_Text.pdf.

United Nations Development Fund for Women (UNIFEM). 2010a. *A Life Free of Violence Is Our Right! The UN Trust Fund to End Violence Against Women.* http:// www.unifem.org/materials/item_detail.php?ProductID=83.

United Nations Development Fund for Women (UNIFEM). 2010b. Women in Cities International and Red Mujer y Habitat Safe Cities Module. In *Virtual Knowledge Centre to End Violence Against Women and Girls.* http://www.endvawnow.org/ ?safe-cities.

United Nations Development Programme (UNDP). 2007. *Human Development Report 2007. Fighting Climate Change: Human Solidarity in a Divided World.* New York: UNDP.

United Nations Development Programme (UNDP). 2010. *Power, Voice and Rights: A Turning Point for Gender Equality in Asia and the Pacific.* Asia-Pacific Human Development Report. Colombo, Sri Lanka: UNDP.

United Nations Development Programme (UNDP). n.d. *Millennium Development Goals.* http://www.undp.org/mdg/.

United Nations Economic and Social Commission for Asia and the Pacific. 2007. *Economic and Social Survey of Asia and the Pacific 2007*, 105. http://www.unescap. org/survey2007/.

United Nations Economic Commission for Africa (UNECA). 2006. *International Migration and Development: Implications for Africa.* Addis Ababa: Economic Commission for Africa.

United Nations International Labour Office (ILO). 2004a. *Breaking Through the Glass Ceiling. Women in Management. Update 2004.* Geneva: International Labour Office. http://www.ilo.org/global/What_we_do/Publications/ ILOBookstore/Orderonline/Books/lang--en/WCMS_PUBL_9221108457_ EN/index.htm.

United Nations International Labour Office (ILO). 2004b. *Global Employment Trends for Women.* http://www.ilo.org/empelm/what/pubs/lang--en/ docName--WCMS_114325/index.htm.

United Nations Population Division (UNPD). 2008. *World Population Prospects.* New York: United Nations.

United Nations Population Fund (UNFPA). 2002. *Population Ageing and Development: Operational Challenges in Developing Countries.* New York: UNFPA. http:// www.unfpa.org/upload/lib_pub_file/97_filename_Pop.Dev.Strat%205.pdf.

United Nations Population Fund (UNFPA). 2006. *State of World Population 2006: A Passage to Hope: Women and International Migration.* http://www.unfpa.org/ public/home/publications/pid/379.

United Nations Population Fund (UNFPA). 2007. *State of World Population 2007: Unleashing the Potential of Urban Growth.* New York: UNFPA. http://www. unfpa.org/swp/2007/english/introduction.html.

United Nations Population Fund (UNFPA). 2009. *State of World Population, 2009. Facing a Changing World: Women, Population and Climate.* New York: UNFPA.

U.S. Agency for International Development (USAID). 2004. *Improving the Health of the Urban Poor: Learning from the USAID Experience.* Washington, D.C.: USAID.

U.S. Agency for International Development (USAID). 2010. *Women with Disabilities and International Development.* http://www.usaid.gov/our_work/cross-cutting_ programs/wid/gender/wwd.html.

U.S. Department of Education. 2010. http://www2.ed.gov/policy/elsec/leg/ esea02/index.html.

U.S. Department of Education, Office of Special Education and Rehabilitative Services. n.d. *History: Twenty-Five Years of Progress in Educating Children with Disabilities Through IDEA.* http://www.ed.gov/policy/speced/leg/idea/ history.

U.S. Department of Health and Human Services (US DHHS). 2001. *National Standards for Culturally and Linguistically Appropriate Services in Health Care: Final Report.* Washington, D.C.: US DHHS, Office of Minority Health.

U.S. Department of Health and Human Services (US DHHS). 2004. *Emergency Preparedness Toolkit for Managers.* US DHHS, Office on Disability. http://www. hhs.gov/od/disabilitytoolkit/index.html.

U.S. Department of Health and Human Services (US DHHS). 2007, March. *Community Health Worker National Workforce Study.* US DHHS, Health Resources and Services Administration, Bureau of Health Professions. ftp:// ftp.hrsa.gov/bhpr/workforce/chw307.pdf.

U.S. Department of Health and Human Services (US DHHS). 2009a, September 21–22. *Healthy Community Design Expert Workshop Report.* Atlanta: Centers for Disease Control and Prevention.

U.S. Department of Health and Human Services (US DHHS). 2009b. *Office of Refugee Resettlement Fact Sheet.* http://www.acf.hhs.gov/programs/orr/press/ office_refugee_factsheet.htm.

U.S. Department of Health and Human Services (US DHHS). 2010. *Moving into the Future with New Dimensions and Strategies: A Vision for 2020 for Women's Health Research.* NIH Publication No. 10-7606. Bethesda, Md.: Public Health Service, National Institutes of Health, Office of Research on Women's Health.

U.S. Department of Health and Human Services (US DHHS). n.d. *New Freedom Initiative.* http://www.hhs.gov/newfreedom/.

U.S. Department of Labor. 2005. *Employment Laws: Disability and Discrimination.* http://www.dol.gov/odep/pubs/fact/laws.htm.

U.S. Department of State. 2010. *Secretary's International Fund for Women and Girls: Why Women? Why Now?* http://www.state.gov/s/gwi/womensfund/why/index. htm.

U.S. Federal Transit Administration (FTA). 2010. http://www.fta.dot.gov/ civilrights/civil_rights_2360.html.

U.S. Office of Management and Budget (OMB). 1997. *Directive 15 Revisions to the Standards for the Classification of Federal Data on Race and Ethnicity.* http://www. whitehouse.gov/omb/fedreg_1997standards.

Valdés, X. 2008, December. Haciendo frente a la violencia de género: intervenciones desde la sociedad civil. *Ediciones SUR* 65.

Vital Wave Consulting. 2009. *Health for Development: The Opportunity of Mobile Technology for Healthcare in the Developing World.* Washington, D.C.: UN Foundation-Vodafone Foundation Partnership.

VSO. *Disability and HIV.* 2010. http://www.vsointernational.org/what-we-do/ advocacy/disability-and-hiv/.

Wang'ombe, J. 1994. *Health Care Financing in Kenya. Policy Issues and Potential for Social Financing.* Nairobi, Kenya: University of Nairobi Printer, 1–10.

Water, Our Thirsty World (Special issue). 2010. April. *National Geographic*.

Watts, Charlotte, T. Abramsky, L. Kiss, L. Francisco, L. Michau, T. Musuya, et al. 2010. Baseline Findings from the *SASA!* Study: A Cluster Randomized Controlled Trial in Kampala, Uganda. Unpublished manuscript.

WcP Observer. 2010. *Mexico Bans Junk Food in Schools & Requires Physical Education to Fight Obesity from a Young Age*. http://www.worldculturepictorial.com/blog/content/mexico-bans-junk-food-schools-requires-physical-educ.

The White Ribbon Alliance. n.d. *Global Maternal Mortality Fact Sheet*. http://www.whiteribbonalliance.org/Resources/Documents/WRA%20Global%20Maternal%20Mortality%20Fact%20Sheet%202009.pdf.

Whitzman, C. 2007. The Loneliness of the Long-Distance Runner: Long-Term Feminist Planning Initiatives in London, Toronto, Montreal and Melbourne. *Planning Theory and Practice* 8(2): 203–25.

WICI. 2006. *Moving from the Margins—Actions for Safer Cities for the Full Diversity of Women and Girls: Lessons for Increasing the Visibility of Crime Prevention at the Local Level*. Montreal: WICI.

Wick, I. 2010. *Women Working in the Shadows*. Seigburg, German: SÜDWIND Institut für Ökonomie und Ökumene.

Wild, Sarah, Roglic Gojka, Anders Green, Richard Sicree, and Hilary King. 2004. Global Prevalence of Diabetes: Estimates for the Year 2000 and Projections for 2030. *Diabetes Care* 27(5): 1047–53.

The William and Flora Hewlett Foundation, McKinsey & Company. 2008. *The Nonprofit Marketplace: Bridging the Gap in Philanthropy*. http://givingmarketplaces.org/materials/whitepaper.pdf.

Winter, Carolyn, and Rebecca Macina. 1999. *Girls Education: World Bank Support Through the International Development Association (IDA)*. http://siteresources.worldbank.org/EDUCATION/Resources/278200-1099079877269/547664-1099080014368/Girls_ed_WB_support_through_IDA_En99.pdf.

Women's Initiatives for Safer Environments (WISE). 2005. *Women's Community Safety Audit Guide: Safety for Women, Safety for Everyone, Let's Act on It!* Ottawa: WISE.

Women's Right to Adequate Housing and Land, Middle East/North Africa. 2004. Proceedings of the Alexandria Consultation. http://www2.ohchr.org/english/issues/housing/docs/alexandriaconsultations.pdf.

Wood, Richard. 2002. *Faith in Action: Religion, Race, and Democratic Organizing in America*. Chicago: University of Chicago Press.

World Bank. 2006. Mainstreaming Gender in Transport. *Gender and Transport Resource Guide*.

World Bank. 2007. *Global Monitoring 2007 Millennium Developmental Goals—Confronting the Challenges of Gender Equality and Fragile States*, 107. http://siteresources.worldbank.org/INTGLOMONREP2007/Resources/3413191-1176390231604/1264-FINAL-LO-RES.pdf.

World Bank. 2009. *Girls' Education: A World Bank Priority*. http://web.worldbank.org/WBSITE/EXTERNAL/TOPICS/EXTEDUCATION/0,,contentMDK:20298916~menuPK:617572~pagePK:148956~piPK:216618~theSitePK:282386,00.html.

World Bank. 2010. *Health, Nutrition and Population: Reproductive Health and Disability*. http://web.worldbank.org/WBSITE/EXTERNAL/TOPICS/EXTHEALTHNUTRITIONANDPOPULATION/EXTPRH/0,,contentMDK:20286128~menuPK:632615~pagePK:148956~piPK:216618~theSitePK:376855,00.html.

World Health Organization. 1996. Creating Healthy Cities in the 21st Century (background paper prepared for UN Conference on Human Settlements: Habitat II, Istanbul, June 3–14, 1996).

World Health Organization. 2000. *World Health Report 2000.* Geneva: WHO.

World Health Organization. 2005. *WHO Multi-Country Study on Women's Health and Domestic Violence Against Women: Summary Report of Initial Results on Prevalence, Health Outcomes and Women's Responses.* Geneva: World Health Organization.

World Health Organization. 2007a. *Global Age-Friendly Cities: A Guide.* Geneva: World Health Organization.

World Health Organization. 2007b. *Youth and Road Safety.* Geneva: World Health Organization.

World Health Organization. 2008a. *Closing the Gap in a Generation: Health Equity Through Action on the Special Determinants of Health.* Final report of the Commission on Social Determinants, 145. http://apps.who.int/bookorders/anglais/detart1.jsp?sesslan=1&codlan=1&codcol=15&codcch=741#.

World Health Organization. 2008b. *Healthy Urbanization Learning Circle (HULC).* Geneva: World Health Organization.

World Health Organization. 2009a. *Global Health Risks. Mortality and Burden of Disease Attributable to Selected Major Risks.* Geneva: World Health Organization, 24.

World Health Organization. 2009b. *Women and Health. Today's Evidence, Tomorrow's Agenda.* Geneva: World Health Organization.

World Health Organization. 2010a. *Health Equity in All Urban Policies.* A report on the expert consultation on intersectoral action in the prevention of noncommunicable disease. http://www.who.or.jp/ISA_Report_final_22Feb2010.pdf.

World Health Organization. 2010b. *Progress on Sanitation and Drinking-Water: 2010 Update.* Geneva: World Health Organization.

World Health Organization. 2010c. *Skilled Birth Attendants.* http://www.who.int/making_pregnancy_safer/topics/skilled_birth/en/index.html.

World Health Organization. 2010d. *10 Facts About Diabetes.* http://www.who.int/features/factfiles/diabetes/09_en.html.

World Health Organization. 2010e. *Why Urban Health Matters.* Geneva: World Health Organization.

World Health Organization. 2010f. *Why Urban Health Matters. 2010 World Health Day.* http://www.who.int/world-health-day/2010/.html.

World Health Organization. 2010g. *Women's Mental Health: The Facts.* http://www.who.int/mental_health/prevention/genderwomen/en/.

World Health Organization. 2010h. *Millennium Development Goals. Disability and Rehabilitation Team (DAR)—Achieving the Millennium Development Goals for People with Disabilities.* http://www.who.int/disabilities/media/events/idpdinfo031209/en/index1.html.

World Health Organization, UNICEF, UNFPA, and the World Bank. 2010. *Trends in Maternal Mortality: 1990 to 2008.* http://whqlibdoc.who.int/publications/2010/9789241500265_eng.pdf.

Yamanaka, Keiko. 1993. New Immigration Policy and Unskilled Foreign Workers in Japan. *Pacific Affairs* 66(1): 72–90.

Yang, C., J. Yang, X. Luo, and P. Gong. 2009. Use of Mobile Phones in an Emergency Reporting System for Infectious Surveillance After the Sichuan Earthquake in China. *Bulletin of the WHO* 87: 619–23.

Yonder, A., and M. Tamaki. 2010. *Our Spaces: Grassroots Women Formalize Their Leadership & Access to Essential Services.* New York: Huairou Commission.

Yusuf, S., K. Nabeshima, and W. Ha. 2007. Income and Health in Cities: The Messages from Stylized Facts. *Journal of Urban Health: Bulletin of the New York Academy of Medicine* 84(1): i35–i41.

Zulu, E. M., F. N. Dodoo, and A. C. Ezeh. 2004. Urbanization, Poverty, and Sex: Roots of Risky Sexual Behaviors in Slum Settlements in Nairobi, Kenya. In *HIV and AIDS in Africa: Beyond Epidemiology*, eds. E. Kalipeni, S. Craddock, J. R. Oppong, and J. Ghosh. Oxford: Blackwell.

Contributors

Eugenie L. Birch is Lawrence C. Nussdorf Professor of Urban Research; chair of the Graduate Group of City and Regional Planning, University of Pennsylvania School of Design; co-director, Penn Institute for Urban Research; and series co-editor, City in the Twenty-First Century, University of Pennsylvania Press. Her most recent books are *Global Urbanization* (2011), *Growing Greener Cities* (2008), co-edited with Susan M. Wachter, *Urban and Regional Planning Reader* (2009), and *Local Planning Principles and Practice* (co-edited with Gary Hack, Paul Sedway, and Mitchell Silver). With Christopher Silver, she has recently edited the special centennial issue of *Journal of the American Planning Association* (75[2], 2009) to which she contributed "One Hundred Years of City Planning's Enduring and Evolving Connections." She has been a commissioner, New York City Planning Commission, and a member of the jury to select the designers of the World Trade Center site.

Manupreet Chawla is a medical student at Wayne State University School of Medicine and is a candidate for a Masters of Public Health degree at the Harvard School of Public Health, with a concentration in quantitative methods. She worked with Dr. Claudia Garcia-Moreno on intimate partner violence against women during pregnancy. She is interested in understanding the impact of substance abuse and intimate partner violence on women's mental and reproductive health. She has served as the co-coordinator of Code Blue, a student run organization encouraging medical students to provide education to teenagers in various Detroit public schools on topics relating to teen pregnancy, sexual health, safety, and abuse. She also participated in the Child Family Health International HIV/AIDS and Public Health program in India in 2007, during which she assisted in the efforts of nonprofit organizations providing health care to street children, sex workers, men, women, and children with HIV/AIDS. She also holds a master's degree in Basic Medical Science from Wayne State University School of Medicine and was the recipient of the medical student research symposium award in 2007 for research investigating the redistribution of mRNA following global cerebral ischemia and reperfusion in rat hippocampal neurons.

Diane Cornman-Levy is currently the executive director of the Federation of Neighborhood Centers in Philadelphia. Before working at the federation, she was the founder and executive director of Journey Home, a nonprofit organization that provides health and human services to more than 2,500 children, youth, adults, and families per year. For the past twenty years, she has focused on designing and implementing innovative approaches to building the capacity of youth, families, adults, and communities with the overall goal of breaking the cycle of poverty. Her efforts have culminated in the creation of three innovative community health-training programs for health professional students, the creation of a community center in Lower North Philadelphia, the development of three innovative youth development programs for at-risk youth, and a green job readiness partnership for low-skilled adults.

Rosaly Correa-de-Araujo is a cardiovascular pathologist trained at the National Heart, Lung, and Blood Institute, National Institutes of Health. She currently serves as the deputy director for the Office on Disability, Office of the Secretary (OS), U.S. Department of Health and Human Services. Prior to this position, as director of the Office of the Americas Region, Office of Global Health Affairs/OS, Dr. Correa led a priority secretarial initiative on health diplomacy in Central America that culminated with the establishment of a regional health care training center under the Gorgas Memorial Institute, Ministry of Health of Panama, and for which she received a special recognition by the Ministry of Health of Panama. As the HHS Agency for Healthcare Research and Quality's Director of Women's Health and Gender-based Research, Dr. Correa expanded the agency's portfolio and received AHRQ's Director Award of Excellence for introducing the gender-approach to health services research. She holds the position of adjunct associate professor in the School of Medicine at George Washington University.

Nida Corry is an associate at Abt Associates, Inc., a global research and consulting firm. Previously, she was an American Association for the Advancement of Science Policy Fellow with the Office of Research on Women's Health at the National Institutes of Health. Dr. Corry's research has focused on the evaluation of predictors of functioning and disability following serious injury, assessment and treatment of prevalent conditions among trauma survivors, and determinants of preventative and risky health behaviors. She was the recipient of the American Burn Association 2009 Clinical Research Award for her study of posttraumatic stress, pain, and disability following major burn injury. Dr. Corry received her Ph.D. in clinical psychology from Purdue University and completed her post-doctoral fellowship in behavioral medicine at Johns Hopkins University.

Grace Roberts Dyrness is a private consultant in local and economic development and a part-time professor in the School of Policy, Planning and Development at the University of Southern California, where she teaches in the areas of social context of planning and sustainable development. She has conducted research in Los Angeles, Oakland, San Francisco, Santa Barbara, Philippines, Kenya, and Tanzania, with a focus on homeless women and vulnerable children and the role of faith-based organizations. She has a master's degree in urban anthropology from the Ateneo de Manila University, Philippines, and a doctorate in planning and development studies from the University of Southern California.

Julio Frenk is dean of the faculty at the Harvard School of Public Health (HSPH) and is T & G Angelopoulos Professor of Public Health and International Development, a joint appointment between the Harvard Kennedy School of Government and HSPH. Dr. Frenk served as the minister of health of Mexico from 2000 to 2006, where he introduced universal health insurance. He has also held leadership positions at the National Institute of Public Health of Mexico, the Mexican Health Foundation, the World Health Organization, the Bill & Melinda Gates Foundation, and the Carso Health Institute. In September 2008, Dr. Frenk received the Clinton Global Citizen Award for changing "the way practitioners and policy makers across the world think about health."

Claudia Garcia-Moreno is Coordinator for Gender, Reproductive Rights, Sexual Health and Adolescence in the World Health Organization. A physician from Mexico with a master of science degree in community medicine from the London School of Hygiene and Tropical Medicine, she has over twenty-five years of experience in public health, spanning Africa, Latin America, and parts of Asia. For the past fifteen years her work has focused on women's health and gender in health, including being responsible for gender and women's health work in the World Health Organization. She has led WHO's work on gender and HIV/AIDS and on violence against women, and coordinated the WHO Multi-Country Study on Women's Health and Domestic Violence Against Women. She has led or been a member of several initiatives on violence, including the Sexual Violence Research Initiative and the Violence Against Women Panel of the International Federation of Gynecologists-Obstetricians (FIGO). She is on the editorial board of *Reproductive Health Matters* and reviews and publishes papers on women's health and violence against women for several international journals.

Jane Golden is the executive director of the City of Philadelphia Mural Arts Program. Since the Mural Arts Program began in 1984 as a component of the Philadelphia Anti-Graffiti Network, she has been its driving force, overseeing its growth from a small city agency into the nation's largest mural program, a catalyst for positive social change and a model for community development across the country and around the globe. Under Golden's direction, in partnership with communities, grassroots organizations, city agencies, schools, and philanthropies, the Mural Arts Program has created over 3,000 landmark works of public art, earning Philadelphia international recognition as the "City of Murals." Golden holds a Master of Fine Arts degree from the Mason Gross School of the Arts at Rutgers University and degrees in fine arts and political science from Stanford University. In addition, Golden has received honorary doctoral degrees from Swarthmore College, Philadelphia's University of the Arts, Widener University, Haverford College, and Villanova University. Most recently she received a scholarship through the Social Enterprise Initiative to attend the Harvard Business School Strategic Perspectives in Non-Profit Management Program.

Octavio Gómez-Dantés is researcher at the Center for Health Systems Research of the National Institute of Public Health of Mexico. Between 2001 and 2006 he was director general for performance evaluation at the Ministry of Health of Mexico, and between 2007 and 2008 he worked as director of analysis and evaluation at the CARSO Health Institute (Mexico City). His areas of academic expertise are health policy and international health, and he has published forty-three scientific articles, ten books, and fifteen book chapters. Dr. Gómez-Dantés holds a medical degree from the Autonomous Metropolitan University (Mexico) and two master's degrees, one in public health and the other in health policy and planning, both from the Harvard School of Public Health.

David Gouverneur is a lecturer in landscape architecture and city planning. He received his Master of Architecture degree in urban design from Harvard University and his bachelor's degree in architecture from the Universidad Simón Bolívar in Caracas, Venezuela. He was chair of the School of Architecture at Universidad Simón Bolívar, director of urban development of Venezuela, and co-founder and professor of the Urban Design program and director of the Mayor's Institute in Urban Design at Universidad Metropolitana in Caracas, Venezuela. His professional practice focuses on urban plans and projects for historic districts, rehabilitation of areas affected by extraordinary natural events, new centralities and mixed-use districts, improvement of informal settlements, and tourism/recreational areas. Since 2002 he has lectured at the Department of Landscape Architecture at the University of Pennsylvania. Students working under his supervision have won different awards since he has been at Penn. Dr. Gouverneur received the G. Holmes Perkins Academic Award in 2008.

Jeane Ann Grisso is a professor of public health, nursing, and medicine at the University of Pennsylvania. She has served as principal investigator of many investigations focused on urban women's health issues, including studies of reproductive health, intimate partner violence, menopause, and injuries. Dr. Grisso recently returned to Penn after seven years at the Robert Wood Johnson Foundation, where she and her colleagues developed a portfolio of national programs and initiatives addressing intimate partner violence and policy programs addressing a range of women's health issues. She is currently working with Philadelphia's public health clinics on an intervention for patients who experience intimate partner violence and a separate intervention for employees. She is also co-principal investigator (with Stephanie Abbuhl) of a recently funded National Institutes of Health intervention program to improve the status of junior women faculty in academic medicine. Dr. Grisso was the founder of the program FOCUS on the Health & Leadership of Women. She is a senior scholar and core faculty member of the Center for Public Health Initiatives at Penn, where she teaches epidemiological methods, community-based participatory research, and biostatistics. Dr. Grisso has a joint appointment in the Schools of Nursing and Medicine.

Amy Gutmann became the eighth president of the University of Pennsylvania on July 1, 2004. As Penn's president, she has been a forceful advocate for increasing access to higher education, integrating knowledge across multiple disciplines to address complex problems, and championing civic engagement with communities both domestically and globally. An eminent political scientist and philosopher, Dr. Gutmann is the Christopher H. Browne Distinguished Professor of Political Science in the School of Arts and Sciences at Penn with secondary faculty appointments in philosophy, the Annenberg School for Communication, and the Graduate School of Education. She has authored and edited 15 books as well as more than 100 articles, essays, and book chapters, and she continues to teach and write on ethics and public policy, democracy, and education. In November 2009, she was named by President Barack Obama as chair of the Presidential Commission for the Study of Bioethical Issues. Prior to her appointment at Penn, Dr. Gutmann served as Provost at Princeton University, where she was also the Laurance S. Rockefeller University Professor of Politics. She was the founding Director of the University Center for Human Values, an eminent multidisciplinary center that supports teaching, scholarship, and public discussion of ethics and human values.

Anne Hochwalt is a professional relations and marketing fellow on Procter & Gamble's Global Feminine Care External Relations Team. She has a Ph.D. in environmental medicine from New York University and is board certified in toxicology. She manages scientific communications, professional relations, and issues management for Procter & Gamble's Fem Care brands—Tampax tampons and Always pads and liners. Dr. Hochwalt has been involved with Procter & Gamble's Protecting Futures program since 2007, developing the fundamental basis of understanding and technical support for the program. Protecting Futures, one of Procter & Gamble's Live, Learn, and Thrive initiatives, is a program that works with partner organizations to provide puberty education, sanitary protection, and sanitary facilities to help vulnerable girls stay in school. Protecting Futures also works to raise awareness and build advocacy for vulnerable girls by working with thought-leading organizations to research related issues and interventions.

Brad Kerner works for Save the Children, a nonprofit organization working to inspire breakthroughs in the way the world treats children and to achieve immediate and lasting change in their lives. He holds a master's degree in public health from the Mailman School of Public Health at Columbia University. Kerner has more than a decade of experience dealing with adolescent sexual and reproductive health issues that have led him to work in Armenia, Bangladesh, Egypt, Ethiopia, Gabon, Guinea, Haiti, Malawi, Mali, Mozambique, Nepal, Republic of Georgia, Rwanda, South Africa, Uganda, the United States, and Vietnam. Since 2005, he has been Save the Children's adolescent reproductive health specialist, a role in which he supports a number of strategies that improve an adolescent's ability to attain his or her reproductive rights—including youth-friendly health services, community-based distribution of family planning, school-based puberty and sexuality education, peer education, and HIV prevention. Kerner currently manages programs in South Africa, Ethiopia, and Nepal that explore community attitudes about menstruation and how programmatic interventions can help girls stay in school as they begin puberty.

Ruth Levine is deputy assistant administrator in the Bureau of Policy, Planning and Learning at the United States Agency for International Development (USAID). Before joining USAID in March 2010, she was vice president for programs and operations and senior fellow at the Center for Global Development, a Washington, D.C., think tank focusing on development policy. She joined the Center for Global Development (CGD) soon after it was created in the fall of 2001 and helped to shape the center's unique approach to making the world a better place: conducting independent research to devise practical new policy solutions to reduce global poverty and inequality, and then pushing those ideas into action. An internationally recognized health economist with over fifteen years' experience designing and assessing the effects of social sector programs in Latin America, Eastern Africa, the Middle East, and South Asia, she joined CGD as a senior fellow and later became CGD's vice president for programs and operations. Before joining CGD, Levine designed, supervised, and evaluated loans at the World Bank and the Inter-American Development Bank. Between 1997 and 1999, she served as the advisor on the social sectors in the Office of the Executive Vice President of the Inter-American Development Bank.

Carol A. McLaughlin is the research director for global public health at the Center for High Impact Philanthropy at the University of Pennsylvania. She is a primary care physician and infectious disease/public health specialist with experience in research, community engagement, and program implementation in the United States and the developing world. Dr. McLaughlin received M.D. and M.P.H. degrees from the Johns Hopkins University School of Medicine and School of Public Health, respectively. She completed combined internal medicine and pediatric training through the Harvard Combined Residency Program and infectious diseases training at the University of Pennsylvania. She graduated magna cum laude from Princeton University's Woodrow Wilson School of Public and International Affairs with a bachelor's degree in public and international policy.

Afaf Ibrahim Meleis is the Margaret Bond Simon Dean of Nursing at the University of Pennsylvania School of Nursing, professor of nursing and sociology, and director of the school's WHO Collaborating Center for Nursing and Midwifery Leadership. Prior to coming to Penn, she was a professor on the faculty of nursing at the University of California, Los Angeles and the University of California, San Francisco. She is a member of the Institute of Medicine and a board member of CARE. Dr. Meleis is a fellow of the Royal College of Nursing in the United Kingdom, the American Academy of Nursing, and the College of Physicians of Philadelphia. She is the global ambassador for the Girl Child Initiative of the International Council of Nurses, and she is also president and counsel general Emeriti of the International Council on Women's Health Issues (ICOWHI). Dr. Meleis has held several summits focused on advancing women's health including the Penn Summit on Global Issues in Women's Health, "Safe Womanhood in an Unsafe World" (2005), and the Urban Women's Think Tank Conference (2007), and she co-hosted the Penn-ICOWHI 18th Congress on Cities and Women's Health: Global Perspectives, at the University of Pennsylvania. She has written seven books and over forty chapters about the theoretical development of the nursing discipline, women's health, and diversity, and over 175 articles in multidisciplinary journals. Dr. Meleis graduated magna cum laude from the University of Alexandria, earned an M.S. in nursing, an M.A. in sociology, and a Ph.D. in medical and social psychology from the University of California, Los Angeles.

DeAnne K. Hilfinger Messias is professor in the College of Nursing and Women's and Gender Studies Program at the University of South Carolina. A Brazilian American community health nursing researcher, her expertise includes immigrant women's health, language access issues, health-care interpretation, and community-based participatory research. Her work in Brazil ranged from directing a community health initiative in the Amazon Basin to coordination of nursing education at an urban women's health center. In South Carolina, improving health-care access among limited-English-proficient Spanish speakers has been the focus of her research and community initiatives. She is a founding member of the South Carolina Hispanic/Latino Health Coalition and was instrumental in the formation and development of the South Carolina Partnership for Cancer Prevention. Findings from this participatory research initiative indicated the extent to which Latinas face barriers to preventive services. This led to the development and testing of the Language for Healthcare Access Curriculum, an educational intervention aimed at improving the ability of immigrants to navigate the U.S. health-care system. Dr. Messias currently spearheads the Hispanic Health Research Network, a campus-community-health service partnership aimed at building the cultural, linguistic, and research capacity of primary health-care services in South Carolina and is engaged in community-based participatory research projects with immigrant women in South Carolina and Texas. She earned a B.A.S. in Latin American Studies from the University of Illinois, a B.S.N. in nursing from the University of Arizona, an M.S. in community health nursing from Indiana Wesleyan University, and a Ph.D. in nursing from the University of California, San Francisco.

Tina C. Musuya holds an M.A. in sociology from Makerere University, Kampala, and is the executive director for the Center for Domestic Violence Prevention (CEDOVIP). Musuya oversees CEDOVIP's implementation of SASA! Mobilizing Communities to Prevent Violence Against Women and HIV. Under her guidance, CEDOVIP won the 2010 UNAIDS Red Ribbon Award for innovative work in preventing violence against women and HIV and has gained recognition from civil society leaders, policymakers, community members, and government bodies throughout Uganda. Musuya has six years of experience working with communities, institutions, government, and civil society to create everyday activists who stand up and act to prevent violence against women in their own relationships and communities in Uganda. She led CEDOVIP's development of a Uganda Police Force training module on gender-based violence and a handbook outlining standard protocol for handling cases of domestic violence. She has advocated for legislation on violence against women, engaged in policy formulation at a local level (influencing the enactment of the first-ever domestic violence bylaw in Uganda for Kawempe Division), helped draft the Domestic Violence Bill as part of the Uganda Law Reform Commission, and spearheaded a successful advocacy campaign for passage of the Domestic Violence Act.

Francisca M. Mwangangi is a full-time assistant lecturer in the Department of Nursing at Presbyterian University of East Africa. After completing her B.Sc.N. at the University of Nairobi in 2002, Mwangangi taught in a diploma nursing program in a rural mission teaching hospital. In 2005, she joined Aga Khan University Hospital in Nairobi as a staff nurse in the Department of Surgery. She later assumed management of the Aga Khan University Hospital's Breast Health Program while continuing to teach on a part-time basis at Aga Khan University's Advanced Nursing Studies Program. In 2008, Mwangangi was voted Nurse of the Year in the Oncology Program. She left the Aga Khan University Hospital in 2009 for her present position but continues to volunteer in the Breast Health Program. Mwangangi is a member of the Multinational Association of Supportive Care in Cancer (MASCC) and the Kenya Cancer Association. She is currently completing a master's degree in public health in the University of Nairobi with a specialization in health economics, planning, and policy. Mwangangi is one of the Penn-Rockefeller scholars for 2010 to 2011 involved in an online discussion on urban women's health issues.

Sheela Patel is director of the Society for the Promotion of Area Resource Centers, an India nongovernmental organization (NGO) based in Mumbai that works in partnership with two community-based social movements, Mahila Milan and the National Slum Dwellers Federation, on addressing issues of land tenure, secure housing, and basic services for the squatters living informally in cities in India. She also chairs the board of Shack/Slum Dwellers International, which is a transnational organization with thirty-three country federations of slum dwellers and their support NGOs, which was formed to create a learning alliance that supports communities in learning from one another and negotiating with their cities, national governments, and international organizations to create space for the poor to participate in changing cities to work for all.

Vivian W. Pinn has served as the first full-time director of the Office of Research on Women's Health at the National Institutes of Health (NIH) since 1991 and is also associate director for research on women's health at NIH. Dr. Pinn came to NIH from Howard University College of Medicine, where she had been professor and chair of the Department of Pathology. Dr. Pinn earned her B.A. from Wellesley College in Massachusetts and received her M.D. from the University of Virginia School of Medicine. She received her postgraduate training in pathology at the Massachusetts General Hospital, Harvard Medical School, before assuming faculty positions at the medical schools of Tufts and then Howard Universities. Dr. Pinn currently co-chairs the NIH Working Group on Women in Biomedical Careers with the director of NIH. Dr. Pinn has received numerous honors, awards, and honorary degrees. She is a fellow of the American Academy of Arts and Sciences, was elected to the Institute of Medicine in 1995, and is an elected member of AOA and Sigma Xi. She also served as the eighty-eighth president of the National Medical Association (and the second woman president) in 1989 in addition to leadership positions and membership in many other professional organizations and societies.

Katherina M. Rosqueta is the founding executive director of the Center for High Impact Philanthropy at the University of Pennsylvania. Her work and comments have been cited in numerous mainstream media including the *Wall Street Journal*, *Chronicle of Philanthropy*, CBS News, and the *New York Times*. She is a frequent speaker on issues of social impact and philanthropy and has lectured at the Wharton Business School, Stanford Graduate School of Business, University of California Haas School of Business, and the University of San Francisco's Institute for Nonprofit Organization Management. Previously, she was a consultant at McKinsey & Company. Prior to joining McKinsey, she worked in community development, nonprofit management, and corporate and venture philanthropy. She received her B.A. cum laude from Yale University and her M.B.A. from the Wharton School at the University of Pennsylvania.

Shweta Shukla is head of external relations for Procter & Gamble and part of the company's executive team in India. She is deeply committed to children's education and is responsible for the launch of Project Shiksha in 2004, a national cause-related marketing campaign that helps educate underprivileged children in India. Under her leadership, Project Shiksha has touched the lives of nearly 100,000 children. Since 2007, Shukla has been closely involved with Project Parivartan, Procter & Gamble's public-private partnership with the Ministry of Health in India that currently supports approximately 360,000 menstruating women. This is a unique program where government-appointed community health workers become a bridge between young rural women and essential items of hygiene like sanitary napkins. This program has the potential to reach more than 200 million rural women.

Varina Tjon-A-Ten was a member of the House of Representatives for the Dutch Labour Party from 2003 to 2006. While in Parliament, Tjon-A-Ten was a spokesperson for Development Cooperation, and she was an advocate for women, children, immigrants, and the disabled. Her work has been aimed at empowering disadvantaged groups in Dutch society, and in that capacity she has been managing director for the Foundation on Work and Enterprise, managing director of the Regional Office for Multicultural Development in Eindhoven, and project manager at the Institute for Multicultural Development in Utrecht. Tjon-A-Ten is also an expert on the negative impacts that lack of sanitary napkins and other menstrual protection materials have on the lives of women and girls in developing countries, and the impact these problems have on reaching the United Nation's Millennium Development Goals. She is currently a teacher at The Hague University.

Susan M. Wachter is the Richard B. Worley Professor of Financial Management and professor of real estate and finance at The Wharton School of the University of Pennsylvania; professor of city and regional planning at the University of Pennsylvania's School of Design; co-director of the Penn Institute for Urban Research; and series co-editor, City in the Twenty-First Century, University of Pennsylvania Press. Dr. Wachter served as assistant secretary for policy development and research at the U.S. Department of Housing and Urban Development, a presidentially appointed and Senate confirmed position, from 1998 to 2001. She has been president of the American Real Estate and Urban Economics Association and co-editor of *Real Estate Economics*, the leading academic real estate journal. Dr. Wachter was chair of the Wharton Real Estate Department from 1996 to 1998. She received the Lifetime Achievement Award from the American Real Estate and Urban Economics Association in 2005. Recent publications include "Immigration and the Neighborhood," *American Economic Journal*; *Economic Policy* (forthcoming); "Subprime Lending and Real Estate Prices," *Real Estate Economics* (39[1], 2011); "Explaining the House Bubble," *Social Science Resource Network* (2010); "Mortgage Put Options and Real Estate Markets," *Journal of Real Estate Finance and Economics* (2009); "The Inevitability of Market-Wide Underpriced Risk," *Real Estate Economics* (34[4], 2006); and "The American Mortgage in Historical and International Context," *Journal of Economic Perspectives* (19[4], 2005). At Penn, Dr. Wachter co-chairs the Academic Committee for the Master of Urban Spatial Analytics degree and is a recipient of the Lindback Award for Teaching Excellence. Dr. Wachter is frequently called upon to appear on national media and to testify before Congress on real estate and housing policy issues.

Index

Acknowledgments

To produce a volume such as this, particularly in an area that has received little scholarly attention—that is, the intersection of women's health issues with the urban conditions in which women live—required the collaboration of many people. Though they are far too numerous to recognize individually, we thank them as a group, and we will highlight a few because of the depth and/or longevity of their contributions. First and foremost, the national planning committee for the Penn-ICOWHI (International Council on Women's Health Issues) 18th Congress, whose members include academics, community activists, artists, administrators, and government officials, worked tirelessly to organize the four-day meeting that inspired this book. Drawn from nursing, medicine, epidemiology, public health, anthropology, and urban planning, the committee members identified the critical areas of scholarship and the experts to address them.

The Board of Governors of the ICOWHI has had a long history of fostering dialogue about women and their health. It has sponsored eighteen conferences to disseminate research and practice on the topic throughout the world. The results have advanced the science in women's health, enhanced government commitment, and created an advocacy voice for women and their issues.

The leadership of the University of Pennsylvania provided unwavering support for this project. President Amy Gutmann believed in our plans and contributed her knowledge and voice to the project as well as other intangible support. Her able team, Provost Vincent Price and Senior Vice Provost for Research Steven Fluharty, were not only instantly convinced and conversant about our goals, but also led the way in securing resources to bring this volume to fruition. We view this book as a demonstration of our mutual commitment to integrating knowledge across fields.

The generous intellectual and financial support of foundations was transformative for our thinking and that of our colleagues. In particular, Judith Rodin, president, and Darren Walker, former vice president, of The Rockefeller Foundation had the vision and leadership to begin the conversation about interdisciplinary approaches to addressing global urbanization at the Global Urban Summit in Bellagio, Italy, in 2007, which we attended to our great benefit. Along with Robert Buckley, managing director of the Rockefeller Foundation, Rodin and Walker helped us deepen that dialogue. This book is one of the many outcomes of that initial work.

The Board of Overseers of the School of Nursing and the Advisory Board of the Penn Institute for Urban Research provided counsel and funding. Dean Kehler and Lawrence and Melanie Nussdorf, have been critical to the success of a shared cities and women's health initiative that has led to this volume.

Among our team, Caroline Glickman and Janet Tomcavage managed the 18th ICOWHI Congress, Cities and Women's Health: Global Perspectives, as well as the details of this book with unparalleled energy and commitment. Without Cara Griffin's expert editorial support we would not have been able to produce this volume. Her professional expertise, wisdom, and cultural sensitivity are appreciated by all the authors.

We are indebted to the editorial staff at the University of Pennsylvania Press, who have made this book possible. Peter Agree, editor-in-chief, believed in this project from its inception. He ensured that the manuscript was carefully critiqued and instigated many revisions to bring it to this high level of contribution. The positive and constructive comments of anonymous reviewers were extraordinarily valuable. Our editors at Penn Press are much appreciated for having helped smooth the rough edges of the manuscript. Finally, the authors have given unstinted commitment and considerable expertise in each of their chapters. They aspire, as we do, to improve the quality of women's lives through better health in the cities of today and tomorrow.

Afaf I. Meleis
Eugenie L. Birch
Susan M. Wachter